Lu's Basic Toxicology

Lu's Basic Toxicology

Fundamentals, Target Organs, and Risk Assessment

Sixth Edition

Sam Kacew
*University of Ottawa,
Ontario, Canada*

Byung-Mu Lee
*College of Pharmacy,
Sungkyunkwan University,
Seoul, South Korea*

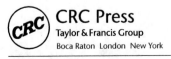

CRC Press
Taylor & Francis Group
Boca Raton London New York

CRC Press is an imprint of the
Taylor & Francis Group, an **informa** business

CRC Press
Taylor & Francis Group
6000 Broken Sound Parkway NW, Suite 300
Boca Raton, FL 33487-2742

© 2013 by Taylor & Francis Group, LLC
CRC Press is an imprint of Taylor & Francis Group, an Informa business

Visit the Taylor & Francis Web site at
http://www.taylorandfrancis.com

and the CRC Press Web site at
http://www.crcpress.com

Printed and bound in Great Britain by CPI Group (UK) Ltd, Croydon, CR0 4YY injury, or damage caused to any person or property arising in any way from the use of this book.

A CIP record of this book is available from the British Library.

ISBN: 978-1-84184-953-9
eISBN: 978-1-84184-954-6

Orders may be sent to: Informa Healthcare, Sheepen Place, Colchester, Essex CO3 3LP, UK
Telephone: +44 (0)20 7017 6682
Email: Books@Informa.com
Website: http://informahealthcarebooks.com

For corporate sales please contact: CorporateBooksIHC@informa.com
For foreign rights please contact: RightsIHC@informa.com
For reprint permissions please contact: PermissionsIHC@informa.com

Typeset by Exeter Premedia Services Private Ltd., Chennai, India
Printed and bound in the United Kingdom

Frank C. Lu
1915–2011

Consulting Toxicologist in Food Additives, Pesticides, and Environmental Chemicals, Consulting Toxicology, Miami, Florida, USA, and Managing Editor of the journal Biomedical and Environmental Sciences, published from China. Dr. Lu's work in the field of toxicology has been recognized on numerous occasions. He was a recipient of the International Achievement Award from the International Society of Pharmacology and Toxicology. He also received the Magnolia Award from the Shanghai Municipal Government for his work in the advancement of preventive medicine, specifically in the promotion of occupational safety and environmental health. In addition, the Frank C. Lu Foundation for Advancement of Preventive Medicine was established in China to honor him. In conjunction with his work in toxicological testing and assessment, Dr Lu taught toxicology courses in several countries, notably Canada, China, the United Kingdom, and the United States.

Table of Contents

Preface   *ix*

PART I: General Principles of Toxicology

1. **General considerations**   **1**

2. **Absorption, distribution, and excretion of toxicants**   **12**

3. **Biotransformation of toxicants**   **27**

4. **Toxic effect**   **42**

5. **Modifying factors of toxic effects**   **59**

**PART II: Testing Procedures for Conventional
      and Nontarget Organ Toxicities**

6. **Conventional toxicity studies**   **73**

7. **Carcinogenesis**   **87**

8. **Mutagenesis**   **109**

9. **Developmental toxicology**   **125**

10. **Lactation**   **137**

PART III: Target Organs and Systems

11. **Toxicology of the immune system**   **149**

12. **Respiratory system inhalation toxicology**   **160**

13. **Toxicology of the liver**   **170**

14. **Toxicology of the kidney**   **181**

15. **Toxicology of the skin**   **192**

16. Toxicology of the eye   202

17. Toxicology of the nervous system   213

18. Reproductive and cardiovascular systems   229

19. Toxicology of the endocrine system   244

PART IV: Toxic Substances and Risk Assessment

20. Food additives and contaminants   262

21. Toxicity of pesticides   277

22. Nanotoxicity   293

23. Toxicity of metals   305

24. Over-the-counter preparations   327

25. Environmental pollutants   335

26. Occupational toxicology   347

27. Toxicological evaluation   361

Chemical index   *379*
Subject index   *390*

Preface

Toxicology is an important science. It provides a sound basis for formulating measures to protect the health of workers against toxicants in factories, farms, mines, and other occupational environments. It is also valuable in the protection of public health hazards associated with toxic substances in food, air, and water. Toxicology has played and will continue to play a significant role in the health and welfare of the world. World Health Organization, being cognizant of the importance of toxicology, organized a toxicology training course in China in 1982, as part of the ongoing China–WHO collaborative program on medical sciences. One of the authors (FCL) was invited to lectures on basic toxicology. The first edition of this book originated from those lecture notes.

Over the years, a number of important developments have occurred in toxicology. Furthermore, some readers of the book have suggested that discussions on certain groups of important chemicals and toxicants would not only provide some general knowledge of these substances, but also facilitate a deeper appreciation of the various aspects of toxicology. The book has received worldwide acceptance, as evidenced by its repeated editions and reprintings, and by the appearance of its version in six foreign languages (Chinese, French, Indonesian, Italian, Spanish, and Taiwan Chinese).

This new edition has been further updated and expanded to include new chapters on toxicology of the endocrine system and nanotoxicology. Thus, there are chapters on lactation, over-the-counter products, and occupational toxicology, as well as a section describing the symptomatology of the Gulf War Syndrome and the probable toxicants implicated. The other chapters have been updated/expanded, notably those on carcinogenesis, developmental toxicology, immunology, food additives and contaminants, environmental toxicology, and safety/risk assessment. However, details of some toxicity tests have been abbreviated to keep the size of the book within bounds; the retained material is intended to portray more clearly the effects of toxicants.

It is hoped that these additions and updates will enhance the usefulness of the book. In making these changes, the authors have kept in mind the broad aim of the first edition, namely, brevity and relatively comprehensive coverage of the subjects. Thus the book continues to serve as an updated introductory text for toxicology students and for those in the stream of allied sciences who require a background in toxicology. Furthermore, as toxicology is a vast subject and is fast expanding, the book is likely to be useful to those who have become specialized in one or more areas in toxicology but wish to brush up in some other areas. The extensive chemical index and subject index will facilitate the retrieval of specific topics.

Sam Kacew
Byung-Mu Lee

1

General considerations

People are exposed to a great variety of natural and synthetic substances. Under certain conditions such exposures produce adverse health effects, ranging in severity from subtle biological changes to death. Society's ever-increasing desire to identify and prevent these effects has prompted the dramatic evolution of toxicology as a study of poisons to the present-day complex science.

DEFINITION AND PURPOSE OF TOXICOLOGY

Toxicology is the study of the nature and mechanisms underlying toxic effects exerted directly or indirectly by substances such as biological, chemical, physical, genetic or psychological agents on living organisms and other biological systems. Toxicology also deals with quantitative or qualitative assessment of the adverse effects in relation to the concentration or dosage, duration, and frequency of exposure of the organisms.

The assessment of health hazards of industrial chemicals, environmental pollutants, and other substances represents an important element in the protection of the health of the workers and members of communities. In-depth studies of the nature and mechanism of the effects of toxicants are invaluable in the invention of specific antidotes and other ameliorative measures. Along with other sciences, toxicology contributes to the development of safer chemicals used as drugs, food additives, and pesticides, as well as many useful industrial chemicals for computers, cellular phones, televisions, and electronic equipment. Even the adverse effects per se are exploited in the pursuit of more effective insecticides, anthelmintics, antimicrobials, antivirals, and warfare agents. The purpose of toxicology is to protect human health or ecosystems from the exposure to hazardous substances.

SCOPE AND SUBDISCIPLINES

Toxicology is a science that has a broad scope. It deals with toxicity studies of substances used (*i*) in medicine for diagnostic, preventive, and therapeutic purposes; (*ii*) in the food industry as direct and indirect additives; (*iii*) in agriculture as pesticides, growth regulators, artificial pollinators, and animal feed additives; and (*iv*) in the chemical industry as solvents, components, and intermediates of plastics, components of electronic devices and many other types of chemicals. It is also concerned with the health effects of metals (as in mines and smelters), radiation, petroleum products, paper and pulp, flame retardants, toxic plants, and animal toxins. Overall, toxicology covers general safety issues in our life.

Because of its broad scope as well as the need to accomplish different goals, toxicology has a number of subdisciplines. For example, a person may be exposed, accidentally or otherwise, to excessively large amounts of a toxicant and become severely intoxicated. If the identity of the toxicant is not known, *Analytical Toxicology* will be called upon to identify the toxicant through analysis of body fluids, stomach contents, suspected containers, etc. Those engaged in *clinical toxicology* administer antidotes, if available, to counter some specific toxicity, and take other measures to ameliorate the symptoms and signs and hasten the elimination of the toxicant from the body. There may also be legal implications, and that will be the task of *forensic toxicology*.

Intoxication may occur as a result of occupational exposure to toxicants. This may result in acute or chronic adverse effects. In either case, the problem is in the domain of *occupational toxicology*. The general public is exposed to a variety of toxicants, via air, water, and soil, contact with skin as well as from food as additives, pesticides, and contaminants, often at low levels that may be harmless acutely but may have long-term adverse effects. In pregnancy, the fetus is exposed via the maternal circulation while a lactating infant is exposed via breast milk. The sources of these substances, their transport, degradation, and bioconcentration in the environment, and their effects on humans are dealt with in *environmental toxicology*. *Regulatory toxicology* attempts to protect the public by setting laws, regulations, and standards to limit or suspend the use of very toxic chemicals as well as defines use conditions for others. Some of the relevant laws in the United States are listed in Appendix 1.

To set meaningful regulations and standards, extensive profiles of the toxic effects are essential. Such profiles can be established only with a great variety of relevant and comprehensive toxicological data derived from in-vitro, in-vivo, and human studies, which form the foundation of regulatory toxicology.

The basic part of such studies is referred to as *conventional toxicology*. In addition, knowledge of the mechanism of action, provided by *mechanistic toxicology*, enhances the toxicological evaluation and provides a basis for other branches of toxicology. The knowledge gained is then utilized to assess the risk of adverse effects to the environment and humans and is termed as risk assessment. A health risk assessment constitutes a written document that is based upon all pertinent scientific information regarding toxicology, human experiences, environmental fate, and exposure scenario. These data are subject to critique and interpretation. The aim of risk assessment is to estimate the potential of an adverse effect that occurs in humans and wildlife ecological system posed by exposure to a specific amount of toxic substances. Risk assessments include several elements such as (*i*) description of the potential adverse health effects based on an evaluation of results of epidemiological, clinical, preclinical, and environmental research; (*ii*) extrapolation from these results to predict the type and estimate the extent of adverse health effects in humans under given conditions of exposure; (*iii*) judgments as to the number and characteristics of individuals exposed at various intensities and durations; (*iv*) and summary judgments on the existence and overall magnitude of the public health problem (Paustenbach, 2002). Risk characterization represents the final and the most critical step in the risk assessment process whereby data on the dose–response relationship of a chemical are integrated with estimates of the degree of exposure in a population to characterize the likelihood and severity of a health risk outcome (Williams and Paustenbach, 2002).

EARLY DEVELOPMENTS

The ancient man was well aware of the toxic effects of a number of substances, such as venom of snakes, the poisonous plants like hemlock and aconite, and the toxic heavy metals such as arsenic, lead, and antimony. Some of these were actually used intentionally for their toxic effects to commit homicide and suicide. For centuries, homicides with toxic substances were common in Europe. To protect against poisoning, there were continual efforts directed toward the discovery and development of preventive and antidotal measures. However, a more critical evaluation of these measures was only begun by Maimonides (1135–1204) with his famous medical work *Poisons and Their Antidotes*, published in 1198.

More significant contributions to the evolution of toxicology were made in the sixteenth century and later. Paracelsus stated: "No substance is a poison by itself. It is the dose (the amount of the exposure) that makes a substance a poison" and "the right dose differentiates a poison from a remedy." These statements laid the foundation for the concept of the "dose–response relation" and the "therapeutic index" developed later. In addition, he described in his book *Bergsucht* (1533–1534) the clinical manifestations of chronic arsenic and mercury poisoning as well as miner's disease. He might be considered the forefather of occupational toxicology. Orfila wrote an important treatise (1814–1815) describing a systematic correlation between the chemical and biological information on certain poisons.

He also devised methods for detecting poisons and pointed to the necessity for chemical analysis for legal proof of lethal intoxication. The introduction of this approach ushered in a specialty area of modern toxicology, namely, forensic toxicology.

RECENT DEVELOPMENTS

In the face of growing population, modern society demands improvements in health and living conditions, including nutrition, clothing, dwelling, and transportation. To meet this goal, a great variety of chemicals, many of them in large quantities, must be manufactured and used. It has been estimated that tens of thousands of different chemicals are in commercial production in industrialized countries. In one way or another, these chemicals come in contact with various segments of the population: individuals are engaged in their manufacture, handling, use (e.g., painters, applicators of pesticides), consumption (e.g., drugs, food additives, natural food products or neutraceuticals), or misuse (e.g., suicide, accidental poisoning, and environmental disasters). Furthermore, people may be exposed to more persistent chemicals via various environmental media and be affected more insidiously. To illustrate the devastating effects of toxicants, some examples of massive acute and long-term poisonings are listed in Appendix 2. In some of these episodes, a considerable amount of sophisticated toxicological investigation was conducted before the etiology was ascertained. These and other tragic outbreaks of massive chemical poisonings have resulted in intensified testing programs, which have revealed the great diversity of the nature and site of toxic effects. This revelation, in turn, has called for more studies using a greater number of animals, a greater number of indicators of toxicity, biomonitoring of chemicals, etc. There is, therefore, a need to render the task of toxicologically assessing the vast number of chemicals by using increasingly more complex testing procedures to be made more manageable. As an attempt to fulfill this need, criteria have been proposed and adopted for the selection of chemicals to be tested according to their priority. In addition, the "tier systems" allow decisions to be made at different stages of toxicological testing, thus avoiding unnecessary studies. If a chemical is found to be exceedingly toxic using a simplified tier 1 screen such as loss of renal creatinine excretion and histopathology damage, then the compound is removed from the market and does not require more sophisticated tier 2 or 3 testing. This procedure is particularly remarkable because the current testing system for carcinogenicity, mutagenicity, and immunotoxicity, and reproductive capacity is quite expensive and involves a multitude of tests (chaps. 7, 8, 11, and 18, respectively).

Because the number of individuals exposed to these chemicals being large, society cannot defer appropriate control until serious injuries have appeared. The modern toxicologist, therefore, must attempt to identify, where possible, indicators of exposure, and early, reversible signs of adverse health effects. These will permit the formulation of decisions at the appropriate step to safeguard the health of individuals, either as occupational workers or in exposed communities. The achievements in these areas have assisted responsible personnel in instituting appropriate medical surveillance of occupational workers and other exposed populations. Notable examples are the use of cholinesterase inhibition as an indicator of exposure to organophosphorous pesticides or various biochemical parameters to monitor exposure to lead. Such "biological markers" or "biomarkers" are intended to measure exposure to toxicants or their effects as well as to detect susceptible population groups (NRC, 1987); they are used for clinical diagnosis, monitoring of occupational workers, and facilitating safety/risk assessment (WHO, 1993). Recently, systems toxicology (i.e., toxicogenomics, toxicoproteomics, and toxicometabolomics) has been considered a promising approach to develop new biomarkers comprehensively for predicting stage-dependent toxicity of substances and risk assessment (McHale et al., 2010; Yang et al., 2010).

Advances made in biochemical and toxicokinetic studies as well as those in genetic toxicology, immunotoxicology, reproductive toxicology, morphological studies on a subcellular level, and biochemical studies on a molecular and genetic level have all contributed to a better understanding of the nature, site, and mechanisms of action of toxicants. For example, technological breakthroughs enabled in-vitro studies to demonstrate whether hepatocytes or nonparenchymal cells affected by a chemical carcinogen are related to differences in their ability to repair the DNA damage induced by the chemical. Studies using isolated nephrons have provided insight into the site and mode of action of nephrotoxicants (chap. 14). Various other types of in-vitro studies have demonstrated the possibility of their use in screening toxicants for specific effects such as mutagenicity and dermal irritancy. Numerous studies have shown that the responses to toxicants are better correlated with the effective dose, that is, the concentration of the toxicant at the target site of action, rather than the administered dose. Furthermore, it is important that we know whether the effects observed result mainly or entirely from an active metabolite, or from the concentration of the metabolite formed rather than that of the parent chemical.

An important function of toxicology is to determine safe levels of exposure to natural and synthetic chemicals (see the section "Scopes and Subdisciplines" that discusses risk assessment), thereby preventing the adverse effects of exposures to toxicants. One of the earliest official actions in this field was taken by the U.S. Food and Drug Administration. It stipulated that a 100-fold margin was required for a food additive to be permitted for use. In other words, a chemical additive should not occur in the total human diet in a quantity greater than one-hundredth of the amount that is the maximum safe dosage in long-term animal experiments (Lehman and Fitzhugh, 1954). For several reasons this approach was not practicable on an international level (chap. 20). While evaluating a number of food additives in 1961, WHO coined the term "acceptable daily intake (ADI)" (WHO, 1962). Using the ADI procedure, WHO has since convened annual meetings of experts on food additives, contaminants, residues of veterinary drugs, and pesticide residues. Assessment of these chemicals resulted, where appropriate, in the assignment of ADIs (chap. 20). The term "ADI" and the WHO evaluations have been adopted by regulatory agencies in many nations. The inception, evolution, and application of ADI have been outlined by Lu (1988). For toxicants in the occupational settings, quantitative assessments are provided in terms of "threshold limit values" (Federal Register, 1971).

These determinations involve comprehensive studies of the toxic properties, demonstration of dosages that produce no observable adverse effects, establishment of dose–effect and dose–response relationships, and toxicokinetic and biotransformation studies. The greatly increased scope and the multiplicity of subdisciplines as outlined above provide a vivid view of recent progress in toxicology.

SOME CHALLENGES AND SUCCESSES

The so-called aniline tumors were reported by Rehn (1895), a German surgeon, in the urinary bladders of three men who had worked in an aniline factory. The role of aniline and aniline dyes as etiological agents was confirmed only some 40 years later, after much experimental investigation in animals (e.g., Hueper et al., 1938), and extensive epidemiological studies by Case et al. (1954) had been carried out. This discovery led to improved occupational standards and more stringent controls of food colors derived from coal tar.

In the late 1950s, thalidomide was widely used as a sedative. It has a very low acute toxicity and readily met the toxicity-testing protocol prevailing at that time. However, a rare form of congenital malformation, phocomelia (the virtual absence of extremities), was observed among some offspring of mothers who had taken this drug during the first trimester (Lenz and Knapp, 1962). This tragedy led to the explosive development of teratology (developmental toxicology), an important specialty area of toxicology. The importance of modifying factors has been dramatized by the tragic effect of cobalt among heavy beer drinkers (chap. 5).

The once prevalent lead poisoning in certain areas of industrialized countries has now largely disappeared. This great accomplishment in the field of public health has resulted from the implementation of control measures devised on the basis of the knowledge gained from the numerous toxicological studies of lead. However, this has now raised new concerns. Lead has been replaced by the gasoline additive methylcyclopentadienyl manganese tricarbonyl (MMT). Combustion of MMT-containing gasoline generates tailpipe emissions of manganese and studies have shown that manganese produces central nervous system disturbances (Gwiadza et al., 2007). Thus, it should be borne in mind that removal of one chemical and replacement with another does not necessarily reduce the risk for development of adverse effects.

Many cases of serious illness that culminated in permanent paralysis and death were reported in Minamata and Niigata in Japan in the 1950s and 1960s, respectively (Study Group of Minamata Disease, 1968; Tsubaki and Irukayama, 1977). The cause of the illness was eventually traced to methyl mercury in the fish caught locally. The fish were contaminated with this chemical, which had been discharged as such, that is, untreated into the water by a factory, or the contaminant was derived from elemental mercury discharged by the factory and methylated through microorganisms in the mud. Measures to rehabilitate the surviving patients and legal control of the factories have been instituted.

On the other hand, the cause of another mysterious illness in Japan, known as *itai-itai* disease, remains unsolved, although cadmium apparently played a role. The patients had resided for many years in areas that were in the vicinity of mines and where the cadmium levels in rice and water were excessive.

A more solid foundation in the assessment of risks of chemical carcinogens resulted from recent advances in epidemiological studies, long-term animal studies, short-term mutagenesis/carcinogenesis tests, and mechanistic studies, as well as the realization that carcinogens differ in their potency, latency, and mode of action depending on species, strains, and sex (chaps. 7 and 25).

TOXICITY VS. OTHER CONSIDERATIONS

In general, exposure to toxic substances is to be avoided. However, the severity of the effects varies greatly; some chemicals induce mild, transient, reversible effects, whereas those of others may be irreversible, serious, and even fatal. Exposure to the former type of substances might thus be acceptable, but, as a rule, not the latter. Examples of the exceptions: methyl mercury, which is extremely toxic, is present in many species of fish. Because of the nutritional value of fish, permissible levels of methyl mercury are established to minimize the risk, yet not deny this valuable source of nutrients. Aflatoxin B_1 is one of the most potent carcinogens but is present in a variety of foods. Yet the contaminated food is not banned as long as the toxin does not exceed the permissible levels.

The complex nature of assessing the toxicity of a substance in light of its benefits is also exemplified by the toxicology seen in lactation and over-the-counter (OTC) products. The former involves weighing the benefits of breast feeding versus the toxicity of certain potential contaminants. OTC products, when improperly used, present toxicological problems. However, the value of these products in general cannot be ignored. There is a growing debate of natural food products (nutraceuticals), where the benefits are accepted by some, yet these products have not been assessed toxicologically and there are reports of adverse effects. The therapeutic value of these products is subject to debate and needs extensive study as the number of consumers is in the millions, but the toxicity remains unknown.

The perception of risk and the benefits to society are crucial. It is clearly documented that with the introduction of chemicals to control infectious diseases and diminished occupational exposure through the use of protective gear have increased the life expectancy (or benefit) for humans. However, to completely eliminate any risk at all requires excessively high costs. Hence, it may not be realistic to derive any benefits if society demands that all risk be removed no matter what the cost is. In essence, by completely removing all chemicals and potential risks, the life expectancy will decrease and mortality will rise. The concept of acceptable risk and benefit ratio needs to be borne in mind. The dilemmas involved in these topics are further described and discussed in other chapters.

FUTURE PROSPECTS

The need of new substances will undoubtedly continue. Some of them will treat or prevent a variety of diseases, which are currently untreatable or unpreventable. Others will render food more plentiful, tastier, and hopefully healthier. Still others will improve living conditions in various ways. At the same time, people are more conscious of subtle adverse effects on health and expect the new substances to be "absolutely safe." Furthermore, the disposal of these substances and their by-products is expected to produce no environmental hazards, adversely affecting humans and the ecosystem.

To satisfy these seemingly irreconcilable societal demands, a toxicologist must carry out a series of studies on each substance: is it readily absorbed, distributed to specific organs, stored, and/or readily excreted? Is it detoxicated or bioactivated? What kind of adverse effects does it induce and what are the host and environmental factors, termed confounding factors, which can alter these effects? How does it produce the effect on a cellular and molecular level? What type of "general toxicity" does it produce? What organs are its targets? What is its predominant mechanism of action? How or can it be eliminated from the organism? Answers to these and other questions will provide a scientific basis for assessing its safety and risk for the intended use.

It is evident that the multitude of studies involved will place an increasing demand on the limited facilities for toxicological testing and on the short supply of qualified personnel. It is of utmost importance, therefore, that toxicity data generated anywhere be accepted internationally. However, to ensure general acceptance, the data must meet certain standards. The "Good Laboratory Practice" promulgated by the U.S. Food and Drug Administration (FDA, 1980) and the Organization of Economic Cooperation and Development (OECD, 1982) should be adopted by all countries involved in toxicological testing.

To streamline the long and costly testing of each chemical separately, there have been schemes that test a representative chemical extensively and verify the results on other members of the group with minimal testing. This practice has been adopted successfully when the substances included in a group are essentially similar. A proposal to ban all chlorine compounds, however, appears to have gone too far in ignoring the great diversity of the toxic nature and potency of such a large group of substances (Karol, 1995). Similar calls for the ban of substances containing bromine, especially flame retardants present in furniture, computers, and televisions, which are crucial for protection against hazards from fire damage, have been instituted by a segment of the population based on the adverse effects of these chemicals. It will be a major challenge to determine how diverse a variety of chemicals can be rationally grouped for toxicological testing and assessment purposes.

Other trends designed to simplify and hasten the testing include a reduction in the use of laboratory animals and supplement or supplant them with in-vitro studies. This is done partly in response to a societal call on humane grounds.

Isolated organs, cultured tissues and cells, and lower forms of life will be increasingly used. Furthermore, such test systems will likely be faster and less expensive, and will augment the variety of studies, especially those related to the mechanism of toxicity. An understanding of the mechanism of action of a chemical is often valuable in providing a sounder basis for the assessment of its safety and risk. Other types of improvements of the testing procedure with respect to simplicity and reliability will continue to be made. Currently there is a major movement termed "Toxicity Testing in the 21st Century" where computational models are being developed to predict the toxicity of chemicals based upon some in-vitro data (Rhomberg, 2010; Roggen, 2011). Although this will go a long way in reducing animal usage, the computational model cannot always predict effects in vivo in animals and humans. One must bear in mind that this is only a model and can have a useful function as a tier 1 screen as in-vivo testing will still be required.

As noted earlier, to provide a basis for proper assessment of the safety or risk of a chemical and for a variety of other purposes, toxicology is increasingly becoming a multifaceted science. To facilitate the acquisition of a broad knowledge of toxicology, this book covers four major areas.

Part I describes general topics related to absorption, distribution, and excretion of toxicants, their transformation in the body, the various types of toxic effects they exert, and the host and environmental factors that modify these effects.

Procedures used in determining the general and specific effects are described in Part II.

Part III describes the organ/system-specific toxicants and the procedures commonly used to detect their effects. Part IV discusses several major groups of toxicants such as food additives and contaminants, pesticides, metals, OTC preparations, various environmental pollutants, and toxicants in the workplace. The last chapter outlines the widely adopted approaches to the assessment of safety and risk of noncarcinogenic and carcinogenic chemicals. In addition, two indices are appended listing chemicals and subjects, respectively, to assist the reader in retrieving relevant parts of the text.

REFERENCES

Case RAM, Hosker ME, McDonald DB, et al. (1954). Tumours of the urinary bladder in workmen engaged in the manufacture and use of certain dyestuff intermediates in the British chemical industry. Br J Ind Med 11, 75–104.

FDA. (1980). Code of Federal Regulations, Title 21, Food and Drugs. Part 58. Washington, DC: US. Government Printing Office.

Federal Register. (1971). Threshold Limit Values Adopted by the American Conference of Governmental Industrial Hygienists, 1968, vol. 36, no. 105, May 29. Washington, DC: US. Government Printing Office.

Gwiadza R, Lucchini R, Smith D (2007). Adequacy and consistency of animal studies to evaluate the neurotoxicity of chronic low-level manganese exposure in humans. J Toxicol Environ Health A 70, 594–605.

Hueper WC, Wiley FH, Wolfe HD (1938). Experimental production of bladder tumors in dogs by administration of beta-naphthylamine. J Ind Hyg Toxicol 20, 46–84.

Karol MH (1995). Toxicologic principles do not support the banning of chlorine: a society of toxicology position paper. Fundam Appl Toxicol 24, 1–2.

Lehman AJ, Fitzhugh OG (1954). 100-fold margin of safety. Q Bull Assoc Food Drug Officials U.S. 18, 33–5.

Lenz W, Knapp K (1962). Thalidomide embryopathy. Arch Environ Health 5, 100–5.

Lu FC (1988). Acceptable daily intakes: inception, evolution and application. Regul Toxicol Pharmacol 8, 45–60.

McHale CM, Zhang L, Hubbard AE, et al. (2010). Toxicogenomic profiling of chemically exposed humans in risk assessment. Mutat Res. 705, 172–83.

NRC Committee on Biological Markers. (1987). Biological markers in environmental health research. Environ Health Perspect 74, 3–9.

OECD. (1982). Good Laboratory Practice in the Testing of Chemicals. Paris Cedex, France: Organization of Economic Cooperation and Development.

Paustenbach DJ (2002). Human and Ecological Risk Assessment. Theory and Practice. New York, NY: John Wiley and Sons, Inc.

Rehn L (1895). Blasengeschwulste bei fuchsin-arbeiten. Arch Klin Chir 50, 588.

Rhomberg LR (2010). Toxicity testing in the 21st century: how will it affect risk assessment? J Toxicol Environ Health B Crit Rev. 13,361–75.

Roggen EL (2011). In vitro toxicity testing in the twenty-first century. Front Pharmacol. 2, 1–3.

Study Group of Minamata Disease. (1968). Minamata Disease. Minamata, Japan: Minamata University.

Tsubaki T, Irukayama K (1977). Minamata Disease: Methyl Mercury Poisoning in Minamata and Niigata, Japan. New York, NY: Elsevier Scientific.

WHO. (1962). Sixth Report of the Joint FAD/WHO Expert Committee on Food Additives. Geneva, Switzerland: World Health Organization.

WHO. (1993). Biomarkers and risk assessment: concepts and principles. Environ Health Criteria 155.

Williams PRD, Paustenbach DJ (2002). Risk characterization: principles and practice. J Toxicol Environ Health B 5, 337–406.

Yang B, Wang Q, Lei R, et al. (2010). Systems toxicology used in nanotoxicology: mechanistic insights into the hepatotoxicity of nano-copper particles from toxicogenomics. J Nanosci Nanotechnol 10, 8527–37.

Appendix 1   U.S. Laws that have a Basis in Toxicology

Responsible Agency	Law
Food and Drug Administration	Federal Food, Drug, and Cosmetic Act
Environmental Protection Agency	Federal Insecticide, Fungicide, and Rodenticide Act
	Clean Air Act
	Safe Drinking Water Act
	Toxic Substances Control Act
Consumer Product Safety Commission	Consumer Product Safety Act
	Federal Hazardous Substances Act
Occupational Safety and Health Administration	Occupational Safety and Health Act

Appendix 2   Examples of Outbreaks of Mass Poisoning in Humans

Location and Year	Toxicant	Adverse Effect	Number Affected
Detroit, MI., 1930	Tri-*o*-cresyl phosphate in "ginger jake"	Delayed neurotoxicity	16,000
London, UK, 1952	Sulfur dioxide and suspended particulate matter Win air	Increased deaths from heart and lung diseases	3000
Toyama, Japan, 1950s	Cadmium in rice	Severe kidney and bone disease ("*itai-itai* disease")	200[a]
Minamata, Japan, 1950s	Methyl mercury in fish	Severe neurological disease ("Minamata disease")	200[a,b]
Southeast Turkey, 1956	Hexachlorobenzene in wheat	Porphyria, neurological diseases	4000
Morocco, 1959	Tri-*o*-cresyl phosphate in adulterated oil	Delayed neurotoxicity	10,000
Japan, 1956–1977	Clioquinol	Subacute myelo-opticoneuropathy	10,000
Western Europe, late 1950s and early 1960s	Thalidomide	Phocomelia	10,000
Fukuoka, Japan, 1968	Polychlorinated biphenyls	Skin disease, general weakness	1700
Iraq, 1972	Methyl mercury in wheat	Deaths from neurological disease	500
		Nonfatal cases	50,000
Madrid, Spain, 1981	Toxic oil in food	Deaths with various symptoms and signs	340
		Nonfatal cases	20,000
Bhopal, India, 1984	Methyl isocyanate released into air	Deaths from acute lung disease	6000
		Nonfatal cases	200,000
Chernobyl	Radioactivity release	Deaths	31
		Childhood leukemia	75[a]
			Normally less than 1

[a]Many more cases with mild or moderate symptoms and signs of intoxication.
[b]Hundreds of cases occurred in Niigata, Japan, in the 1960s from the same source, fish.

2

Absorption, distribution, and excretion of toxicants

INTRODUCTION

A toxicant, apart from causing local effects at the site of contact, can be detrimental only after it is absorbed by the organism. Absorption can occur systematically through the skin, the gastrointestinal (GI) tract, the lungs, and several minor routes. Furthermore, the nature and intensity of the effects of a chemical on an organism depend on its concentration in the target organs. The concentration depends not only on the administered dose but also on other factors, including absorption, distribution, metabolism, receptor binding, storage, and excretion. For a chemical to be absorbed, distributed, degraded, and eventually excreted, a toxicant must pass through a number of cell membranes. A cell membrane generally consists of a biomolecular layer of lipid molecules with proteins scattered throughout the membrane (Fig. 2.1).

There are four mechanisms by which a toxicant may pass through a cell membrane; the most important of them is passive diffusion through the membrane. The others are filtration through the membrane pores, carrier-mediated transport, and engulfing by the cell. The last two mechanisms are different in that the cell takes an active part in the transfer of a toxicant across its membranes.

Passive Diffusion

Most toxicants cross cell membranes by simple, passive diffusion. The rate of passage is related directly to the concentration gradient across the membrane and to the lipid solubility. For example, mannitol is hardly absorbed (<2%), acetylsalicylic acid is fairly well absorbed (21%), and thiopental is even more readily absorbed (67%). It is noteworthy that the chloroform:water partition of the non-ionized forms of these chemicals is, respectively, <0.002, 2, and 100. For references to this and other examples, see Hogben et al. (1958).

Many toxicants are ionizable. The ionized form is often unable to penetrate the cell membrane because of its low lipid solubility. On the other hand, the

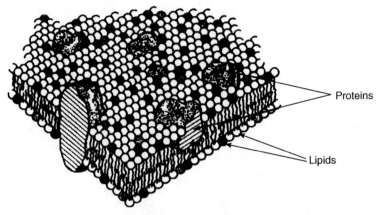

Figure 2.1   Schematic diagram of a biological membrane. Spheres represent head groups (phosphatidylcholine) and zigzag lines indicate tail ends of lipids. Black, white, and stippled spheres indicate different kinds of lipids. Large bodies represent proteins; some are located on the surface, others within the membrane. *Source*: From Singer and Nicholson (1972).

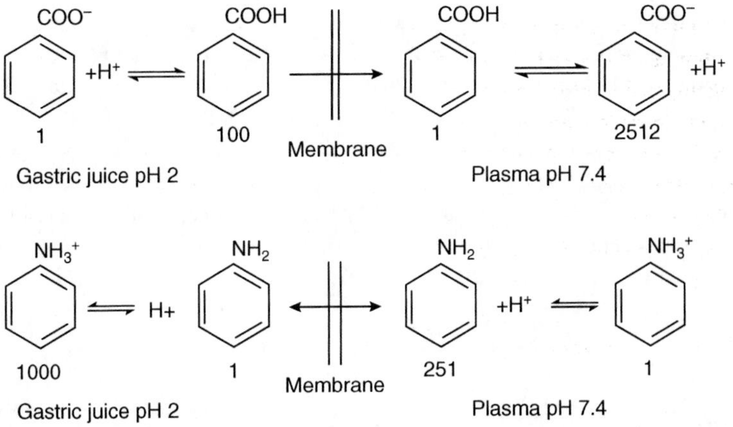

Figure 2.2   Disposition of benzoic acid and aniline in gastric juice and plasma. Figures immediately below the structural formulas represent proportions of ionized and non-ionized forms. *Source*: From Timbrell (1991).

non-ionized form is likely lipid-soluble enough to do so, and its rate of penetration depends on the lipid solubility. The extent of ionization of weak organic acids and bases depends on the pH of the medium. Thus, for the former, such as benzoic acid, diffusion is facilitated in acidic environment, where they exist mainly in the non-ionized form; for the latter, such as aniline, diffusion is facilitated in basic environment (Figs. 2.2 and 2.3).

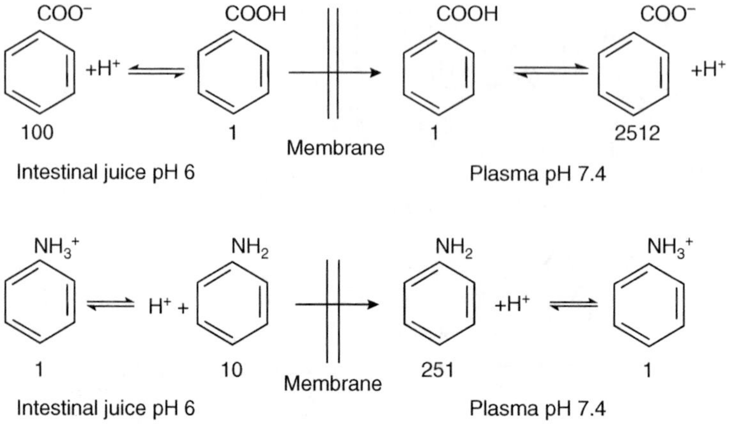

COO⁻   COOH   COOH   COO⁻

+H⁺ ⇌   ⇌   +H⁺

100   1   1   2512

Membrane

Intestinal juice pH 6   Plasma pH 7.4

NH₃⁺   NH₂   NH₂   NH₃⁺

⇌ H⁺ +   +H⁺ ⇌

1   10   251   1

Membrane

Intestinal juice pH 6   Plasma pH 7.4

Figure 2.3   Disposition of benzoic acid and aniline in intestinal juice and plasma. *Source*: From Timbrell (1991).

Filtration

The membranes of the capillaries and the glomeruli have relatively large pores (about 70 nm) and allow molecules smaller than albumin (molecular weight 60,000 Da) to pass through. Bulk flow of water through these pores results from hydrostatic and/or osmotic pressure and can act as a carrier of toxicants. The pores in most cells, however, are relatively small (about 4 nm) and allow chemicals only up to a molecular weight of 100–200 Da to pass through. Chemicals of larger molecules, therefore, can filter into and out of the capillaries. They can, therefore, establish equilibrium between the concentrations in the plasma and in the extracellular fluid, but they cannot do so by filtration between the extracellular and intracellular fluids.

Carrier-Mediated Transport

This involves the formation of a complex between the chemical and a macromolecular carrier on one side of the membrane. The complex then diffuses to the other side of the membrane, where the chemical is released. Thereafter, the carrier returns to the original surface to repeat the transport process. The carrier has a limited capacity. When it is saturated, the rate of transport is no longer dependent on the concentration of the chemical and assumes zero order kinetics. Structure, conformation, size, and charge are important in determining the affinity of a chemical for a carrier site, and competitive inhibition can occur among chemicals with similar characteristics.

Active transport involves a carrier that moves molecules across a membrane against a concentration gradient, or, if the molecule is an ion, against an electrochemical gradient. It requires the expenditure of metabolic energy and can be inhibited by poisons that interfere with cell metabolism.

Facilitated diffusion is similar to active transport but does not move molecules against a concentration gradient. Furthermore, it is not energy-dependent, and metabolic poisons will not inhibit this process. Therefore, facilitated diffusion is classified as passive transport system.

Engulfing by the Cell (Endocytosis)

Particles may be engulfed by cells. When the particles are solid, the process is called phagocytosis and when they are liquid, it is called pinocytosis. This process is also called active transport and requires energy. Such special transport systems are important for the removal of particulate matter from the alveoli and of certain toxic substances from the blood by the reticuloendothelial system. Carrageenans (molecular weight about $10,000 \sim 40,000$ Da) are also absorbed from the gut by this process.

ABSORPTION

The main routes by which toxicants are absorbed are the GI tract, lungs, and skin. However, in toxicologic studies, special routes such as intravenous, intraperitoneal, intradermal, intramuscular, and subcutaneous injections are also used. Other minor routes include intracardiac and intra-articular injection, and intraosseous infusion.

Gastrointestinal Tract

Many toxicants can enter the GI tract along with food and water or alone as drugs or other types of chemicals. With the exception of those that are caustic or very irritating to the mucosa, most toxicants do not exert any toxic effect unless they are absorbed. Absorption can take place along the entire GI tract. For example, certain drugs are administered as sublingual tablets and suppositories to be absorbed in the mouth and the rectum, respectively. However, the mouth and rectum are, in general, insignificant sites of absorption of environmental chemicals.

The stomach is a significant site of absorption, especially for weak acids, which will exist in the diffusible, non-ionized, and lipid-soluble form. On the other hand, weak bases will be highly ionized in the acidic gastric juice and therefore not readily absorbable. The difference in absorption is further amplified by the circulating plasma. Weak acids will exist mainly in ionized form in plasma and be carried away, whereas weak bases will exist in non-ionized form and can diffuse back to the stomach. The influence of these factors, using benzoic acid and aniline as examples, is shown in Figure 2.2.

In the intestine, weak acids will exist mainly in the ionized form; hence they are less readily absorbable. However, upon entering the blood, they become ionized and thus will not readily diffuse back. On the other hand, weak bases will exist mainly in the non-ionized form; hence more readily absorbable, as shown in Figure 2.3. It should be noted that intestinal absorption is further enhanced by the long contact time and the large surface area provided by the villi and microvilli.

In the intestine, there are special carrier-mediated transport systems that are responsible for the absorption of nutrients, such as monosaccharides, amino acids, and elements such as iron, calcium, and sodium. However, a few toxicants, such as 5-fluorouracil (5-FU), thallium, and lead, are known to be absorbable from the intestine by active transport systems. In addition, particulate matters such as those of the azo dyes and polystyrene latex can enter the intestinal cell by pinocytosis.

Respiratory Tract

The main site of absorption in the respiratory tract is the alveoli in the lungs. This is especially true for gases such as carbon monoxide, nitrogen oxides, and sulfur dioxide, and for vapors of volatile liquids such as benzene and carbon tetrachloride. Their ready absorption is related to the large alveolar area, high blood flow, and proximity of the blood to the alveolar air.

The rate of absorption is dependent on the solubility of the gas in the blood—the more soluble it is, the faster the absorption. However, equilibrium between the air and the blood is reached more slowly for more soluble chemicals, such as chloroform, compared with less soluble chemicals, such as ethylene. This is because the more soluble a chemical, the more of it can be dissolved in the blood. As the alveolar air can carry only a limited amount of the chemical, more respirations and hence a longer time will be required to attain equilibrium. It will take even longer if the chemical is also deposited in the fat tissue.

In addition to gases and vapors, liquid aerosols and airborne particles may also be absorbed. In general, large particles ($>10\,\mu m$) do not enter the respiratory tract; when they do, they are deposited in the nose and disposed of by wiping, blowing, and sneezing. Very small particles ($<0.01\,\mu m$) are likely to be exhaled. Those in the range of $0.01–10\,\mu m$ are deposited in various parts of the respiratory tract. The larger ones are likely to be deposited in the nasopharynx and absorbed either through the epithelium of this region or through the GI tract epithelium after they are swallowed along with the mucus. Smaller particles are deposited in the trachea, bronchi, and bronchioli, and are then either aspirated onto the mucociliary escalator or engulfed by phagocytes. The particles carried up by the escalator will be coughed up or swallowed. The phagocytes with engulfed particles will be absorbed into the lymphatics. Some free particles can also migrate into the lymphatics. Soluble particles may be absorbed through the epithelium into the blood.

A detailed examination of the deposition of particles of various sizes in different parts of the respiratory tract is provided by a Task Group on Lung Dynamics (1966). However, as a rough estimate, 25% of inhaled particles are exhaled, 50% are deposited in the upper respiratory tract, and 25% are deposited in the lower respiratory tract (Morrow et al., 1966).

Skin

In general, the skin is relatively impermeable, and therefore it constitutes a good barrier, separating the organism from its environment. However, some chemicals can be absorbed through the skin in sufficient quantities to produce systemic effects.

A chemical may be absorbed via the hair follicles or through the cells of the sweat glands or those of the sebaceous glands. These are, however, minor routes for absorption because they constitute only a small surface area of the skin. Therefore, the percutaneous absorption of a chemical is essentially through the skin proper, which consists of the epidermis and dermis (Fig. 15.1 of chap. 15).

The first phase of percutaneous absorption is diffusion of the toxicant through the epidermis, the most important barrier, and especially its stratum corneum. The stratum corneum consists of several layers of thin, cohesive, dead cells that contain chemically resistant material (protein filament). Small amounts of polar substances appear to diffuse through the outer surface of the protein filaments of the hydrated stratum corneum; non-polar substances dissolve in and diffuse through the lipid matrix between the protein filaments.

In the human stratum corneum, there are significant differences in structure and chemistry from one region of the body to another, which are reflected in the permeability to chemicals. For example, toxicants cross the scrotum readily, cross the abdominal skin less readily, and cross the sole and palm with great difficulty (Zbinden, 1976).

The second phase of percutaneous absorption is diffusion of the toxicant through the dermis, which contains a porous, non-selective, aqueous diffusion medium. Therefore, it is much less effective as a barrier than the stratum corneum; as a consequence, abrasion or removal of the latter causes a marked increase in the percutaneous absorption. Acids, alkalis, and mustard gases will also increase the absorption by injuring this barrier. Some solvents, notably dimethyl sulfoxide, also increase dermal permeability.

DISTRIBUTION

After a chemical enters the blood, it is distributed rapidly throughout the body. The rate of distribution to each organ is related to the speed and the amount of blood that flows through the organ, the ease with which the chemical crosses the local capillary wall and the cell membrane, and the affinity of components of the organ for the chemical.

Barriers

The *blood–brain barrier* (BBB) is located at the brain capillary wall. The capillary endothelial cells are tightly joined, leaving few or no pores between these cells (Bradbury, 1984).Thus, the toxicant has to pass through the capillary endothelium itself. A lack of vesicles in these cells further reduces their transport ability.

Finally, the protein concentration of the interstitial fluid in the brain is low, in contrast to that in other organs; protein binding therefore does not serve as a mechanism for the transfer of toxicants from the blood to the brain. For these reasons, the penetration of toxicants into the brain depends on their lipid solubility. An outstanding example is the toxicant methyl mercury, which enters the brain readily and the main toxicity of which is on the central nervous system. In contrast, inorganic mercury compounds are not lipid soluble, do not enter the brain readily, and exert their main adverse effects not on the brain but on the kidney. Glucose is transported across the brain capillary wall by glucose transporter the glucose transporter 2 (GLUT2).

The *placental barrier* differs anatomically among various animal species. There are six layers of cells between fetal and maternal blood in some species, whereas in others there is only one layer. Furthermore, the number of layers may change as the gestation progresses. Although the relationship of the number of layers of the placenta to its permeability needs quantitative determination, the placental barrier does impede the transfer of toxicants to the fetus, which is therefore protected to some extent. However, the concentration of a toxicant such as methyl mercury may be higher in certain fetal organs, such as the brain, because of the less-effective fetal blood–brain barrier. On the other hand, the fetal concentration of the food coloring amaranth is only 0.03–0.06% of that of the mother (Munro and Willes, 1978).

Other barriers are also present in organs such as the eyes and testes. In addition, the erythrocyte plays an interesting role in the distribution of certain toxicants. For example, its membrane acts as a barrier against the penetration of inorganic mercury compounds but not that of alkyl mercury. Furthermore, there is affinity of the erythrocyte cytoplasm for alkyl mercury compounds. Because of these factors, the concentration of inorganic mercury compounds in the erythrocytes is only about half that in the plasma, whereas that of methyl mercury in the erythrocyte is about 10 times that in the plasma (WHO, 1976).

Binding and Storage

As noted above, binding of a chemical in a tissue can result in a higher concentration in that tissue. There are two major types of binding. The covalent type of binding is irreversible and is, in general, associated with significant toxic effects. The non-covalent binding usually accounts for a major portion of the dose and is reversible. Therefore, this process plays an important role in the distribution of toxicants in various organs and tissues. There are several types of non-covalent binding as outlined by Guthrie (1980). In general, storage of toxicants in non-target organs may be considered as the first step to protect our body, but their chronic release from non-target organs into the body may produce chronic intoxication later.

Plasma proteins can bind normal physiological constituents in the body as well as many foreign compounds. Most of the latter are bound to the albumin and are therefore not immediately available for distribution to the extravascular space. However, since the binding is reversible, it permits the bound chemical to dissociate from the protein, thereby replenishing the level of unbound chemical, which may then cross the capillary endothelium. The toxicologic significance of the binding can be illustrated by the possible induction of coma by the administration of sulfonamide drugs to patients who are taking antidiabetic drugs. The antidiabetic drugs are bound to the plasma proteins but can be replaced by the sulfonamide drugs, which have a greater affinity for the plasma protein. The antidiabetic drugs thus released may precipitate a hypoglycemic coma. Other types of plasma proteins for storage are lipoproteins (for vitamins, cholesterol, steroid, lipid soluble agents, and basic drugs), gamma globulins for antigens, transferrin for iron, and ceruloplasmin for copper.

The *liver* and *kidney* have a higher capacity for binding chemicals. This characteristic may be related to their metabolic and excretory functions. Certain proteins have been identified in these organs for their specific binding property, such as metallothionein (MT), which is important for the binding of cadmium in the liver and kidney, and possibly also for the transfer of the metal from the liver to the kidney. Binding of a substance can increase its concentration in an organ rapidly. For example, 30 minutes after a single administration of lead, its concentration in the liver is 50 times higher than that in the plasma. MTs can be also upregulated in various organs/tissues by inflammatory stimuli, suggesting the possible target of MTs in inflammatory diseases (Inoue et al., 2009). MTs (e.g., MT-I, MT-II, MT-III, and MT-IV, and other isoforms) have various biological effects on heavy metal homeostasis, cancer, circulation, diabetes, immune system, and antioxidative defense (Thirumoorthy et al., 2011).

The *adipose tissue* is an important storage depot for lipid-soluble substances such as dichlorodiphenyltrichloroethane (DDT), dieldrin, and polychlorinated biphenyls (PCBs). They appear to be stored in the adipose tissue by simple dissolution in the neutral fats. There exists the potential that the plasma concentration of the substances stored in the fat may increase sharply as a result of rapid mobilization of fat following starvation. Conjugation of fatty acid to toxicants, such as DDT, may also be a mechanism by which these chemicals are retained in the lipid-containing tissues and cells of the body (Leighty et al., 1980).

Bone is a major site for storage of such toxicants as fluoride, lead, and strontium. The storage takes place by an exchange adsorption reaction between the toxicants in the interstitial fluid and the hydroxyapatite crystals of bone mineral. By virtue of similarities in size and charge, F^- may readily replace OH^-, and calcium may be replaced by lead or strontium. These stored substances can be released by ionic exchange and by dissolution of bone crystals through osteoclastic activity.

EXCRETION

After absorption and distribution in the organism, toxicants are excreted, rapidly or slowly. A generally accepted indicator of the rate of elimination of a toxicant is its "half-life" $(t_{1/2})$, which is the time required to remove 50% of it from the bloodstream.

The toxicants are excreted as the parent chemicals, as their metabolites, and/or as conjugates of them. The principal routes of excretion are the urine and feces, but the liver and lungs are also important excretory organs for certain types of chemicals. In addition, there are a number of other minor routes for excretion, including, sweat, saliva, and milk.

Urinary Excretion

The kidney removes toxicants from the body by the same mechanisms as those used in the removal of end products of normal metabolism, namely, glomerular filtration, tubular diffusion, and tubular secretion.

The glomerular capillaries have large pores (70 nm); therefore, most toxicants will be filtered at the glomerulus, except those that are very large (greater than 60,000 Da) or those that are tightly bound to plasma protein. Once a toxicant enters the glomerular filtrate, it will either be passively reabsorbed across the tubular cells if it has a high lipid/water partition coefficient or remains in the tubular lumen and be excreted if it is a polar compound.

A toxicant can also be excreted through the tubules into the urine by passive diffusion. As urine is normally acidic, this process plays a role in the excretion of organic bases. On the other hand, organic acids are unlikely to be excreted by passive diffusion through the tubular cells. However, weak acids are often metabolized to stronger acids, thereby increasing the percentage of the ionic forms that are not reabsorbed through the tubular cells and are thus excreted.

Certain toxicants can be secreted by the cells of the proximal tubules into the urine. There are two distinct secretory mechanisms, one for organic acids (e.g., glucuronide and sulfate conjugates) and the other for organic bases. Protein-bound toxicants can also be secreted, provided the binding is reversible. Furthermore, chemicals of similar characteristics compete for the same transport system. For example, probenecid can increase the serum level of penicillin and prolong its activity by blocking its tubular excretion.

Biliary Excretion

The liver is also an important organ for the excretion of toxicants, especially for compounds with high polarity (anionic and cationic), conjugates of compounds bound to plasma proteins, and compounds with molecular weights greater than 300 Da. In general, once these compounds are in the bile, they are not reabsorbed into the blood and are excreted via the feces. However, there are exceptions, such as the glucuronide conjugates, which can be hydrolyzed by intestinal flora, enabling the reabsorption of the free toxicants.

The importance of the biliary route of excretion for some chemicals has been well demonstrated in experiments that showed a several-fold increase of the acute toxicity in animals with ligated bile ducts. Such chemicals include digoxin, indocyanine green, ouabain, and, most dramatically, diethylstilbestrol (DES).

The toxicity of DES is increased by a factor of 130 in rats with ligated bile ducts (Klaassen, 1973).

Lungs

Substances that exist in the gaseous phase at body temperature are excreted mainly by the lungs. Volatile liquids are also readily excreted via the expired air. Highly soluble liquids such as chloroform and halothane are excreted slowly because of their storage in the adipose tissue and the limited ventilation volume. Excretion of toxicants from the lung is accomplished by simple diffusion through cell membranes. The breakdown of compounds to constituents such as carbon dioxide results in excretion of this gas via the lungs.

Other Routes

The *gastrointestinal tract* is not a major route of excretion of toxicants. However, because the human stomach and intestine, each secretes about 3 L of fluid per day, some toxicants are excreted along with the fluid. The excretion is mainly by diffusion and thus the rate depends on the pK_a of the toxicant and the pH of the stomach and intestine.

The excretion of toxicants in mother's *milk* is not important as far as the host organism is concerned. However, the presence of toxic substances in milk may be toxicologically significant because they can be passed in the milk from the mother to the nursing child and from cows to humans. The excretion is also via simple diffusion. As milk is slightly acidic, basic compounds will reach a higher level in milk than in plasma, while the opposite is true with acidic compounds. Lipophilic compounds such as DDT and PCB also reach a higher level in milk because of its higher fat content.

Sweat and *saliva* are also minor routes of excretion of toxicants. The excretion also occurs by diffusion; thus it is confined to the non-ionized, lipid-soluble forms of the toxicants. Substances excreted in the saliva are usually swallowed and then become available for reabsorption in the GI tract.

PHYSIOLOGICALLY BASED PHARMACOKINETIC MODELING

Physiologically based pharmacokinetic (PBPK) models represent the body as a set of functional compartments, for example blood, brain, liver, muscle, skin, and the remainder of the body. A schematic PBPK model for manganese is illustrated in Figure 2.4. All compartments need not necessarily be involved as shown in Figure 2.5, as a PBPK model for methyl ethyl ketone, where brain as opposed to manganese, is not a significant target. PBPK facilitates simulation of pharmacokinetic profiles of chemicals on the basis of available information on relevant physiological, physicochemical, and biochemical factors (Thompson et al., 2008). These models utilize biological information to predict the disposition of

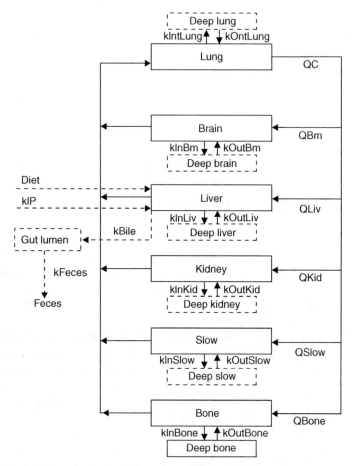

Figure 2.4 Schematic of physiologically based pharmacokinetic model for assessing tracer doses of radiolabeled and total manganese. *Source*: From Teeguarden et al. (2007).

chemicals for which limited human data are available. It is essential to understand that the chemical is present at low or pharmacological levels and the responses are linear. PBPK models are becoming increasingly important in chemical health risk assessment. In order to construct PBPK models to predict the disposition of chemicals, it is important to take into account genetic makeup, life stage, and health status, because these are confounding factors that may affect the disposition and subsequently the risk assessment. The PBPK model for an infant will be markedly different from an adult and thus the risk for a child in general is greater than that for an adult (Price et al., 2003). Governmental agencies have come to rely in recent years on PBPK modeling as an essential tool in the overall assessment of a chemical hazard for humans.

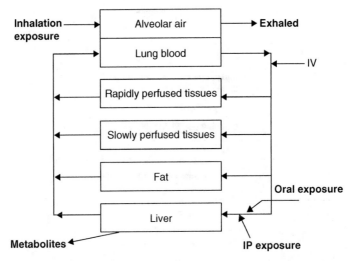

Figure 2.5   Schematic diagram of physiologically based pharmacokinetic model for methyl ethyl ketone. *Source*: From Thrall et al. (2002).

A further step is the use of physiologically based toxicokinetic (PBTK) models where the chemical is present in excessive or toxic levels and where the responses do not follow a linear pattern (Dixit et al., 2003). Toxicokinetic models are often defined based upon the nature of the rate processes, be it absorption across the GI tract, hepatic metabolism, or elimination by the kidney. A conceptual representation of a PBTK model for volatile organic chemicals is illustrated in Figure 2.6. At toxic concentrations, the solubility of chemicals is altered leading to different absorption patterns, excess bioavailability, and accumulation, and the predictability of chemical disposition becomes less reliable. A toxicokinetic model is only a tool to estimate chemical concentrations and generates parameters that are useful for further analysis and quantification of biological processes under study. Toxicokinetics serves as a bridge for extrapolating chemical concentrations across different species, from in-vitro to in-vivo studies, from chemical exposure to systemic dose in risk assessment, or as a link between physiology or genetics and chemical disposition in populations of animals and humans.

LEVELS OF TOXICANTS IN THE BODY

As noted above, the nature and intensity of the effects of a chemical depend on its concentration at the site of action, namely, the effective dose rather than the administered dose. The level in the target organ is, in general, a function of the blood level. However, binding of a toxicant in a tissue will increase its level, whereas tissue barriers tend to reduce the level. As the blood level is more readily

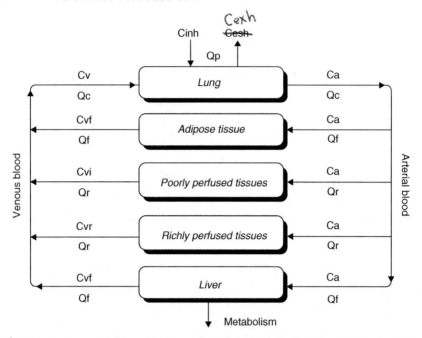

Figure 2.6   Conceptual representation of PBTK model for volatile organic chemicals. Qp and Qc refer to alveolar ventilation rate and cardiac output. Cinh, Cexh, Cv, and Ca refer to chemical concentration in inhaled air, exhaled air, venous blood, and arterial blood, respectively. Cvf and Qf refer to venous blood concentrations leaving tissue compartments and blood flow to tissues (i.e., f, adipose tissue; s, slowly perfused tissues; r, richly perfused tissues; and l, liver). *Source*: From Haddad et al. (2000).

determined, especially over a time period, it is the parameter often used in toxico-kinetic studies.

While the toxicant is being absorbed, its blood level rises. In the meantime, the rates of its excretion, biotransformation (chap. 3), and the distribution to other organs and tissues also increase. The curve depicting the blood level against time and the area under that curve (AUC) are useful tools in toxicokinetics. In a series of experimental studies, Smyth and Hottendorf (1980) demonstrated that the AUC for a solution of a chemical is, in general, greater than that for its suspension, and it is greater for acidic than basic chemicals. They also illustrated the effects of the route of administration, dose level, and dosing vehicle on the AUC.

The influence of the rate of excretion on the blood level is vividly shown in Figure 2.7. Saccharin is rapidly excreted; hence its blood level drops rapidly, even after repeated administration. On the other hand, methyl mercury is excreted very slowly; its gradual accumulation culminates in a near plateau only after 270 days (Munro and Willes, 1978). It should be noted that the blood level of a chemical does not necessarily correlate with toxicity. In the case of blood lead levels, the concentration found was high but did not appear to correlate with any adverse

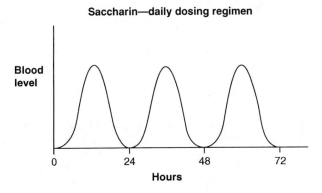

Figure 2.7 Comparative chemobiokinetics of saccharin and methyl mercury chloride. *Source*: From Munro and Willes (1978).

effects, especially in children. The blood chemical concentration is simply a marker of exposure and not necessarily toxicity.

Methods for determining the rate and extent of absorption, distribution, binding, storage, and excretion at various organs and tissues are readily found in the literature. A summary of some of them is given in a WHO publication and OECD guideline (WHO, 1986; OECD, 2009).

REFERENCES

Bradbury MWB (1984). The structure and function of the blood–brain barrier. Fed Proc 43, 186–90.

Dixit R, Riviere J, Krishnan K, et al. (2003). Toxicokinetics and physiologically based toxicokinetics in toxicology and risk assessment. J Toxicol Environ Health B 6, 1–40.

Guthrie FE (1980). Absorption and distribution. In: Hodgson E, Guthrie FE, eds. Introduction to Biochemical Toxicology. New York, NY: Elsevier.

Haddad S, Charest-Tardif G, Krishnan K (2000). Physiologically based modeling of the maximal effect of metabolic interactions on the kinetics of components of complex chemical mixtures. J Toxicol Environ Health A 61, 209–23

Hogben CAM, Tocco DJ, Brodie BB, et al. (1958). On the mechanism of intestinal absorption of drugs. J Pharmacol Exp Therap 125, 275–82.

Inoue K, Takano H, Shimada A, et al. (2009). Metallothionein as an anti-inflammatory mediator. Mediators Inflamm 2009, 7.

Klaassen CD (1973). Comparison of the toxicity of chemicals in newborn rats to bile duct-ligated and sham-operated rats and mice. Toxicol Appl Pharmacol 24, 37–44.

Leighty EG, Fentiman AF Jr, Thompson RM (1980). Conjugation of fatty acids to DDT in the rat: Possible mechanism for retention. Toxicology 15, 77–82.

Morrow PE, Hodge HC, Newman WF, et al. (1966). Deposition and retention models for internal dosimetry of the human respiratory tract. Health Phys 12, 173–207.

Munro IO, Willes AF (1978). Reproductive toxicity and the problems of in vitro exposure. In: Galli A, Paoletti R, Veterazzi G, eds. Chemical Toxicology of Food. Amsterdam, The Netherland: Elsevier/North Holland.

OECD. (2009). OECD guideline for the testing of chemicals draft proposal for a revised TG: 417 "Toxicokinetics". [online] Available from: http://www.oecd.org/dataoecd/26/32/44216274.pdf.

Price K, Haddad S, Krishnan K (2003). Physiological modeling of age-specific changes in the pharmacokinetics of organic chemicals in children. J Toxicol Environ Health A 66, 417–33.

Singer SJ, Nicolson GC (1972). The fluid mosaic model of the structure of cell membranes. Science 175, 720–31.

Smyth AD, Hottendorf GH (1980). Application of pharmacokinetics and biopharmaceutics in the design of toxicological studies. Toxicol Appl Pharmacol 53, 179–95.

Task Group on Lung Dynamics. (1966). Deposition and retention models for internal dosimetry of the human respiratory tract. Health Phys 12, 173–207.

Thirumoorthy N, Shyam Sunder A, Manisenthil Kumar K, et al. (2011). A review of Metallothionein isoforms and their role in pathophysiology. World J Surg Oncol 20, 9–54.

Timbrell JA (1991). Principles of Biochemical Toxicology. London, UK: Taylor & Francis.

Thompson CM, Sonawane B, Barton HA, et al. (2008). Approaches for applications of physiologically based pharmacokinetic models in risk assessment. J Toxicol Environ Health B 11, 519–47.

WHO. (1976). Mercury: Environmental Health Criteria 1. Geneva, Switzerland: World Health Organization, p. 70.

WHO. (1986). Principles of Toxicokinetic Studies. Environmental Health Criteria 57. Geneva, Switzerland: World Health Organization.

Zbinden G (1976). Percutaneous drug permeation. In: Progress in Toxicology, vol. 2. New York, NY: Springer-Verlag.

Teeguarden JG, Gearhart J, Clewell HJ, et al. (2007). Pharmacokinetic modeling of manganese. III. Physiological approaches accounting for background and tracer kinetics. J Toxicol Environ Health A 70, 1515–26.

Thrall KD, Soelberg JJ, Weitz KK, et al. (2002). Development of a physiologically based pharmacokinetic model for methyl ethyl ketone in F344 rats. J Toxicol Environ Health A 65, 881–96.

3

Biotransformation of toxicants

GENERAL CONSIDERATIONS

As noted in the previous chapter, a toxicant can be absorbed into an organism through different routes. After absorption it is distributed to various parts of the body, including the excretory organs, and is thus available for excretion. Many chemicals are known to undergo biotransformation (metabolic transformation or metabolism), which occurs in the organs and tissues. The most important site of such reactions is the liver; the others being the lungs, stomach, intestine, skin, and kidneys. During the process of biotransformation, "xenobiotics" (foreign substances to an organism or toxic substances) can be either activated (toxic form) or inactivated (nontoxic form) to become reactive or nonreactive to biomolecules such as DNA, RNA, proteins, and lipids.

There are two types of biotransformation:

1. Phase I involving oxidation, reduction, and hydrolysis may be considered degradation reactions
2. Phase II involving the production of a compound (a conjugate) that is biosynthesized from the toxicant, or its metabolite, plus an endogenous metabolite may be considered conjugation reactions

Biotransformation is, therefore, a process that, in general, converts the parent compounds into metabolites and then forms conjugates, but it may involve only one of these reactions. For example, benzene undergoes oxidation, a phase I reaction, to form phenol, which conjugates with sulfate, a phase II reaction. However, when the administered chemical is phenol, it will conjugate with sulfate without a phase I reaction. The metabolites and conjugates are usually more water-soluble and more polar, hence more readily excretable. Biotransformation mediated by phase I and II metabolizing enzymes can, therefore, be considered a mechanism of detoxication (detoxication or bioinactivation) by the host organism.

However, it must be noted that in certain cases the metabolites are more toxic than the parent compounds. Such reactions are known as "bioactivation."

This is frequently noted with chemicals that induce cancer where the metabolite and not the parent compound is the culprit.

The rate of biotransformation and the type of biotransformation of a toxicant often differ from one species of animal to another and even from one strain to another, a fact that often accounts for the difference of toxicity in these animals (see chap. 5). The age and sex of the animal and its exposures to other chemicals may also alter the biotransformation. Genetic polymorphisms in xenobiotic-metabolizing enzymes and transporter have been considered a critical factor for individual susceptibility or variation in toxic responses (Ginsberg et al., 2009; Johansson and Ingelman-Sundberg, 2011). Knowledge of such factors is important in the design of toxicological studies and in the interpretation of health hazards of toxicants to humans.

PHASE I (DEGRADATION) REACTIONS

The three types of phase I reactions, namely, oxidation, reduction, and hydrolysis, are briefly described.

Oxidation

The biotransformation of a great variety of chemicals involves oxidative processes. The most important enzyme systems catalyzing the processes involve cytochrome P-450 and NADPH cytochrome P-450 reductase. In these reactions, one atom of molecular oxygen is reduced to water and the other is incorporated into the ~~where~~ substrate as follows: $SH + O_2 + NADPH + H \rightarrow SOH + HO + NAPD$, S is the substrate.

The cytochrome-linked monooxygenases (oxidases) are located in the endoplasmic reticulum. When a cell is homogenized, the endoplasmic reticulum breaks down to small vesicles known as microsomes. Because of the location of these enzymes and the great variety of chemicals that they may catalyze, they are also known as microsomal, mixed-function oxidases (MFOs). The human P-450 MFO system consists of more than 30 isozymes. They catalyze a great variety of chemicals as shown in this chapter. In addition, oxidation of a number of toxicants is catalyzed by nonmicrosomal oxidoreductases that are located in the mitochondrial fraction in the $100,000 g$ supernatant of tissue homogenates.

Oxidation may take place in a variety of reactions, and often more than one metabolite is formed. The following are some examples.

Microsomal Oxidation

1. Aliphatic oxidation involves oxidation of the aliphatic side chains of aromatic chemicals: for example, *n*-propylbenzene → 3-phenylpropan-1-ol, 3-phenylpropan-2-ol, and 3-phenylpropan-3-ol, as well as aliphatic compounds such as *n*-hexane.

2. Aromatic hydroxylation generally proceeds through an epoxide intermediate: for example, naphthalene $\rightarrow$ naphthalene-1, 2-epoxide $\rightarrow$ 1-naphthol + 2-naphthol.
3. Epoxidation: for example, aldrin $\rightarrow$ dieldrin.
4. Oxidative deamination: for example, amphetamine $\rightarrow$ phenylacetone.
5. N-dealkylation: for example, *N,N*-dimethyl-*p*-nitrophenyl $\rightarrow$ carbamate *N*-methyl-*p*-nitrophenyl carbamate.
6. O-dealkylation: for example, *p*-nitroanisole $\rightarrow$ *p*-nitrophenol.
7. S-dealkylation: for example, 6-methylthiopurine $\rightarrow$ 6-mercaptothiopurine.
8. N-oxidation: for example, trimethylamine $\rightarrow$ trimethylamine oxide.
9. N-hydroxylation: for example, aniline $\rightarrow$ phenylhydroxylamine.
10. P-oxidation: for example, diphenylmethylphosphine $\rightarrow$ diphenylmethylphosphine oxide.
11. Sulfoxidation: for example, methiocarb $\rightarrow$ methiocarb sulfone.
12. Desulfuration involves the replacement of Sby O: for example, parathion $\rightarrow$ paraoxon.

Nonmicrosomal Oxidations Catalyzed by Enzymes in Mitochondria, Cytosol, and Nuclei

1. Amine oxidation: Monoamine oxidase is located in mitochondria and diamine oxidase is a cytosolic enzyme. Both are involved in the oxidation of the primary, secondary, and tertiary amines, such as 5-hydroxytryptamine and putrescine into their corresponding aldehydes.
2. Alcohol and aldehyde dehydrogenations are catalyzed, respectively, by alcohol dehydrogenase and aldehyde dehydrogenase: for example, ethanol $\rightarrow$ acetaldehyde $\rightarrow$ acetic acid.

Reduction

Toxicants may undergo reductions through the function of reductases. These reactions are less active in mammalian tissues but more so in intestinal bacteria. A notable example is the reduction of prontosil to sulfanilamide converting an inactive chemical to an effective antibacterial drug.

Microsomal Reduction

1. Nitro reduction: for example, nitrobenzene $\rightarrow$ nitrosobenzene $\rightarrow$ phenyl hydroxylamine -aniline.
2. Azo reduction: for example, azobenzene aniline.

Nonmicrosomal reductions occur via the reverse reaction of alcohol dehydrogenases (see the section, "Nonmicrosomal Oxidations Catalyzed by Enzymes in Mitochondria, Cytosol, and Nuclei").

Hydrolysis

Many toxicants contain ester-type bonds and are subject to hydrolysis. These are essentially esters, amides, and compounds of phosphate. Mammalian tissues, including the plasma, contain a large number of nonspecific esterases and amidases, which are involved in hydrolysis. The esterases, usually located in the soluble fraction of the cell, may be broadly categorized into four classes:

1. arylesterases, which hydrolyze aromatic esters;
2. carboxyl esterases, which hydrolyze aliphatic esters;
3. cholinesterases, which hydrolyze esters in which the alcohol moiety is choline; and
4. acetyl esterases, which hydrolyze esters in which the acid moiety is acetic acid.

In contrast to esterases, amidases cannot be classified according to substrate specificity. Furthermore, enzymatic hydrolysis of amides proceeds much more slowly than that of esters, probably a result of the lack of substrate specificity.

PHASE II (CONJUGATION) REACTIONS

Phase II reactions involve several types of endogenous metabolites that, as noted above, may form conjugates with the toxicants per se or their metabolites. These conjugates are generally more water soluble and more readily excretable. This is because the physiological transport mechanisms for the endogenous metabolites also recognize the conjugates and hence facilitate their excretion.

Glucuronide Formation

This is the most common and the most important type of conjugation. The enzyme catalyzing this reaction is uridine diphosphate -glucuronyl transferase and the coenzyme is uridine-5′-diphospho-α-d-glucuronic acid. This enzyme is also located in the endoplasmic reticulum. There are four classes of chemical compounds that are capable of forming conjugates with glucuronic acid: (*i*) aliphatic or aromatic alcohols, (*ii*) carboxylic acids, (*iii*) sulfhydryl compounds, and (*iv*) amines.

Sulfate Conjugation

This reaction is catalyzed by sulfotransferases. These enzymes are found primarily in the cytosolic fraction of liver, kidney, and intestine. The coenzyme is 3-phosphoadenosine-5′-phosphosulfate. The functional groups of the foreign compounds for sulfate transfer are phenols and aliphatic alcohols as well as aromatic amines.

Methylation

This reaction is catalyzed by methyl transferases. The coenzyme is S-adenosyl-methionine. Methylation is not a major route of biotransformation of toxicants because of the broader availability of uridine-5′-diphospho-α-d-glucuronic acid, which leads to the formation of glucuronides. Furthermore, it does not always increase the water solubility of the methylated products. The enzymes are located in both the mitochondrial and cytosolic fractions.

Acetylation

Acetylation involves transfer of acetyl groups to primary aromatic amines, hydrazines, hydrazides, sulfonamides, and certain primary aliphatic amines. The enzyme and coenzyme involved are, respectively, N-acetyl transferases and acetyl coenzyme A. In certain cases, such as isoniazid, acetylation results in a decrease in water solubility of an amine and an increase in toxicity.

Amino Acid Conjugation

This conjugation is catalyzed by amino acid conjugates and coenzyme A. Aromatic carboxylic acids, arylacetic acids, and aryl-substituted acrylic acids can form conjugates with not only α-amino acids, mainly glycine, but also with glutamine in humans and certain monkeys and ornithine in birds.

Glutathione Conjugation

This important reaction is affected by glutathione S-transferases and the cofactor glutathione (GSH, a tripeptide; γ-glu-cys-gly). Glutathione conjugates subsequently undergo enzymatic cleavage and acetylation, forming N-acetylcysteine (mercapturic acid) derivatives of the toxicants, which are readily excreted. Examples of chemicals such as epoxides and aromatic halogens that conjugate with glutathione are shown in Figure 3.1. In addition, glutathione can conjugate unsaturated aliphatic compounds and displace the nitro groups in chemicals.

In the process of biotransformation of toxicants, a number of highly reactive electrophilic metabolites are formed. In particular, the generation of reactive oxygen species (ROS) is believed to be responsible for the cancer produced by diesel exhaust particles. Some of these metabolites can react with cellular constituents and cause cell death, induce tumor formation, or affect immune function. The role of glutathione is to react with the electrophilic metabolites such as ROS and thus prevent their harmful effects on the cells. However, exposure to very large amounts of such reactive substances can deplete the glutathione, thereby resulting in marked toxic effects. An example of the depletion of glutathione by acetaminophen and the concomitant increase in covalent binding

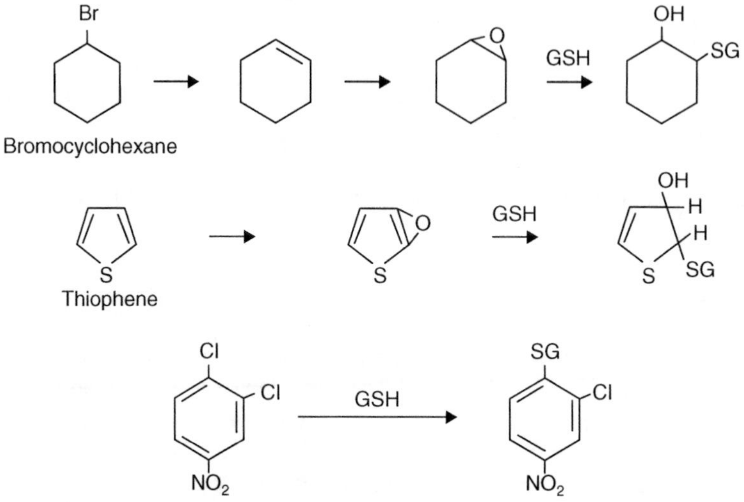

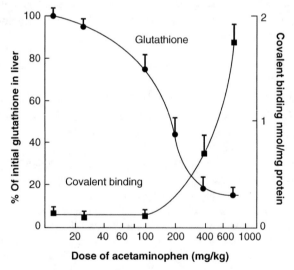

Br

Bromocyclohexane

GSH

OH
SG

Thiophene

GSH

OH
H
H
S SG

Cl
Cl

GSH

SG
Cl

NO$_2$

NO$_2$

3, 4-Dichloronitrobenzene

Figure 3.1 Conjugation of epoxide and dehalogenation catalyzed by glutathione (GSH) transferase. *Source*: From Timbrell (1991).

Figure 3.2 Protective effect of glutathione against covalent binding of acetaminophen to liver proteins. *Source*: From Wills (1981).

to macromolecules is shown in Figure 3.2. Similarly, 3-methylindole is bio-activated mainly in lungs and, after depleting the glutathione, will induce lung damages (Adams et al., 1988). Furthermore, certain glutathione conjugates may become toxic (Anders et al., 1988).

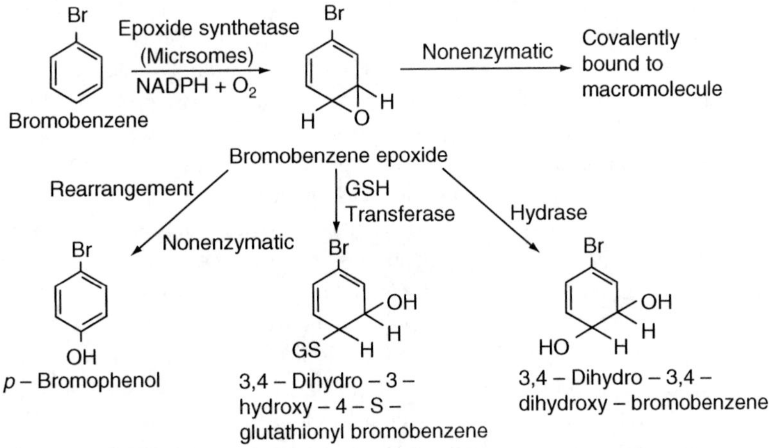

Figure 3.3   The bromobenzene epoxide formed from the parent chemical may covalently bind to macromolecules, but such binding may be minimal when the other metabolic routes are predominant. *Source*: From Gillette and Mitchell (1975).

For additional information on the biological functions of glutathione in the conjugation of electrophiles and as antioxidant, see DeLeve and Kaplowitz (1991) and Commandeur et al. (1995).

BIOACTIVATION

Certain chemically stable compounds can be converted into chemically reactive metabolites. The reactions are generally catalyzed by cytochrome P-450–dependent monooxygenase systems, but other enzymes, including those of the intestinal flora, are involved in certain cases. Furthermore, additional phase I or phase II reactions may be required. The reactive metabolites, such as epoxides, can become covalently bound to cellular macromolecules and cause necrosis and/or cancer. Others, such as free radicals, can cause lipid peroxidation resulting in tissue damage. Descriptions of the bioactivation of various classes of chemicals are available in the literature, such as the book edited by Anders (1985). The following are some notable examples. Appendix 1 lists a number of chemicals that are known to be bioactivated.

Epoxide Formation

Many aromatic compounds are converted to epoxides by microsomal mixed-function oxygenase systems. The biotransformation of bromobenzene to its epoxide and subsequent reactions serves as an interesting example of bioactivation and its consequences. These are depicted in Figure 3.3.

Although bromobenzene epoxide may become covalently bound to tissue macromolecules and cause injury, the alternative routes of metabolism may prevent or reduce the injury. The most important of these routes is the conjugation with glutathione. This reaction is important in that it serves as a protective mechanism. Only after the hepatic levels of reduced glutathione have been greatly depleted will the bromobenzene epoxide significantly bind to macromolecules and result in hepatic necrosis. Depletion of glutathione occurs when a huge dose of bromobenzene is present or when there has been an induction of microsomal enzymes; both conditions increase the amount of bromobenzene epoxide. Other reactions include a non-enzymatic arrangement to form p-bromophenol and the formation of 3,4-dihydro-3,4-dihydroxy-bromobenzene catalyzed by hydrase.

Other chemicals that undergo epoxidation include aflatoxin B_1, benzene, benzo(a)pyrene, furosemide, olefins, polychlorinated, and polybrominated biphenyls, trichloroethylene, and vinyl chloride. Bioactivation takes place mainly in the liver, and the resulting reactive metabolites induce toxicity through covalent binding with macromolecules in the tissue, resulting in necrosis or cancer formation.

N-Hydroxylation

Microsomal enzymes from many tissues can N-hydroxylate a variety of chemicals. Some of the N-hydroxy metabolites, such as those of acetaminophen, 2-acetylaminofluorene, urethane, and certain aminoazo dyes, can cause cancer or tissue necrosis through covalent binding, whereas others, such as certain aromatic amines, can induce hemolysis or methemoglobinemia.

N-hydroxy metabolites are also subject to conjugation reactions. Their conjugates with glucuronic acid are readily excreted; those formed with sulfuric or acetic acid, however, may be unstable and thus can be mutagenic, carcinogenic, and highly toxic (Weisburger and Weisburger, 1973).

Free Radical and Superoxide Formation

Free radicals are unstable and highly reactive molecules that are capable of independent existence, contain one or more unpaired electrons, have an extremely short half-life, and seek to gain additional electrons to have complete pairs or to bind to other molecules to increase their stability. Certain halogen-containing compounds undergo metabolism to form free radicals. For example, carbon tetrachloride forms trichloromethyl radical, which causes peroxidation of polyunsaturated lipid as well as covalently binds to protein and unsaturated lipid. These initial reactions are followed by disturbances of various cellular components, as described in chapter 12. Halothane and bromotrichloromethane are other examples of chemicals that may form free radicals. The herbicide paraquat is known to produce superoxide radicals (Halliwell et al., 1992).

It should be noted that during the metabolic process some chemicals produce not only their reactive metabolites, but generate free radicals such as ROS (radical forms: superoxide anion, hydroxyl radical, peroxyl and alkoxyl radical; non-radical forms: O_3, H_2O_2, hypochlorous acid, and singlet oxygen) or chemical radicals. For example, benzo(a)pyrene (BaP) produces an ultimate metabolite [e.g., benzo(a)pyrene 7,8-diol 9,10-epoxide (BPDE)], ROS, and BaP radical cation (Jiang et al., 2007). Free radicals such as ROS, reactive nitrogen species (radical forms: nitric oxide and nitrogen dioxide; non-radical forms: peroxynitrite, nitroxyl anion, nitrosyl cation, nitronium anion, nitrous acid, etc.), and organic radicals can activate nonreactive toxicants to form biologically reactive intermediates or reactive toxicants without metabolizing enzymes. Free radicals play a central role in toxicological sciences and they are involved in various kinds of toxic manifestations and common mechanisms of toxic actions (Choi and Lee, 2004). Therefore, toxic effects may be ameliorated or prevented by scavenging free radicals with antioxidants, such as antioxidant vitamins, curcumin, isoflavonoids, resveratrol, and plant polysaccharides.

Other Pathways

Ethanol can be oxidized by a dehydrogenase to acetaldehyde, which has been implicated in some of the manifestations of alcohol toxicity. Pyrrolizidine alkaloids are dehydrogenated to reactive pyrrole derivatives, which are carcinogenic. There is evidence confirming that the acute toxicity of aliphatic nitriles is attributable to the cyanide released through hepatic microsomal enzyme activities (Willhite and Smith, 1981).

Activation in the GI Tract

Nitrites and certain amines can react in the acidic environment of the stomach to form nitrosamines, many of which have been shown to be potent carcinogens, and nitrates, which, under certain conditions, can be converted to nitrites that may induce methemoglobinemia. The artificial sweetener cyclamate is converted by intestinal bacteria to cyclohexylamine, which can induce testicular atrophy. Cycasin is converted to its aglycone, methylazoxymethanol, which is hepatotoxic and can induce tumors.

COMPLEX NATURE OF BIOTRANSFORMATION

Toxicants generally undergo several types of biotransformation, resulting in a variety of metabolites and conjugates. Some of the various metabolites and conjugates of bromobenzene are shown in Figure 3.3. Organophosphorous insecticides, such as fenitrothion, chlorofenvinphos, and omethoate, can be metabolized through dealkylation, oxidation, desulfuration, or hydrolysis, yielding 10 or more different metabolites.

Parathion, an organophosphorous pesticide, is bioactivated in the liver to paraoxon, which is a much more potent cholinesterase inhibitor. Infusion of parathion by way of the vena cava, bypassing the liver, therefore produced little cholinesterase inhibition, but a moderate effect was induced following infusion by way of the portal vein. On the other hand, infusion of paraoxon via the vena cava nearly completely blocked the cholinesterase activity, whereas it had negligible effect after an infusion via the portal vein, since it is detoxicated in the liver (Westermann, 1961).

A reactive metabolite formed in a phase I reaction can be further metabolized, such as carbon tetrachloride and halothane. Such a metabolite may also be followed by a phase II reaction to produce another reactive metabolite. For example, 2-acetylaminofluorene after N-hydroxylation can undergo acetylation or form sulfate or glutathione conjugates, all of which are highly reactive.

The relative importance of various types of biotransformation of a toxicant depends on many host, environmental, and chemical factors as well as the dose of the toxicant. Since the metabolites resulting from different types of biotransformation are often markedly different in their effects, the toxicity of a chemical can be greatly altered by these factors, as will be discussed in chapter 5.

Some of the metabolic reactions take place in sequence; hence interference with the normal metabolic pathway may have considerable influence on the toxic effects. For example, ethanol is normally metabolized through the intermediary product acetaldehyde. In normal humans the acetaldehyde formed is rapidly further metabolized to acetate, which in turn is converted to carbon dioxide and water. However, if the aldehyde dehydrogenase is inhibited, such as after the administration of disulfiram, the level of acetaldehyde rises and results in distress symptoms such as nausea, vomiting, headache, and palpitations.

A toxicant may be transformed in one organ to a stable proximate metabolite, which is transported to another organ and metabolizes to the ultimate toxic metabolite (Cohen, 1986).

Reeves (1981) provides a number of examples of biotransformation of "typical" chemicals, as well as a limited generalization of the typical routes of foreign compound metabolism in humans (Fig. 3.4).

Developmental and Children Considerations

The ability to handle chemicals in the fetus, infant, and child varies distinctly from that in the adult. Makri et al. (2004) described the metabolic characteristics of neonates to the adolescent, which would ultimately affect the susceptibility of the subject to various chemicals. In general, a neonate, infant, or child is more susceptible to chemical exposure. The age categories are as follows: neonate is 0–1 month, infant from 1 month to 2 years, preschool from 2 to 6 years, the child from 6 to 12 years, and adolescent from 12 to 16 years. Cytochrome P-450 is low from zero to one year, which indicates that a chemical half-life is longer and elimination is prolonged. In essence, this manifests as a higher susceptibility to chemical effects. Alcohol dehydrogenase is barely detectable in the infant and is present at five years of age, indicating an inability to handle alcohol and thus toxic consequences to the infant. Glucuronidation pathways and acetylation capacity are not available until

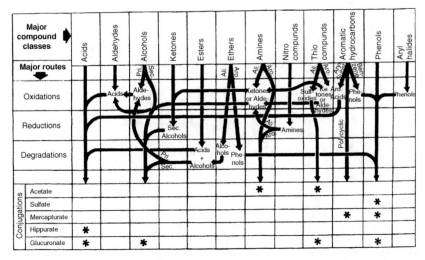

Figure 3.4 Typical routes of foreign compound metabolism in humans. *Source:* From Reeves (1981).

3 years of age, again indicating an enhanced susceptibility. Although sulfate conjugation is higher from 0 to 3 years, the capacity falls to the adult level 3 to 10 years. The difficulty here is that sulfation is not a predominant route for elimination of various compounds and thus results in enhanced chemical susceptibility.

The U.S. Environmental Protection Agency cancer risk assessment guidance recommends a default assumption that children are inherently up to 10-fold more sensitive than adults to carcinogen exposures. However, as pointed out by Pyatt et al. (2007), there is no evidence that children are at increased risk for chemically induced acute myelogenous leukemia development. In fact it would appear that the risk for drug-induced leukemia development is actually lower in younger children. These findings clearly demonstrate that generalized observations in toxicology can result in miscalculations of risk and unnecessary concerns. The need for extensive data in making decisions, especially as it pertains to sensitive subpopulations is warranted.

Elderly

It must also be borne in mind that the metabolic pathways are age dependent and less reliable in the elderly, which also manifests as increased susceptibility to toxicity in the elderly. The elderly are generally a population that is exposed to multidrug therapy, resulting in drug interactions and reduced capacity of the liver to handle these agents. With concurrent environmental chemical exposure and multidrug administration in a subject with compromised ability to eliminate chemicals, the occurrence of toxicity attributed to environmental chemicals can be additive or synergistic.

REFERENCES

Adams JD Jr, Laegreid WW, Huijzer JC, et al. (1988). Pathology and glutathione status in 3-methylindole-treated rodents. Res Commun Chem Pathol Pharmacol 60, 323–36.

Anders MW, ed (1985). Bioactivation of Foreign Compounds. New York, NY: Academic Press.

Anders MW, Lash L, Dekant W, et al. (1988). Biosynthesis and biotransformation of glutathione S-conjugates to toxic metabolites. CRC Crit Rev Toxicol 18, 311.

Choi SM, Lee BM (2004). An alternative mode of action of endocrine-disrupting chemicals and chemoprevention. J Toxicol Environ Health B Crit Rev 7, 451–63.

Cohen GM (1986). Basic principles of target organ toxicity. In: Cohen GM, ed Target Organ Toxicity. Boca Raton, FL: CRC Press.

Commandeur JNML, Stijntjes GJ, Vermeulen NPE (1995). Enzymes and transport systems involved in the formation and disposition of glutathione S-conjugates. Pharmacol Revs 47, 271–330.

DeLeve LD, Kaplowitz N (1991). Glutathione metabolism and its role in hepatotoxicity. Pharmacol Ther 52, 287–305.

Gillette JR, Mitchell JR (1975). Drug actions and interactions: theoretical considerations. In: Eichler O, Farah A, Herken H, Welch AD, eds. Handbook of Experimental Pharmacology. New Series, vol. 28. New York, NY: Springer-Verlag, 359–82.

Ginsberg G, Smolenski S, Hattis D, et al. (2009). Genetic Polymorphism in Glutathione Transferases (GST): Population distribution of GSTM1, T1, and P1 conjugating activity. J Toxicol Environ Health B Crit Rev 12, 389–439.

Halliwell B, Gutteridge JMC, Cross CE (1992). Free radicals, antioxidants and human diseases—Where are we now? J Lab Clin Med 119, 598–620.

Jiang H, Gelhaus SL, Mangal D, et al. (2007). Metabolism of benzo[a]pyrene in human bronchoalveolar H358 cells using liquid chromatography-mass spectrometry. Chem Res Toxicol 20, 1331–41.

Johansson I, Ingelman-Sundberg M (2011). Genetic polymorphism and toxicology—with emphasis on cytochrome p450. Toxicol Sci 120, 1–13.

Makri A, Goveia M, Balbus J, et al. (2004). Children's susceptibility to chemicals: A review by developmental stage. J Toxicol Environ Health B 7, 417–35.

Pyatt DW, Aylward LL, Hays, SM (2007). Is age an independent risk factor for chemically induced acute myelogenous leukemia in children? J Toxicol Environ Health B 10, 379–400.

Reeves AL (1981). The metabolism of foreign compounds. In: Reeves AL, ed Toxicology: Principles and Practices, Vol 1. New York, NY: John Wiley.

Timbrell JA (1991). Principles of Biochemical Toxicology. London, UK: Taylor & Francis.

Westermann EO (1961). Bioactivation of parathion. Proceedings of International Pharmacology Meeting 6: 205. In: Ariens EJ, Simmonis AM, Offermeier J, eds Introduction to General Toxicology. New York, NY: Academic Press,147.

Weisburger JH, Weisburger EK (1973). Biochemical formation and pharmacological, toxicological and pathological properties of hydroxylamines and hydroxyamic acids. Pharmacol Rev 25, 166.

Willhite CC, Smith RP (1981). The role of cyanide liberation in the acute toxicity of aliphatic nitriles. Toxicol Appl Pharmacol 59, 589–602.

Wills ED (1981). The role of glutathione in drug metabolism and the protection of the liver against toxic metabolites. In: Gorrod JW, ed Testing for Toxicity. London, UK: Taylor & Francis.

Appendix 1 Examples of Bioactivation[a]

Parent Compound	Toxic Metabolite	Mechanism of Toxicity	Toxic Effect
Acetaminophen	N-acetyl-p-benzoquinone imine	Covalent binding	Hepatic necrosis, GI bleeding, nephrotoxicity
2-Acetylaminofluorene (AAF)	N-hydroxy-AAF, sulfate ester	Covalent binding	Cancers (liver, kidney, bladder)
Aflatoxin B_1	Aflatoxin-8,9-epoxide	Covalent binding	Hepatic cancer
Allyl formate	Acrolein	Covalent binding	Hepatic necrosis, lung toxicity
Amiodarone	Des ethyl amiodarone	Ethylation	Pulmonary fibrosis, thyroid abnormalities, ophthalmological effects, neurological changes
Amygdalin	Mandelo nitrile, hydrogen cyanide	Cyanide formation	Cytotoxic hypoxia, toxicity of nervous, cardiovascular, and respiratory systems
N-arylsuccinimide	3,5-Dichlorophenyl-2-hydroxysuccinimide	Oxidation and hydrolysis	Nephrotoxicity
Benzene	Benzene epoxide→ hydroquinone, 1,2,4-trihydroxybenzene	Covalent binding	Bone marrow depression, leukemia
Benzo (a)pyrene (BaP)	BaP-7,8-epoxide → (+)BaP-7,8-diol-9, 10-epoxide [(+)BPDE-I]	Covalent binding	Cancers (lung, stomach, cervix, skin)
Bromobenzene	2-Bromoquinone, 4-bromoquinone, bromobenzene epoxides	Covalent binding	Hepatic, renal, bronchiolar toxicity
1,3-Butadiene	3,4-Epoxy-1-butene (EB) 1,2:3,4-diepoxybutane (DEB), 3,4-epoxy-1,2-butanediol (EB diol)	Covalent binding	Cancer (stomach, blood, lymphatic system), hepatic necrosis, narcosis, reproductive toxicity
2-Butoxyethanol	2-Butoxyacetic acid	Oxidation	Hemolytic disorders
Carbon tetrachloride	Trichloro methane free radical	Covalent binding	Hepatic necrosis, hepatic cancer, neurotoxicity

(continued)

Appendix 1 Examples of Bioactivation[a] (*continued*)

Parent Compound	Toxic Metabolite	Mechanism of Toxicity	Toxic Effect
Carcinogenic alkyl nitrosamines	α-Hydroxylation	Alkylation	Cancer (liver, esophagus, many organs)
Carcinogenic aminoazo dyes	N-hydroxy derivatives	Covalent binding	Hepatic cancer, bladder cancer
Carcinogenic Polycyclic aromatic hydrocarbons (PAHs)	PAH-diolepoxide	Covalent binding	Cancers (lung, skin, stomach)
Chloroform	Phosgene	Covalent binding	Hepatic, renal necrosis
Cycasin	Methyl azoxy methanol, gut flora	Alkylation	Cancers (liver, kidney, intestine), hepatic necrosis
Cyclophosphamide	Phosphoramide	Alkylation	Cytotoxic, nephrotoxicity
Formaldehyde	—	Covalent binding	Nasal cancer, leukemia?
Fluoroacetate	Fluoro citrate	Enzyme inhibition	General toxicity
Furosemide	Epoxide?	Covalent binding	Hepatic, renal necrosis
Halothane	Free radical	Covalent binding	Hepatic necrosis
Isoniazid	Acetyl hydrazine	Covalent binding	Hepatic necrosis
Metam sodium	(Metabolite of) methyl isothiocyanate	Reduction	Immunosuppression, spontaneous abortion with increased frequency, asthma
Methemoglobin-producing aromatic amines and nitro compounds	N-hydroxy metabolites	Cyclic oxidoreduction	Methemoglobinemia
Methoxyflurane	Inorganic fluoride	Enzyme inhibition	Renal failure
Monocrotaline	Monocrotaline pyrrole	Electrophile monocrotaline pyrrole → formation of free radical	Lung and liver damage
Naphthylamine	N-hydroxy naphthylamine	Covalent binding	Bladder cancer

(*continued*)

Appendix 1   Examples of Bioactivation[a] (*continued*)

Parent Compound	Toxic Metabolite	Mechanism of Toxicity	Toxic Effect
Nitrates	Nitrites	Hemoglobin oxidation	Methemoglobinemia
Nitrites plus secondary or tertiary amines	Nitrosamines	Alkylation	Hepatic, pulmonary cancers
Parathion	Paraoxon	Covalent binding to cholinesterase	Neuromuscular paralysis
Purine and pyrimidine base analogues	Mononucleotides, nucleotide triphosphates	Lethal synthesis, lethal incorporation	Cytotoxicity
Safrole (also known as shikimol)	1'-Hydroxy safrole	Covalent binding	Cancers
Styrene	Styrene oxide	Covalent binding	Lung tumors
Urethane (ethyl carbamate)	N-hydroxy urethane, vinyl carbamate?	Alkylation	Cancers (liver, lung), cytotoxicity
Vinyl chloride	Chloroethylene epoxide	Covalent binding	Liver cancer

[a]The site of bioactivation is the liver, except as otherwise noted. Covalent binding refers to DNA, protein, or lipid adduct formation with reactive metabolites of chemicals or reactive chemicals themselves.

4

Toxic effect

GENERAL CONSIDERATIONS

Toxic effects are greatly variable in nature, potency, target organ, and mechanism of action. A better understanding of their characteristics can improve the assessment of the associated health hazards. It can also facilitate the development of rational preventive and therapeutic measures.

All toxic effects result from biochemical interactions between the toxicants (and/or their metabolites) and certain structures of the organism. The structure may be nonspecific, such as any tissue in direct contact with corrosive chemicals. More often it is specific, involving a particular subcellular structure. A variety of structures may be affected.

The nature of effects may also vary from organ to organ. The organ-specific effects will be discussed in some detail in the chapters in Part III of this book. In some cases, the reason for a particular organ being affected is known. This knowledge is useful in many ways. A few examples are described in this chapter.

SPECTRUM OF TOXIC EFFECTS

The great variety of toxic effects can be grouped according to the target organ, mechanism of action, or other characteristics such as those discussed next.

Local and Systemic Effects

Certain chemicals can produce injuries at the site of first contact with an organism. These local effects can be induced by caustic substances on the gastrointestinal tract, by corrosive materials on the skin, and by irritant gases and vapors on the respiratory tract.

Systemic effects result only after the toxicant has been absorbed and distributed to other parts of the body. Most toxicants exert their main effects on one or a few organs. These organs are referred to as the "target organs" of these toxicants.

A target organ does not necessarily have the highest concentration of the toxicants in the organism. For example, the target organ of dichlorodiphenyltrichloroethane (DDT) is the central nervous system, but it is concentrated in adipose tissues.

Reversible and Irreversible Effects

Reversible effects of toxicants are those that will disappear following cessation of exposure to them. Irreversible effects, in contrast, will persist or even progress after exposure is discontinued. Certain effects are obviously irreversible. These include carcinomas, teratogenesis, damage to neurons, and liver cirrhosis. In toxicology, irreversible effects are more important than reversible effects because irreversible effects are chronic and hard to be cured.

Certain effects are considered irreversible even though they disappear sometime after cessation of exposure. For example, the "irreversible" cholinesterase-inhibiting insecticides inhibit the activity of this enzyme for a period of time that approximates the time required for the synthesis and replacement of the enzyme.

The effect produced by a toxicant may be reversible if the organism is exposed at a low concentration and/or for a short duration, whereas irreversible effects may be produced at higher concentrations and/or for longer durations of exposure.

Immediate and Delayed Effects

Many toxicants produce immediate toxic effects, which develop shortly after a single exposure, a notable example being cyanide poisoning. Delayed effects occur after a lapse of some time. Carcinogenic effects generally become manifest 10–20 years after the initial exposure in humans; even in rodents, a lapse of many months is required. In some cases, for example, diethylstilbestrol was taken by pregnant mothers to prevent miscarriages (Roy et al., 1997; Dean, 1998). However, vaginal adenocarcinomas occurred in the daughters of mothers taking diethylstilbestrol. This effect took 15–20 years to develop not in the target subject but was found in the offspring. In addition, in men there was evidence of reproductive dysfunctions and increased occurrence of prostatic and testicular cancers. To determine these and other delayed effects of toxicants, long-term studies are essential not only in the directly exposed individual but also in the fetus or offspring.

Morphological, Functional, and Biochemical Effects

Morphological effects refer to gross and microscopic changes in the morphology of the tissues. Many of these effects, such as necrosis and neoplasia, are irreversible and serious. Functional effects usually represent reversible changes in the functions of target organs. Functions of the liver and kidney (e.g., rate of excretion of dyes) are commonly tested in toxicological studies.

Functional effects are in general reversible, whereas morphological effects are not, and functional changes are generally detected earlier or in animals exposed to lower doses than those with morphological changes. In addition, functional tests are valuable in following the progress of effects on target organs in long-term studies in animals and humans. It is worthwhile noting that functional tests can be positive for an adverse effect, yet there is no morphological evidence. An example is the presence of depleted uranium producing proteinuria, indicative of a renal functional alteration, but there are no apparent morphological changes (NAS, 2008). The role of concentration of depleted uranium at the target site may be important as lower amounts of metal may produce the effect seen, but the concentration is not sufficient to induce morphological alterations. This is of particular concern for veterans of the Gulf War and for the assessment of hazard characterization. However, the results are often more variable.

Although all toxic effects are associated with biochemical alterations, in routine toxicity testing, "biochemical effects" usually refer to those without apparent morphological changes. An example of such effects is the cholinesterase inhibition following exposure to organophosphate and carbamate insecticides. Another example is δ-aminolevulinic acid dehydratase inhibition in lead poisoning (see chaps. 19 and 21).

Allergic and Idiosyncratic Reactions

Allergic reaction (also known as hypersensitivity and sensitization reaction) to a toxicant results from previous sensitization to that toxicant or a chemically similar one. The chemical acts as a hapten and combines with an endogenous protein to form an antigen, which in turn elicits the formation of antibodies. A subsequent exposure to the chemical will result in an antigen–antibody interaction, which provokes the typical manifestations of allergy. Thus, this reaction is different from the usual toxic effects, first because a previous exposure is required, and second because a typical sigmoid dose–response curve is usually not demonstrable with allergic reactions. Nevertheless, threshold doses were demonstrable for the induction as well as the challenge in dermal sensitization (Koschier et al., 1983). In addition to the immune response described above, humans can also generate self- or autoantigens, constituents of the body's own tissues in response to a specific humoral or cell-mediated immune response termed as autoimmunity. An example of an autoimmune disease is systemic lupus erythematosus (SLE), and a chemical implicated in SLE occurrence is trichlorothene (Wang et al., 2007).

Generally an idiosyncratic reaction is a genetically determined abnormal reactivity to a chemical. Some patients exhibit prolonged muscular reaction and apnea following a standard dose of succinylcholine. These patients have a deficiency of serum cholinesterase, which normally degrades the muscle relaxant rapidly. Similarly, people with a deficiency of NADH methemoglobinemia reductase

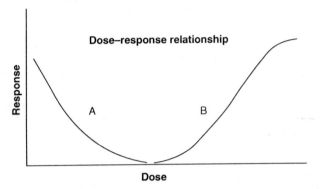

Figure 4.1 Schematic representation of dose–response relationship. *Curve A*: certain essential nutrients, with which the response (deficiency syndrome) increases along with decreased intake. *Curve B*: most chemicals with which the response (toxic effects) increases along with increased intake. Certain substances, for example, selenium, exhibit both types of responses.

are abnormally sensitive to nitrites and other chemicals that produce methemoglobinemia. Recent studies have shown that the susceptibility to arsenic-induced cancer development was dependent on genetic polymorphism. Arsenic metabolism is dependent on methylene tetrafolate reductase and glutathione S-transferases. Polymorphisms in these enzymes result in differences in arsenic metabolism and thus differences in susceptibility to cancer induction (Steinmaus et al., 2007).

Graded and Quantal Responses

Effects on body weight, food consumption, and enzyme inhibition are examples of graded responses. On the other hand, mortality and tumor formation are examples of quantal (all-or-none) responses. Both types of responses can be statistically analyzed as illustrated in chapter 6.

The relationship between dose and response usually follows an S-shaped curve. Figure 4.1A and B is a schematic representation of most chemicals and that of certain essential nutrients, respectively. The latter is exemplified by thiamine and ascorbic acid. Insufficient intake of these vitamins will induce deficiency syndromes, but higher intakes will be readily eliminated in the urine. Selenium is an essential element but an excessive intake will be toxic (see chap. 21); therefore its dose–response relationship is represented by curves A and B.

Another type of dose–response relationship (J-shaped or inverted U-shaped) consists of an effect observable at doses lower than the NOAEL (no-observed-adverse-effect level) (see chap. 25) and is opposite to the main toxic effect (e.g., stimulation vs. inhibition). This is known as "hormesis" and has been reported for a number of chemicals (Calabrese and Baldwin, 2001). Postconditioning hormesis refers to the phenomenon that a beneficial effect of applying mild stress to cells or organisms, that were initially exposed to a high dose of stress (Wiegant et al., 2011).

As the dose of a toxicant increases, so does the response, either in terms of the proportion of the population responding or in terms of the severity of graded responses. Furthermore, additional toxic effects may also appear along with increased doses. For example, methyl mercury induces paresthesia at low doses, but it also induces ataxia, dysarthria, deafness, and death at higher doses, as shown in Figure ~~2.23~~ of chapter 23, which depicts both *dose–response* and *dose–effect* relationships. 23.2

TARGET ORGANS

Toxicants do not affect all organs to the same extent. An understanding of the mechanisms that determine organ specificity will assist in the advancement of various aspects of toxicology. Although the reason is not always clear, the probable mechanisms by which many toxicants act specifically on certain organs are known. In general, the underlying mechanism is either a greater susceptibility of the target organ or a higher concentration of the chemical and/or its metabolite at the site of action. The higher concentration may arise under a variety of conditions. It should be noted that higher concentrations of a compound may be present, for example, in adipose tissue for DDT, yet the effect produced is in the brain at the lower amount. The concentration at the target tissue and receptor must be sufficient for a period of time to produce an effect but this amount may not be the highest in the body.

Sensitivity of the Organ

Neurons and myocardium depend primarily on adenosine triphosphate (ATP) generated by mitochondrial oxidation with little capacity for anaerobic metabolism, and there are rapid ionic shifts through the cell membrane. They are, therefore, especially sensitive to lack of oxygen resulting from disorders of the vascular system or of hemoglobin (e.g., carbon monoxide poisoning).

Rapidly dividing cells, such as those in the bone marrow and the intestinal mucosa, are more susceptible to mitotic poisons (e.g., methotrexate).

Distribution

The respiratory tract and the skin are target organs of industrial and environmental toxicants because these are the sites of absorption. An example is provided by bis(chloromethyl) ether. It produces skin tumors in humans when applied topically, but will induce tumors in the respiratory tract after exposure by inhalation.

On a unit weight basis, the liver and kidney have a higher volume of blood flow, and thus they are in general exposed to toxicants to a greater extent. In addition, these organs have greater metabolic and excretory functions, which also render them more susceptible to toxicants. Being lipophilic, methyl mercury can cross the blood–brain barrier and exert its toxic effects on the nervous system. Inorganic mercury compounds, in contrast, are not able to cross the blood–brain barrier and are not neurotoxic.

Radiation may oxidatively damage DNA by free radical generation and induce tumors. Ultraviolet light has little penetrating power and therefore will only produce skin tumors, whereas ionizing radiation may penetrate tissues and cause leukemia and other types of cancer.

Selective Uptake

Certain cells have a high affinity for selected chemicals. For example, in the respiratory tract, the type I and type II alveolar epithelial cells, which have an active uptake system for endogenous polyamines, will take up paraquat, a structurally similar chemical. This process can result in the damage of the local tissue even when paraquat is administered orally.

Melanin is present in the eye, inner ear, etc. Drugs such as chloroquine and kanamycin that have an affinity for melanin may accumulate, after prolonged administration, in these organs and cause damage. Strontium-90 (Sr-90) with a half-life of 28 years is selectively deposited in the bone and can induce tumors of the bone.

Biotransformation

As a result of *bioactivation*, reactive metabolites are formed. Liver, being a major site of biotransformation, is susceptible to the action of many toxicants. However, there are exceptions. For example, certain metabolites are sufficiently stable; they may affect other organs after being transported there. Thus bromobenzene, though bioactivated in the liver, can affect the kidney.

With some toxicants, bioactivation at certain sites is predominately responsible for the observed effects. For example, the organophosphorothioate insecticides, such as parathion, are bioactivated mainly in the liver, but the abundance of detoxifying enzymes and of reactive but noncritical binding sites there prevents any overt signs of toxicity. On the other hand, nervous tissue has much less bioactivating enzymes, but because the bioactivation takes place near the critical target sites, that is, the synapses, the main toxic manifestations of this group of toxicants arise from the nervous system.

The bioactivating enzymes are not necessarily evenly distributed in an organ or tissue. For example, the Clara cells (non-ciliated bronchiolar epithelial cells) constitute only 1% of the cells in the lung, yet they contain a major portion of the pulmonary cytochrome P-450. The lung is therefore more susceptible to damage by such toxicants as 4-ipomeanol and CCl_4. Recently, Clara cells were found to metabolize styrene to styrene oxide that ultimately resulted in lung carcinoma. A similar situation exists in the kidney. The proximal tubules, especially the S_3

cells, which are located in the pars recta portion of these tubules, have the highest concentrations of this enzyme system, hence the most susceptible parts of the kidney are the proximal tubules, especially its pars recta portion. The nephrotoxicity of haloalkenes is attributed to renal metabolites generated in the kidney.

Repair Mechanism

A toxicant may affect a specific organ because of lack of the required repair mechanism. For example, N-methyl-N-nitrosourea (MNU) produces tumors in the rat mainly in the brain, occasionally in the kidney, but not in the liver. Kleihues and Cooper (1976) demonstrated that the liver is capable of enzymatically excising the O_6-alkyl-guanine induced by MNU from the DNA, whereas the brain is deficient in this respect. The capacity of the kidney falls between that of the liver and brain.

MECHANISMS OF ACTION

Although the mechanisms of action of all toxicants are not fully understood, a number of biochemical reactions are likely involved. The underlying processes/subcellular sites are listed, along with some exemplary toxicants, in Table 4.1.

The table clearly shows the diverse nature of the mechanisms as well as the multiple processes/sites that are involved in the action of a number of toxicants. For many of the toxicants listed in Table 4.1, the mechanisms will be described, along with their toxic manifestations, in the relevant chapters.

Of the various mechanisms of action, disturbance of calcium homeostasis merits special mention because of its importance and complexity. The extracellular level of $Ca2^+$ is more than 10-fold higher than that in the cytosol. The ionic differential is maintained by a variety of mechanisms including the $Ca2^+$ transporting ATPase at the plasma membrane, the store in the endoplasmic reticulum, mitochondria, and nucleus as well as the binding with intracellular calmodulin. Increase in cytosolic $Ca2^+$ may be produced via different mechanisms. For example, CCl_4 and bromobenzene act through inhibition of $Ca2^+$ ATPase, acetaminophen, and CCl_4 through damage of plasma membrane, and cadmium by release of $Ca2^+$ from mitochondria. The rise in cytosolic $Ca2^+$ may affect cytoskeleton thereby damaging cellular integrity either directly or through $Ca2^+$-activated proteases. Oxidant stress produces injury in lungs through an increase in $Ca2^+$ in alveolar macrophages by a Ca-mediated signaling (Hoyal et al., 1998). In addition, 2,3,7,8-tetrachlorodibenzo-p-dioxin (TCDD) may promote "apoptosis" (programmed cell death) by combining with Ah receptor, increasing intracellular $Ca2^+$ activating endonuclease and inducing DNA breakdown (Timbrell, 1991; Halliwell and Cross, 1994).

Most of the reactions take place at various subcellular sites. Table 13.1 in chapter 13 lists a number of hepatotoxicants along with the organelles that they affect.

Table 4.1 Some Mechanisms of Toxic Action[a]

Mechanism of Action	Process/Subcellular Site	Examples of Toxicants
Interference with normal receptor–ligand interaction	Neurotransmitters	Botulinum toxin, organophosphate pesticides
	Hormone receptors	Amitrole, DES, retinoic acid, TCDD
	Enzymes	Fluoroacetate, cyanide, organophosphate pesticides
	Transport proteins	CO, nitrites
Interference with membrane function	Excitable membrane: ion influx	DDT, saxitoxin, tetrodotoxin
	Membrane: fluidity	Organic solvents (e.g., CCl_4, chloroform), ethanol
	Lysosomal membranes	CCl_4, phosphorus, phalloidin
	Mitochondrial membranes	CCl_4, organotins, phosphorus
Interference with cellular energy production	Hemoglobin	CO, nitrites
	Oxidative phosphorylation: uncoupling	Dinitrophenol, organotins
	Electron transport: inhibition	Cyanide, rotenone
	Carbohydrate metabolism: inhibition	Fluoroacetate
Covalent binding to biomolecules	Lipids: peroxidation	CCl_4, ozone, paraquat, phenytoin, free radicals
	Glutathione: depletion	Acetaminophen
	Protein thiols: oxidation	Acetaminophen, phenytoin
	Nucleic acids	Reactive carcinogens, mutagens, teratogens
Perturbation of calcium homeostasis	Cytoskeleton, etc.	Arsenic, cobalt, doxorubicin, microcystin, paraquat, phalloidin
	Apoptosis	TCDD

[a]The toxic effects of a number of the toxicants are described in other sections. For the relevant page, refer to the Chemical Index.
Abbreviations: TCDD, (2,3,7,8-tetrachlorodibenzo-p-dioxin), DDT, dichlorodiphenyltrichloroethane; DES, diethylstilbestrol.

MOLECULAR TARGETS: CHEMICAL NATURE

Proteins

Receptors

Receptors are located across plasma membrane, or in cytosol, or nucleus, and serve to transmit physical or chemical signals to the cell. There are many types of receptors that serve a variety of functions. Some of them are known to be affected by toxicants (see the section "Receptors" at the end of this chapter).

Enzymes

Enzymes are common targets of toxicants. The enzyme effects may be specific, such as the inhibition of acetylcholinesterase (AChE). They may be reversible, such as the case with a number of carbamate insecticides on AChE. Irreversible enzyme inhibition is exemplified by di-isopropyl fluorophosphate, which covalently bind with the enzymes.

The effects may be nonspecific. For example, lead and mercury are inhibitors of a great variety of enzymes. However, some enzymes are more susceptible: for example, δ-aminolevulinic acid dehydrase is especially sensitive to lead, and its activity in erythrocytes is used as an early indicator of lead poisoning.

The last step of the oxidation of many chemicals is catalyzed by the cytochrome oxidase chain. Hydrocyanic acid can bind with the iron in these enzymes and block their redox function. The aerobic respiration of cells is then arrested and biochemical asphyxia ensues.

An enzyme can also be inhibited by a chemical derived by synthesis from the toxicant such as fluoroacetic acid and its derivatives. The process is known as *lethal synthesis*. Fluoroacetic acid is metabolized as acetic acid in the citric acid cycle and fluorocitric acid is synthesized, instead of citric acid. Since fluorocitric acid is an inhibitor of aconitase, further metabolism, and consequently the energy production, is blocked.

In a somewhat similar manner, amino acid antagonists (e.g., azaserine and fluorophenylalanine) can interfere with the utilization of specific amino acids in the synthesis of proteins.

The energy that is liberated by biochemical oxidation is normally stored in the form of high-energy phosphates. *Uncoupling agents* such as dinitrophenol interfere with the synthesis of energy-rich phosphates, and thus the energy is liberated as heat instead of being stored.

Carriers

Carriers such as hemoglobin can be affected by a toxicant through preferential binding. For example, carbon monoxide can bind hemoglobin at the site where oxygen is normally bound. Because of its greater affinity for hemoglobin, it can inactivate hemoglobin and cause manifestations of oxygen deficiency in tissues.

Oxygen transport can also be impaired by an accumulation of methemoglobin, which is an oxidation product of hemoglobin with no oxygen binding ability. In normal individuals, the trace amount of methemoglobin is readily reduced to hemoglobin. Certain toxicants, such as nitrites and aromatic amines, can enhance the formation of methemoglobin and overwhelm the normal process of its reduction to hemoglobin. People with glucose-6-phosphatase dehydrogenase deficiency have a lower capacity to regenerate hemoglobin from methemoglobin and are thus prone to have methemoglobinemia.

P-glycoprotein is a transmembrane protein expressed by small intestine, kidneys, liver, placenta, and the blood–brain barrier (Abu-Qare et al., 2003).

The function of P-glycoprotein is to bind to a chemical and then transport the agent from the cell; in essence, it serves as a carrier of xenobiotic from the cell. Compounds such as ivermectin, chlorpyrifos, and endosulfan showed decreased effectiveness due to increased expression of P-glycoprotein, which acts as a protective transporter.

Structural Proteins

Extracellular structural proteins such as collagen are unlikely to be affected by toxicants. However, toxicants such as ozone and asbestos may cause an increase in fibroblasts and deposition of collagen in the lungs (chap. 12). Intracellular structural proteins, such as cytoskeleton, may be damaged by toxicants such as arsenic (Li and Chou, 1992) paraquat (Li et al., 1987), benzene (Ross, 2000), styrene (Cohen et al., 2002), and deoxynivalenol (Pestka and Smolinski, 2005).

Coenzymes

Coenzymes are essential for the normal function of enzymes. Their levels in the body can be diminished by toxicants that inhibit their synthesis. For example, pyrithiamine can inhibit thiamine kinase, which is responsible for the formation of the coenzyme thiamine pyrophosphate. NADPH can be destroyed in the presence of free radicals, which can be produced by such toxicants as carbon tetrachloride.

Metal-dependent enzymes can be inhibited by chelating agents (e.g., cyanides and dithiocarbamates) through removal of metal coenzymes such as copper and zinc.

Lipids

Peroxidation of polyenoic fatty acids has been suggested as a mechanism of the necrotizing action of a number of toxicants, such as carbon tetrachloride, ozone, and estrogen (Roy et al., 2007). The culprit is believed to be reactive oxygen species (ROS) that is generated by the transformation of the chemical with subsequent ROS interaction with membrane lipid. The resulting outcome is cellular death or necrosis. Covalent binding of bezo(a)pyrene diolepoxide to triglyceride may be associated with the epigenetic mechanism of bezo(a)pyrene carcinogenesis (Kwack and Lee, 2000; Park et al., 2002).

Cell membrane derangement may result after exposure to various types of toxicants. The general anesthetics, ether and halothane, as well as many other lipophilic substances can accumulate in the cell membranes and thereby interfere with transport of oxygen and glucose into the cell resulting in narcosis. The cells of the central nervous system are especially susceptible to a lowering of oxygen tension and glucose level and are therefore among the first to be deleteriously affected by these substances. Membrane dissolution can follow contact with organic solvents and amphoteric detergents. The ions of mercury and cadmium can complex with phospholipid bases and expand the surface area of the membrane, thereby altering its function. Lead ion can increase the fragility of erythrocytes and result in hemolysis. The oxygen-carrying function of hemoglobin is lost after it escapes from the hemolyzed erythrocytes.

Nucleic Acids

Covalent binding between a toxicant (such as alkylating agents) and replicating DNA and RNA can induce cancer, mutations, and teratogenesis. Such toxicants may also exert immunosuppressive effects.

Antimetabolites such as aminopterin and methotrexate may be incorporated into DNA and RNA and then interfere with their replication.

Others

Hypersensitivity reactions result from repeated exposure to a particular substance or to its chemically related substances. The latter phenomenon is referred to as cross sensitization. The substance, if it is a large polypeptide, acts as an antigen and stimulates the body to form antibodies. Otherwise, the substance acts as a hapten and combines with proteins in the body to form antigens. The reaction between an antigen from a later exposure and the corresponding antibodies results in the release of histamine, bradykinin, and others. The reaction has a typical pattern irrespective of the nature of the antigen. Photosensitization reaction is somewhat similar except sunlight is also required for its induction (see chaps. 11, 12, and 15).

Corrosive agents such as strong acids and bases can destroy local tissues by precipitating cellular proteins. Irritation of the underlying tissues occurs as a consequence.

Blockade of renal and biliary tubules may follow the precipitation of relatively insoluble toxicants or their metabolites. For example, acetyl sulfapyridine, a metabolite of sulfapyridine, may block renal tubules; harmol glucuronide from harmol may produce cholestasis.

RECEPTORS

Historical Notes

It has long been observed that a number of poisons and toxins exert certain specific biological effects. John N. Langley proposed in 1905 the concept of a "receptive substance." That the receptors are protein in nature was first suggested by Welsh and Taub (1951).

To demonstrate the protein nature of acetylcholine receptors, Lu (1952) showed that the stimulant effect of acetylcholine on isolated rabbit ileum was lost after the ileum was treated with the proteolytic enzyme trypsin (10 mg/100 mL, for 30 minutes). That the effect was on the receptor rather than the muscle was demonstrated by the fact that the treated ileum still responded to barium chloride, a direct-acting muscle stimulant. In 1971, Cuatrecasas observed that trypsin, at the same concentration as that used by Lu, eliminated the activity of insulin receptor (Cuatrecasas, 1971).

In the 1970s, cholinergic receptors (ChR) were solubilized, isolated, and characterized by several groups of investigators. The amino acid composition of ChR was reported by Heilbronn et al. (1975). They also found that ChR contained about 6% carbohydrates. Although it has been generally agreed that the ligand–receptor complex would initiate responses in the cells, it was Rodbell et al. (1971) who proposed that a "transducer" was required to act between the receptor and the effector. This "transducer" was later confirmed as the G-proteins (Gilman, 1987).

Functional Categories

There are many types of receptors, located either in the cell membrane, the cytosol, or the nucleus. They serve a variety of functions such as metabolism, secretion, muscular contraction, neural activity, and proliferation. In general they are placed in different categories listed in the following text.

Neurotransmitter receptors include the cholinergic (nicotinic, located in ganglia and skeletal muscles, and muscarinic in smooth muscles and brain), α- and β-adrenergic, dopamine, opiates (e.g., endorphin), and histamine (H_1 and H_2) receptors.

Hormone receptors are for insulin, cortisone, ACTH, thyrotropin, estrogen, progesterone, angiotensin, glucagon, prostaglandin, and others.

Certain chemicals such as antidepressants and antitumor agents bind with specific macromolecules that may be considered as "drug receptors." These receptors may well have endogenous messengers (such as endorphins and enkephalins for opiates) but these are as yet undiscovered. Another example of such agents is benzodiazepine, for which receptors, and possible endogenous effectors, have been discovered. Furthermore, antagonists have been synthesized (Lal et al., 1988).

Other receptors are located on *enzymes* and *carrier proteins*. They may also be affected by toxicants as shown in Table 4.1.

Structure and Signal Transduction

The various functional categories of receptors described earlier exert their biological effects upon binding with an appropriate ligand, which may be an endogenous or exogenous substance. These effects are preceded by a series of biochemical activities, the signaling, which vary according to the structural characteristics of the receptor. Structurally they may be placed in four classes of receptors. These are (*i*) G-protein coupled receptors, (*ii*) ligand-gated ion channels, (*iii*) voltage-gated channels, and (*iv*) intracellular receptors.

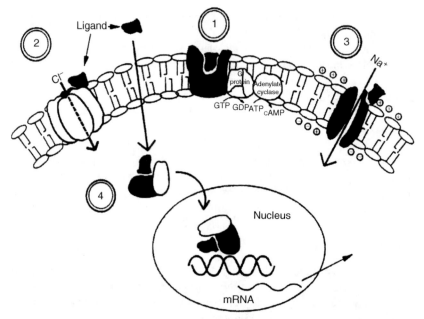

Figure 4.2   Schematic representation of the four classes of receptors. 1. G-protein coupled receptor, 2. ligand-gated ion channel, 3. voltage-gated ion channel, and 4. intracellular receptor. *Source*: From Mailman and Lawler (1994).

With the G-protein coupled receptors (Fig. 4.2: 1), binding with a ligand results in the activation of the G-protein, converting guanosine triphosphate to guanosine diphosphate, which activates or inhibits a specific enzyme (adenylate cyclase or phospholipase C), followed by the formation of a "second messenger," for example, cAMP (from ATP), diacylglycerol, or phosphoinositol. The second messenger then initiates the cellular response—the biological effect. Adrenergic, muscarinic, cholinergic, and dopaminergic neurotransmitters and their analogs are typical ligands for this class of receptors (e.g., ephedrine), as well as others such as diphtheria toxin.

The second class of receptors is transmembrane proteins with an ion channel (Fig. 4.2: 2). Upon binding with a ligand, the receptor undergoes conformational changes resulting in the opening of the channel. This process allows changes of Na^+, K^+, Cl^-, or Ca^{2+} concentrations across the plasma membrane. Nicotinic cholinergic and $GABA_A$ receptors belong to this class. In addition, glutamate and chemicals such as kainate, diazepam, barbiturates, and picrotoxin also act on this type of ion-channel receptors.

The voltage-gated conductance channels (Fig. 4.2: 3) are located across plasma membranes of excitable cells such as neurons and their axons. At present, no endogenous ligands are known. However, the neurotoxins, namely tetrodotoxin and saxitoxin (see chap. 17), bind to a site near the extracellular opening of the

Na^+ channel and block the entry of Na^+ through the channel, thereby interfering with the conduction of nerve impulse.

Intracellular receptors are located in the cytosol or nucleus (Fig. 4.2: 4). The main endogenous ligands are estrogens, androgens, progestins, glucocorticoids, and mineralocorticoids. A representative toxicant that binds with this type of receptor is TCDD. It binds with the Ah receptor in the cytosol, but moves to the nucleus after the binding. For additional details see Mitchell (1992) and Mailman and Lawler (1994).

The ligand that binds with the receptor may be an "agonist" or an "antagonist." An agonist induces the "physiological" function of the receptor, whereas an antagonist blocks its functions. For example, methacholine is an agonist interacting with certain cholinergic receptors, mimicking the effects of acetylcholine, whereas atropine, an antagonist, blocks these effects. Both types have adverse health effects. In addition, an agonist may cause a toxic effect by failing to dissociate from the receptor readily enough, thereby preventing further action of the endogenous messenger, and an antagonist can compete with the messenger for the site on the receptor and block the action of the latter. In addition, a toxicant may induce tolerance to its toxicity by reducing the number of receptors, as shown by Costa et al. (1981) with the chronic treatment with an organophosphate AChE inhibitor.

Receptors in Toxicology

The receptor concept has been valuable in advancing our understanding of certain biochemical, physiological, and pharmacological effects, as well as facilitating the development of drugs. Its role in toxicology is evidenced by an increasing number of receptors being recognized as mediators of effects of toxicants.

Poland and Knutson (1982) reviewed the extensive literature on TCDD and related halogenated aromatic hydrocarbons with respect to their toxicity, their ability to induce aryl hydrocarbon hydroxylase, and their affinity for a cytosol receptor. It was suggested that TCDD binds with the Ah (aromatic hydrocarbon) receptor. The TCDD–receptor complex translocates to the nucleus and there it interacts with specific genomic recognition sites. This initiates the transcription and translation of the specific genes that code for aryl hydrocarbon hydroxylase. A preponderance of evidence suggests that most of the TCDD toxicities are receptor mediated. It was also noted that the concentration of this cytosol receptor is much higher in the liver of C57 BL/6 mice than that of DBA/2 mice, and that the former strain of mice was much more susceptible than the latter with respect to TCDD-induced thymus involution, teratogenesis, and hepatic porphyria. Furthermore, the genetic evidence indicated that the *Ah* locus in mice was the structural gene for the cytosol receptor (see also Whitlock, 1990; Okey et al., 1994).

Many neurotoxicants act through receptors on central nervous system, peripheral nervous system, and autonomic nervous systems. For example, certain organophosphorus compounds act not only through acetylcholine but also on muscarinic receptors (Huff et al., 1994). The receptors for 12,0-tetradecanoyl phorbol 13-acetate (TPA) and retinoic acid are worth noting. TPA, a tumor promoter, binds with a receptor that initiates a chain of events leading to selected replication of initiated cells (Blumberg et al., 1983). Retinoic acid, as TCDD, acts on an estrogen receptor to exert teratogenic and other effects (Lu et al., 1994). A few examples of toxicants that act through receptors are mentioned in the previous section. Peroxisome proliferators such as the hypolipidemic drug clofibrate and the plasticizers phthalate esters are active on the peroxisome proliferator- activated receptors (PPARα, PPARβ/δ, and PPARγ) that are involved in the metabolism of polyunsaturated fatty acids and anti-inflammation (Varga et al., 2011). Furthermore, many immunotoxicants act through specific receptors on T cell, B cell, cytokine, polymorphonuclear cells, and monocytes (Lad et al., 1995). Aberrant expression and regulation of insulin-like growth factor binding protein 3 regulates normal and malignant cell growth (Zou et al., 1998).

REFERENCES

Abu-Qare AW, Elmasry E, Abou-Donia MB (2003). A role for P-glycoprotein in environmental toxicology. J Toxicol Environ Health B 6, 279–288.

Blumberg PM, Delcos BK, Dunn JA, et al. (1983). Phorbol ester receptors and the in vitro effects of tumor promoters. Ann N Y Acad Sci 407, 303–315.

Calabrese EJ, Baldwin LA (2001). The frequency of U-shaped dose responses in the toxicological literature. Toxicol Sci 62, 330–338.

Cohen JT, Carlson G, Charnley G, et al. (2002). A comprehensive evaluation of the potential health risks associated with occupational and environmental exposure to styrene. J Toxicol Environ Health B 5, 1–263.

Costa LG, Schwab BW, Hand H, et al. (1981). Reduced [H3] quinuclidinyl benzilate binding to muscarinic receptors in disulfoton-tolerant mice. Toxicol Appl Pharmacol 60, 441–450.

Cuatrecasas P (1971). Perturbation of the insulin receptor of isolated fat cells with proteolytic enzymes. J Biol Chem 246, 6522–6531.

Dean BS (1998). Diethylstilbesterol. In: Wexler P, ed. Encyclopedia of Toxicology. New York, NY: Academic Press, 477–478.

Gilman AG (1987). G-proteins: Transducers of receptor-generated signals. Ann Rev Biochem 56, 615–649.

Halliwell B, Cross CE (1994). Oxygen-derived species: their relation to human disease and environmental stress. Environ Health Persp 102(Suppl 10), 5–12.

Heilbronn E, Mattsson C, Elfman L (1975). Biochemical and physical properties of the nicotinic ACh receptor from Torpedo marmorata. In: Wollemann M, ed. Properties of Purified Cholinergic and Adrenergic Receptors, vol. 37. New York, NY: Elsevier.

Hoyal CR, Giron-Calle J, Forman HJ (1998). The alveolar macrophage as a model of calcium signaling in oxidative stress. J Toxicol Environ Health B 1, 117–134.

Huff RA, Corcoran JJ, Anderson JK, et al. (1994). Chloropyrifos oxon binds directly to muscarinic receptors and inhibits cAMP accumulation in rat striatum. J Pharmacol Exp Therap 269, 329–335.

Kleihues P, Cooper HK (1976). Repair excision of alkylated bases from DNA in vivo. Oncology 33, 86–88.

Koschier FJ, Burden EJ, Brunkhorst CS, et al. (1983). Concentration-dependent elicitation of dermal sensitization in guinea pigs treated with 2,4-toluene diisocyanate. Toxicol Appl Pharmacol 67, 401–407.

Kwack SJ, Lee BM (2000). Correlation between DNA or protein adducts and benzo[a] pyrene diol epoxide I-triglyceride adduct detected in vitro and in vivo. Carcinogenesis 21, 629–632.

Lad PM, Kapstein JS, Lin CE, eds. (1995). Signal Transduction in Leukocytes. G-Protein-Related and Other Pathways. Boca Raton, FL: CRC Press.

Lal H, Kumer B, Forster MJ (1988). Enhancement of learning and memory in mice by a benzodiazepine antagonist. FASEB J 2, 2707–2711.

Li W, Chou IN (1992). Effects of sodium arsenite on the cytoskeleton and cellular glutathione levels in cultured cells. Toxicol Appl Pharmacol 114, 132–139.

Li W, Zhao Y, Chou IN (1987). Paraquat-induced cytoskeletal injury in cultured cells. Toxicol Appl Pharmacol 91, 96–106.

Lu FC (1952). The effects of proteolytic enzymes on the isolated rabbit intestine. Br J Pharmacol 7, 624–640.

Lu Y, Wang X, Safe S (1994). Interaction of 2,3,7,8-tetrachlorodibenzo-p-dioxin and retinoic acid in MCF-7 human breast cancer cells. Toxicol Appl Pharmacol 127, 1–8.

Mailman RB, Lawler CP (1994). Toxicant-receptor interactions: fundamental principles. In: Hodgson E, Levi PE, eds. Introduction to Biochemical Toxicology. Norwalk, CT: Appleton & Lange.

Mitchell RH (1992). Inositol lipids in cellular signalling mechanisms. Trends Biochem Sci 17, 274–276.

NAS (National Academy of Sciences). (2008). Review of the Toxicologic and Radiologic Risks to Military Personnel from Exposure to Depleted Uranium During and After Combat. Washington, DC: National Academies Press.

Okey AB, Riddick DS, Harper PA (1994). The Ah receptor: mediator of the toxicity of 2,3,7,8-tetrachlorodibenzo-p-dioxin (TCDD) and related compounds. Toxicol Lett 70, 1–22.

Park HS, Park YA, Lee BM (2002). Effects of pH and temperature on benzo[a]pyrene-DNA, -protein, and -lipid adducts in primary rat hepatocytes. J Toxicol Environ Health A 65, 205–214.

Pestka JJ, Smolinski AT (2005). Deoxynivalenol: toxicology and potential effects on humans. J Toxicol Environ Health B 8, 39–69.

Poland A, Knutson JC (1982). 2,3,7,8-Tetrachlorodibenzo-p-dioxin and related halogenated aromatic hydrocarbons: examination of the mechanism of toxicity. Annu Rev Pharmacol Toxicol 22, 517–554.

Rodbell M, Birnbaumer L, Pohl SL, et al. (1971). The glucagon sensitive adenyl cyclase system in plasma membranes of rat liver. V. An obligatory role of guanyl nucleotides in glucagon action. J Biol Chem 246, 1877–1887.

Ross D (2000). The role of metabolism and specific metabolites in benzene-induced toxicity: evidence and issues. J Toxicol Environ Health A 61, 357–372.

Roy D, Cai Q, Felty Q, et al. (2007). Estrogen-induced generation of reactive oxygen and nitrogen species, gene damage and estrogen-dependent cancers. J Toxicol Environ Health B 10, 235–257.

Roy D, Palangat M, Chen C-W, et al. (1997). Biochemical and molecular changes at the cellular level in response to exposure to environmental estrogen-like chemicals. J Toxicol Environ Health 50, 1–29.

Steinmaus C, Moore LE, Shipp M, et al. (2007). Genetic polymorphisms in MTHFR 677 and 1298, GSTM1 and T1 and metabolism of arsenic. J Toxicol Environ Health A 70, 159–170.

Timbrell JA (1991). Principles of Biochemical Toxicology. London, UK: Taylor & Francis.

Varga T, Czimmerer Z, Nagy L (2011). PPARs are a unique set of fatty acid regulated transcription factors controlling both lipid metabolism and inflammation. Biochim Biophys Acta 1812, 1007–1022.

Wang G, Ansari GAS, Khan MF (2007). Involvement of lipid peroxidation-derived aldehyde–protein adduct in autoimmunity mediated by trichloroethene. J Toxicol Environ Health A 70, 1977–1985.

Welsh JH, Taub R (1951). The significance of the carbonyl group and ether oxygen in the reaction of acetylcholine with receptor substance. J Pharmacol Exp Ther 103, 62–73.

Whitlock JP Jr (1990). Genetic and molecular aspects of 2,3,7,8-tetrachlorodibenzo-*p*-dioxin action. Ann Rev Pharmacol Toxicol 30, 251–277.

Wiegant FA, Prins HA, Van Wijk R (2011). Postconditioning hormesis put in perspective: an overview of experimental and clinical studies. Dose Response 9, 209–224.

Zou T, Fleisher AS, Kong D, et al. (1998). Sequence alterations of insulin-like growth factor binding protein 3 in neoplastic and normal gastrointestinal tissues. Cancer Res 58, 4802–4804.

5

Modifying factors of toxic effects

GENERAL CONSIDERATIONS

Toxicity is an inherent property of a toxic substance; however, the nature and extent of the toxic manifestations in an organism that is exposed to the substance depend on a variety of factors. The obvious ones are the dose of the substance and duration of exposure. However, they also include less obvious host factors such as the species and strain of the animal, gender and age, nutritional and hormonal status as well as the presence of medical conditions such as hypertension or compromised function as in AIDS. Various environmental (physical and social) factors also play a part. In addition, the toxic effect of a chemical may be influenced by simultaneous, concurrent, or prior exposure to other chemicals.

The toxic effects may be modified in a number of ways: alterations of the absorption, distribution, and excretion of a chemical; an increase or a decrease of its biotransformation; and changes of the sensitivity of the receptor at the target organ. An example is the combination of N,N-diethyl-m-toluamide (DEET), an insect repellent; pyridostigmine (PB), an antinerve agent; and permethrin, an insecticide used in the Gulf War. PB by itself did not produce any adverse effects but when combined with DEET, the veterans complained of neurotoxicity. Studies showed that DEET application to skin changed dermal properties such that PB was absorbed to a greater extent and thus toxicity was seen.

A clear understanding of the existence of these factors and of their mode of action is important in designing the protocols of toxicological investigation. It is equally important in evaluating the significance of the toxicological data and in assessing the safety/risk to humans under specified conditions of exposure.

The most common mechanism underlying various modifying factors is differences in the rate of detoxication. However, differences in bioactivation, and toxicokinetic, toxicodynamic, physiological, psychological, and anatomic characteristics are responsible for a number of modifying factors. Examples are listed in Appendix 1.

HOST FACTORS

Species, Strain, and Individual

In general, different species of animals respond similarly to most toxicants. However, differences in toxic effect from one species to another have long been recognized. This is clearly demonstrated for the most toxic chemical known, dioxin: the LD 50 is 2 μg/kg for guinea pig; 50 μg/kg for rabbit; 200 μg/kg for mouse, and 2000 μg/kg for hamster. Knowledge in this field has been used to develop, for example, pesticides, which are more toxic to pests than to humans and other mammals. Among various species of mammals, most effects of toxicants are somewhat more similar. This fact forms the basis of predicting the toxicity to humans based on results obtained in toxicological studies conducted in other mammals, such as rat, mouse, dog, rabbit, and monkey. There are, however, notable differences in toxicity even among mammals (Williams, 1974).

Some of these differences can be attributed to variations in detoxication mechanisms. For example, the sleeping time induced in several species of laboratory animals by hexobarbital shows marked differences, which are obviously attributable to the activity of the detoxication enzyme as shown in Table 5.1.

Differences in response to hexobarbital, although less marked, also exist among various strains of mice (Jay, 1955). Other examples include ethylene glycol and aniline. Ethylene glycol is metabolized to oxalic acid, which is responsible for the toxicity, or to carbon dioxide. The magnitude of the toxicity of ethylene glycol in animals is in the following order: cat > rat > rabbit and this is the same for the extent of oxalic acid production. Aniline is metabolized in the cat and dog mainly to o-aminophenol, which is more toxic, but it is metabolized mainly to p-aminophenol in the rat and hamster, which are less susceptible to aniline (Timbrell, 1991).

Differences in bioactivation also account for many dissimilarities of toxicity. A notable example is 2-naphthylamine, which produced bladder tumors in the dog and human but not in the rat, rabbit, or guinea pig. Dogs and humans, but not the others, excrete the carcinogenic metabolite 2-naphthyl hydroxylamine (Miller et al., 1964). Acetylaminofluorene (AAF) is carcinogenic to many species of animals but not to the guinea pig. However, the N-hydroxy metabolite of AAF is carcinogenic to all animals including the guinea pig, demonstrating that the

Table 5.1   Species Differences in the Duration of Action and Metabolism of Hexobarbital

Species	Duration of Action (min)	Plasma Half-Life (min)	Relative Enzyme Activity (μg/g/hr)	Plasma Level on Awakening (μg/mL)
Mouse	12	19	598	89
Rabbit	49	60	196	57
Rat	90	140	135	64
Dog	315	260	36	19

Dose of barbiturate 50 mg/kg in dogs and 100 mg/kg in the other animals.
Source: From Ref. Quinn et al. (1958).

difference between the guinea pig and the other animals is not in their response to the toxicant but in the bioactivation (Weisburger and Weisburger, 1973).

Although differences in biotransformation, including bioactivation, account for species variation in susceptibility to a great majority of chemicals; other factors such as absorption, distribution, and excretion also play a part. In addition, variations in physiological functions are important in toxic manifestations in response to such toxicants as squill. This toxic chemical is a good rodenticide because rats cannot vomit, whereas humans and many other mammals can eliminate this poison by vomiting (Doull, 1980). Anatomic differences may also be responsible, such as with butylated hydroxyanisole (see chap. 19).

With the diversity in the number of rat strains available, it should not be surprising that there are differences in chemical-induced sensitivities. In general, each chemical will induce a change in all rat strains, but the degree of the effect will vary among strains (as in all sciences, there are no exceptions). However, there may be no response in humans. Clearly there are hormonal differences between males and females, but the precise role of these hormones in strain-associated chemical-induced outcomes still remains to be established. It should be noted that the reproductive cycle in female F344 rats is dramatically different from that of Sprague-Dawley rats (Kacew et al., 1995) (Appendix 2). Consequently, the incidence of spontaneous and chemical-induced mammary tumorigenicity is markedly higher in Sprague-Dawley rats, as this stock possesses greater estrogen levels. The human does not resemble the Sprague-Dawley strain and thus findings cannot be applied to humans. In comparing both males and females of the same strain, in general, chemicals including nitrosamines, decalin, hydroquinone, chloroform, etc. induce markedly greater responses in the male. It is of interest that in studies where males and females of different strains are compared, the males of certain strains are far more susceptible to adverse effects.

Apart from the differences in susceptibility that exist from one species to another and from one strain to another, there are also variables among individuals of the same species and same strain. Although the magnitude of such individual variations is usually relatively small, there are exceptions. This phenomenon has been widely studied among humans. For example, there are "slow inactivators," who are deficient in acetyltransferase. Such individuals acetylate isoniazid only slowly and are thus likely to suffer from peripheral neuropathy resulting from an accumulation of isoniazid. On the other hand, people with more efficient acetyltransferase require larger doses of isoniazid to obtain its therapeutic effect and are thus more likely to suffer from hepatic damage.

Differences in response to succinylcholine provide another example. Individuals with an atypical or a low level of plasma cholinesterase may exhibit prolonged muscular relaxation and apnea following an injection of a standard dose of this muscle relaxant. Glucose-6-phosphate dehydrogenase deficiency and altered stability of reduced glutathione are responsible for hemolytic anemia in subjects exposed to primaquine, antipyrine, and similar agents. A more extensive list of potentially hemolytic chemicals and drugs has been compiled by Calabrese et al. (1979).

Less dramatic, but more consistently greater susceptibility, to many drugs has been reported to exist among Indonesians, and perhaps also other Asians (Darmansjah and Muchtar, 1992).

Gender, Hormonal Status, and Pregnancy

Male and female animals of the same strain and species usually react to toxicants similarly. There are, however, notable quantitative differences in their susceptibility, especially in the rat. For example, many barbiturates induce more prolonged sleep in female rats than male ones. The shorter duration of action of hexobarbital in male rats is related to the higher activity of the liver microsomal enzymes to hydroxylate this chemical. This higher activity can be reduced by castration or pretreatment with estrogen. Similarly, male rats demethylate aminopyrine and acetylate sulfanilamide faster than females, and the males are thus less susceptible.

Female rats are also more susceptible than the males to such organophosphorus insecticides as azinphos-methyl and parathion. Castration and hormone treatment reverse this difference. Furthermore, weaning rats of both genders are equally susceptible to these toxicants. However, unlike hexobarbital, parathion is metabolized more rapidly in the female than in male rat. This faster metabolism of parathion results in a higher concentration of its metabolite, paraoxon, which is more toxic than the parent compound. This higher toxicity resulting from greater bioactivation in female rats, compared with males, is also true with aldrin and heptachlor, which undergo epoxidation. The female rat is also more susceptible to warfarin and strychnine. On the other hand, male rats are more susceptible than females to ergot and lead.

Differences in susceptibility between the genders are also seen with other chemicals. For example, chloroform is acutely nephrotoxic in the male mouse but not in the females. Castration or the administration of estrogens reduces this effect in the males, and treatment with androgens enhances susceptibility to chloroform in the females. The greater susceptibility of male mice was explained on the basis of a much higher concentration of cytochrome P-450 (Smith et al., 1983). Strain and gender also play an important role in hyaline droplet nephropathy. Administration of decalin to male F-344, SD, Buffalo, or BN rats increased $\alpha 2_u$-globulin content associated with hyaline droplet formation. In contrast, female F-344, SD, Buffalo, and BN rats showed no evidence of hyaline droplet formation or accumulation of $\alpha 2_u$-globulin. It is of interest that both male and female NCI-Black Reiter (NBR) rats resembled female responsiveness, as there was no hyaline droplet nephropathy. Clearly, the decalin-induced hyaline droplet nephropathy is strain related, but the role of male hormones is difficult to decipher due to the lack of response noted in NBR male rats. However, there are marked differences in endogenous circulating testosterone levels among strains and this may account for the differences between NBR and other strains. It is also conceivable that NBR male rats, unlike SD or F-344, lack the gene necessary to synthesize $\alpha 2_u$-globulin. Nicotine is also more toxic to the male mouse, and digoxin is more toxic to the male dog. However, the female cat is more susceptible to dinitrophenol and the female rabbit is more so to benzene.

Imbalances of non-sex hormones can also alter the susceptibility of animals to toxicants. Hyperthyroidism, hyperinsulinism, adrenalectomy, and stimulation of the pituitary–adrenal axis have all been shown to be capable of modifying the effects of certain toxicants (Doull, 1980; Hodgson, 1987).

Age

In general, it has long been recognized that neonates and very young animals are more susceptible to toxicants such as morphine. For a great majority of toxicants, the young are 1.5–10 times more susceptible than adults (Goldenthal, 1971). In the case of DDT the LD 50 for a newborn is greater than 4000 mg/kg which falls to 730 mg/kg at 10 days; 190 mg/kg at 4 months, and is 220 mg/kg in the adult. This clearly shows that the neonate is less susceptible than the adult to DDT lethality. Hence it is important to emphasize that there are exceptions to the general rules that the young are always more sensitive than adults to chemical exposure.

The available information indicates that the greater susceptibility of the young animals to many toxicants can be attributed to deficiencies of various detoxication enzyme systems (Makri et al., 2004). Both phase I and phase II reactions may be responsible. For example, hexobarbital at a dose of 10 mg/kg induced a sleeping time of longer than 360 minutes in one-day-old mice compared with 27 minutes in the 21-day-old mice. The proportion of hexobarbital metabolized by oxidation in three hours in these animals was 0% and 21–33%, respectively (Jondorf et al., 1959). On the other hand, chloramphenicol is excreted mainly as a glucuronide conjugate. When a dose of 50 mg/kg was given to one- or two-day-old infants, the blood levels were 15 µg/mL or higher over a period of 48 hours. In contrast, children aged 1–11 years maintained such blood levels for only 12 hours (Weiss et al., 1960). Further, the route of exposure plays a significant role in the susceptibility of infants to air pollutants. The lung epithelium is not fully developed until the age of 4 (Foos et al., 2008). Children have a larger lung surface area per kilogram than adults and breathe a greater volume of air per kilogram. Hence air pollution may exert persistent effects on respiratory health, especially in the young. It should be borne in mind that the immune system is immature during this period and it has been postulated that the rise in asthma frequency is attributable to the greater inhalation exposure to pollutants in association with immune function immaturity.

However, not all chemicals are more toxic to the young. Certain substances, notably CNS stimulants, are much less toxic to neonates. Lu et al. (1965) reported that the effect of LD_{50} of DDT was more than 20 times greater in newborn rats than in adults, in sharp contrast to the effect of malathion on age (Table 5.2). This insensitivity to the toxicity of DDT may be reassuring in assessing the potential risk of this pesticide, because of the very much larger intake in young babies via breast feeding and cow's milk, especially on the unit body weight basis.

The effect of age on the susceptibility to other CNS stimulants including other organochlorine insecticides (dieldrin) appears less marked (generally in the range of 2–10-fold). Most organophosphorous pesticides such as malathion are

Table 5.2   Effect of Age on Acute Toxicity of Malathion, DDT, and Dieldrin in Rats

Pesticide	Age	LD_{50} (mg/kg) with 95% CI Limits	
Malathion	Newborn	134.4	(94.0–190.8)
	Pre-weaning	925.5	(679.01–261.0)
	Adult	3697.0	(3179.0–4251.0)
DDT	Newborn	>4000.0	
	Pre-weaning	437.8	(346.3–553.9)
	Adult	194.5	(158.7–238.3)
Dieldrin	Newborn	167.8	(140.8–200.0)
	Pre-weaning	24.9	(19.7–31.5)
	Adult	37.0	(27.4–50.1)

Source: From Lu et al. (1965).

more toxic to the young; schradan (octamethyl pyrophosphoramide) and phenyl-thiourea are notable exceptions (Brodeur and DuBois, 1963).

Apart from differences in biotransformation, other factors also play a role. For example, a lower susceptibility at the receptor has been found to be the reason for the relative insensitivity of young rats to DDT (Henderson and Woolley, 1969).

Certain toxicants are absorbed to a greater extent by the young than by the adult. For example, young children absorb four to five times more lead than adults (McCabe, 1979) and 20 times more cadmium (Sasser and Jarbor, 1977). The greater susceptibility of the young to morphine is attributable to a less efficient blood–brain barrier, as is vividly illustrated in Figure 5.1 (Kupferberg and Way, 1963). Penicillin and tetracycline are excreted more slowly and hence are more toxic in the young (Lu, 1970). Ouabain is about 40 times more toxic in the newborn than in the adult rat because the adult rat's liver is much more efficient in removing this cardiac glycoside from the plasma. The higher incidence of methemoglobinemia in young infants has been explained on the basis that their lower gastric acidity allows upward migration of intestinal microbial flora and the reduction of nitrates to a greater extent. Furthermore, they have a higher proportion of fetal hemoglobin, which is more readily oxidized to methemoglobin (WHO, 1977).

There is evidence that the newborn is more susceptible to such carcinogens as aflatoxin B_1. Furthermore, the fetuses, but not the embryos, of rodents are much more susceptible. For example, there was a 50-fold increase in the potency of ethylnitrosourea. This is also true with nonhuman primates, except the maximal effects that occur during the first third of gestation. If this is true with human fetuses, then they may be exposed to carcinogens before the mothers are aware of their pregnancies (Rice, 1979).

Old animals and humans are also more susceptible to certain chemicals. This problem has not been studied as extensively as in the young. However, the available evidence indicates that the aged patients are generally more sensitive to many drugs. The possible mechanisms include reduced detoxication and an impaired

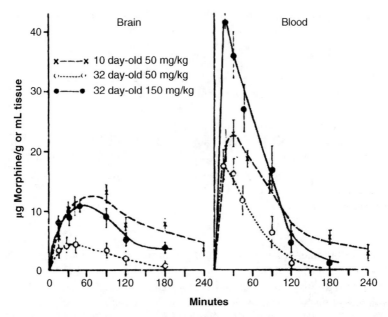

Figure 5.1   Brain and blood levels of free morphine at specific time intervals following intraperitoneal injections of morphine. Bracketed vertical lines show the standard error observed, using four animals per point. *Source*: From Kupferberg and Way (1963).

renal excretion (Goldstein, 1990). In addition, the distribution of chemicals in the body may also be altered because of increased body fat and decreased body water (Jarvik et al., 1981). A number of drugs were found to be likely to induce more severe signs of toxicity. These include most CNS depressants, certain antibiotics, cardiac glycosides, and hypotensive agents (WHO, 1981; Rochon et al., 1999).

Nutritional Status

The principal biotransformation of toxicants, as noted in chapter 3, is catalyzed by the microsomal mixed-function oxidases (MFO). A deficiency of essential fatty acids generally depresses MFO activities. This is also true with protein deficiency. The decreased MFO has different effects on the toxicity of chemicals. For example, hexobarbital and aminopyrine are detoxicated by these enzymes and are thus more toxic to rats and mice with these nutrient deficiencies. On the other hand, the toxicities of aflatoxin A, carbon tetrachloride, and heptachlor are lower in such animals because of their depressed bioactivation of these toxicants. Rats fed low-protein diets were 2–26 times more sensitive to a variety of pesticides (Boyd, 1972). MFO activities are decreased in animals fed high levels of carbohydrates.

A number of carcinogenesis studies demonstrated that restriction of food intake decreases tumor yield. Deficiency of protein generally lowers the tumorigenicity of carcinogens, such as aflatoxin B_1 and dimethyl nitrosamine. The importance of diet on carcinogenesis is further demonstrated by the fact that rats and mice fed diets rich in fats have higher tumor incidences compared with those that are given a restricted diet.

Vitamin A deficiency depresses the MFO. In general, this is also true with deficiencies of vitamins C and E. But thiamine deficiency has the opposite effect. Vitamin A deficiency, in addition, increases the susceptibility of the respiratory tract to carcinogens (Nettesheim et al., 1979).

Some foods contain appreciable amounts of chemicals that are potent inducers of MFO, such as safrole, flavones, xanthines, and indoles. In addition, potent inducers such as DDT and polychlorinated biphenyls are present as contaminants in many foods.

Diseases

The liver is the main organ wherein biotransformation of chemicals takes place. Diseases like acute and chronic hepatitis, cirrhosis of the liver, and hepatic necrosis often decrease the process of biotransformation. The microsomal and nonmicrosomal enzyme systems as well as the phase II reactions may be affected.

Renal diseases may also affect the toxic manifestations of chemicals. This effect stems from disturbances of the excretory and metabolic functions of the kidney. Endocrine disorders such as diabetes mellitus compromise the immune system and thus compromising the ability of individuals to cope with stress induced by chemicals. Heart diseases, when severe, can increase the toxicity of chemicals by impairing hepatic and renal circulation, thus affecting the metabolic and excretory functions of these organs. Respiratory tract disorders such as asthma render the subjects much more susceptible to air pollutants such as SO_2.

ENVIRONMENTAL FACTORS

Physical Factors

Changes in temperature may alter the toxicity. For example, colchicine and digitalis are more toxic to rat than frog, but toxicity to the frog can be increased by raising the environmental temperature. The duration of the response, however, is shorter when the temperature is higher. The effect of environmental temperature on the magnitude and duration of the response is apparently related to the temperature-dependent biochemical reactions responsible for the effect and biotransformation of the chemical.

Researchers' interest in the effect of barometric pressure on the toxicity of chemicals stems from human exposure to these substances in space and in saturation diving vehicles. At high altitudes, the toxicity of digitalis and strychnine is decreased, whereas that of amphetamine is increased. The influence of changes in barometric pressure on the toxicity of chemicals seems attributable mainly, if not entirely, to altered oxygen tension rather than to a direct pressure effect.

Whole-body irradiation increases the toxicity of CNS stimulants but decreases that of CNS depressants. However, it has no effect on analgesics such as morphine. More details and literature citations have been provided by Doull (1980).

The effects of toxicants often show a diurnal pattern that is mainly related to the light cycle. In the rat and the mouse, the activities of cytochrome P-450 are greatest at the beginning of the dark phase.

Social Factors

It is well known that animal husbandry and a variety of social factors can modify the toxicities of chemicals: the handling of the animals, the housing (singly or in groups), the types of cage, the supplier, and bedding materials are all important factors. Some examples of the influence of environmental factors on toxicity are given in chapter 6.

CHEMICAL INTERACTION

Types of Interaction

The toxicity of a chemical in an organism may be increased or decreased by a simultaneous or consecutive exposure to another chemical (Table 6.1 of chap. 6). If the combined effect is equal to the sum of the effect of each substance given alone, the interaction is considered to be *additive*; for example, combinations of most organophosphorous pesticides on cholinesterase activity. If the combined effect is greater than the sum, the interaction is considered to be *synergistic*; for example, carbon tetrachloride and ethanol on the liver, and asbestos exposure and cigarette smoking on the lungs. In the latter example, Selikoff et al. (1968) reported that there was a fivefold increase in lung cancer incidence among asbestos workers, an 11-fold increase among cigarette smokers, and a 55-fold increase among asbestos workers who were cigarette smokers. The term *potentiation* is used to describe the situation in which the toxicity of a substance on an organ is markedly increased by another substance that by itself has no toxic effect on that organ. For example, isopropanol has no effect on the liver, but it can increase considerably the hepatotoxicity of carbon tetrachloride.

Similarly, trichloroethylene (TCE), which exerts little effect on the liver, increases the hepatotoxicity of carbon tetrachloride, as measured by the release of liver enzymes ALT, SDH, and AST (Borzelleca et al., 1990).

The exposure of an organism to one chemical may reduce the toxicity of another. *Chemical antagonism* denotes the situation wherein a reaction between the two chemicals produces a less toxic product, for example, chelation of heavy metals by dimercaprol. *Functional antagonism* exists when two chemicals produce opposite effects on the same physiological parameters, such as the counteraction between CNS stimulants and depressants. *Competitive antagonism* exists when the agonist and antagonist act on the same receptor, such as the blockade of the effects of nicotine on ganglia by ganglionic blocking agents. *Noncompetitive antagonism* exists when the toxic effect of one chemical is blocked by another not acting on the same receptor. For example, atropine reduces the toxicity of acetyl-cholinesterase (AChE) inhibitors not by blocking the receptors on the AChE, but by blocking the receptors for the accumulated acetylcholine.

Mechanisms of Action

Chemical interactions are achieved through a variety of mechanisms. For instance, nitrites and certain amines can react in the stomach to form nitrosamines, the major-ity of which are potent carcinogens, and thus greatly increase the toxicity. On the other hand, the action of many antidotes is based on their interaction with the toxi-cants; for example, thiosulfate is used in cases of cyanide poisoning. Furthermore, a chemical may displace another from its binding site on plasma protein and thereby increase its effective concentration. A chemical may modify the renal excretion of weak acids and weak bases by altering the pH of urine. Competition for the same renal transport system by one chemical can hinder the excretion of another. A nota-ble example is the administration of probenecid along with penicillin to reduce the renal excretion of the antibiotic, thereby prolonging its duration of action.

One important type of interaction involves the binding of chemicals with their specific receptors. An antagonist blocks the action of an agonist, such as a neuro-transmitter or a hormone, by preventing the binding of the agonist to the receptor.

Another important type of interaction results from alterations of the bio-transformation of one chemical by another. Some chemicals are *inducers* of xeno-biotic metabolizing enzymes. They augment the activities of these enzymes, perhaps mainly by de novo synthesis. The common inducers include phenobarbi-tal, 3-methylcholanthrene (3-MC), polychlorinated biphenyl, DDT, and BaP. The inducers may lower the toxicity of other chemicals by accelerating their detoxica-tion; for example, pretreatment with phenobarbital shortens the sleeping time induced by hexobarbital and the paralysis induced by zoxazolamine. Such pre-treatment also reduces the plasma level of aflatoxins (Wong et al., 1981). In addi-tion, 3-MC pretreatment greatly reduces the liver necrosis produced by bromobenzene, probably by increasing the activity of the epoxide hydrase (see Fig. 3.3 of chap. 3). On the other hand, pretreatment with phenobarbital augments the toxicity of acetaminophen and bromobenzene, apparently by increasing the toxic metabolites formed. Repeated administration of a chemical may induce its metabolizing enzymes, as shown with vinyl chloride.

Piperonyl butoxide, isoniazid, and SKF 525 A and related chemicals are inhibitors of various xenobiotic-metabolizing enzymes. For instance, piperonyl butoxide increases the toxicity of pyrethrum in insects by inhibiting their MFO that detoxifies this insecticide. Isoniazid, when taken along with diphenylhydan-toin, lengthens the plasma half-life of the antiepileptic drug and increases its tox-icity. Iproniazid inhibits monoamine oxidase and increases the cardiovascular effects of tyramine, which is found in cheese and which is normally readily metabolized by the oxidase.

Characteristics of Enzyme Induction

Because of the importance of the effect of enzyme induction, much work has been done on certain inducers, notably phenobarbital and polycyclic aromatic hydrocarbons (PAHs). These two types of inducers differ in several aspects. For example, phenobarbital markedly increases the liver weight and the smooth endoplasmic reticulum, but PAHs such as 3-MC and BaP exert little effect on these parameters. Phenobarbital augments mainly the amounts of cytochrome P-450 and NADPH-cytochrome c reductase. PAHs produce little effect on these enzymes, but increase the amounts of cytochrome P-448, which is also known as P_1-450, and aryl hydrocarbon hydroxylase (AHH). These isozymes have different substrate specificity and hence alter the effects of toxicants differently (Sipes and Gandolfi, 1993).

Interactions as Toxicological Tools

Studies on chemical interaction are conducted not only to determine the effects of combinations of chemicals, but the data thereof are also useful in assessing health hazards associated with exposures to such combinations. These studies are also conducted to elucidate the nature and the mode of action of the toxicity of one chemical by the administration of another, as well as to bring out weak or latent effects of chemicals.

It needs to be made abundantly clear that in reality exposure may not be strictly to one compound but to a mixture of chemicals. ATSDR has deemed that exposure to chemical mixtures is one of the priority areas of concern and has significant health implications (DeRosa et al., 2004). Data in this scientific field is sorely lacking and one cannot assume or presume that the compounds will act synergistically or antagonistically. However, it is known that exposure is to a mixture of low levels of benzene, ethyl benzene, toluene, and xylene (BTEX) has severe neurotoxicity consequences.

REFERENCES

Borzelleca JF, O'Hara TM, Gennings C, et al. (1990). Interactions of water contaminants. Fundam Appl Toxicol 14, 477–490.

Boyd EM (1972). Protein Deficiency and Pesticide Toxicity. Springfield, IL: Charles C. Thomas.

Brodeur J, DuBois KP (1963). Comparison of acute toxicity of anticholinesterase insecticides to weanling and adult male rats. Proc Soc Exp Biol Med 114, 509–511.

Calabrese EJ, Moore G, Brown R (1979). Effects of environmental oxidant stressors on individuals with a G-6-PD deficiency with particular reference to an animal model. Environ Health Persp 29, 49–55.

Darmansjah I, Muchtar A (1992). Dose–response variation among different populations. Clin Pharmacol Therap 52, 449–452.

DeRosa CT, El-Masri HA, Pohl H, et al. (2004) Implications of chemical mixtures in public health practice. J Toxicol Environ Health B 7, 339–350.

Doull J (1980). Factors influencing toxicology. In: Doull J, Klaassen CD, Amdur MO, eds. Casarett and Doull's Toxicology. New York, NY: Macmillan.

Foos B, Marty M, Schwartz J, et al. (2008). Focusing on children's inhalation dosimetry and health effects for risk assessment: an introduction. J Toxicol Environ Health A 71, 149–165.

Goldenthal EI (1971). A compilation of LD50 values in newborn and adult animals. Toxicol Appl Pharmacol 18, 185–207.

Goldstein RS (1990). Drug-induced nephrotoxicity in middle-aged and senescent rats. In: Proceedings of the V International Congress of Toxicology. London, UK: Taylor & Francis.

Henderson GL, Woolley DA (1969). Studies on the relative insensitivity of the immature rat to the neurotoxic effects of DDT. J Pharmacol Exp Ther 170, 173–180.

Hodgson E (1987). Modification of metabolism. In: Hodgson E, Levi PE, eds. Modern Toxicology. New York, NY: Elsevier.

Jarvik LF, Greenblatt DJ, Harman D (1981). Clinical Pharmacology and the Aged Patient. New York, NY: Raven Press.

Jay GE Jr (1955). Variation in response of various mouse strains to hexobarbital (Evipal). Proc Soc Exp Biol Med 90, 378–380.

Jondorf WR, Maickel RP, Brodie BB (1959). Inability of newborn mice and guinea pigs to metabolize drugs. Biochem Pharmacol 1, 352–354.

Kacew S, Festing MFW (1995). Role of rat strain in the differential sensitivity to pharmaceutical agents and naturally occurring substances. J Toxicol Environ Health 47, 1–30.

Kacew S, Ruben Z, McConnell RF (1995). Strain as a determinant factor in the differential responsiveness of rats to chemicals. Toxicol Pathol 23, 701–714.

Kupferberg HJ, Way EL (1963). Pharmacologic basis for the increased sensitivity of the newborn rat to morphine. J Pharmacol Exp Ther 141, 105–112.

Lu FC (1970). Significance of age of test animals in food additive evaluation. In: Roe FJC, ed. Metabolic Aspects of Food Safety. Oxford, UK: Blackwell Scientific.

Lu FC, Jessup DC, Lavellee A (1965). Toxicity of pesticides in young versus adult rats. Food Cosmet Toxicol 3, 591–596.

Makri A, Goveia M, Balbus J, et al. (2004). Children's susceptibility to chemicals: a review by developmental stage. J Toxicol Environ Health B 7, 417–435.

McCabe EB (1979). Age and sensitivity to lead toxicity: a review. Environ Health Persp 29, 29–33.

Miller EC, Miller JH, Enomotor M (1964). The comparative carcinogenetics of 2-acetylaminofluorene and its N-hydroxy metabolite in mice, hamsters and guinea pigs. Cancer Res 24, 2018–2032.

Nettesheim P, Snyder C, Kim JCS (1979). Vitamin A and the susceptibility of respiratory tract tissues to carcinogenic insult. Environ Health Persp 29, 89–93.

Quinn GP, Axelrod J, Brodie BB (1958). Species, strain and sex differences in metabolism of hexobarbitone, amidopyrine, antipyrine and aniline. Biochem Pharmacol 1, 152–159.

Rice JM (1979). Perinatal period and pregnancy: intervals of high risk for chemical carcinogens. Environ Health Persp 29, 23–27.

Rochon PA, Anderson GM, Tu JV, et al. (1999). Age and gender-related use of low dose drug therapy. J Am Geriatr Soc 47, 954–959.

Sasser LB, Jarbor GE (1977). Intestinal absorption and retention of cadmium in neonatal rat. Toxicol Appl Pharmacol 41, 423–431.

Selikoff IJ, Hammond EC, Churg J (1968). Asbestos exposure, smoking, and neoplasia. J Am Med Assoc 204, 106–112.

Sipes IG, Gandolfi AJ (1993). Biotransformation of toxicants. In: Amdur MO, Doull J, Klaassen CD, eds. Casarett and Doull's Toxicology. New York, NY: McGraw-Hill.

Smith JH, Maita K, Adler V, et al. (1983). Effect of sex hormone status on chloroform nephrotoxicity and renal drug metabolizing enzymes. Toxicol Lett 28(Suppl 1), 23.

Timbrell JA (1991). Principles of Biochemical Toxicology. London, UK: Taylor & Francis.

Weisburger JH, Weisburger EK (1973). Biochemical formation and pharmacological, toxicological and pathological properties of hydroxylamines and hydroxamic acids. Pharmacol Rev 25, 166.

Weiss CG, Glazko AJ, Weston A (1960). Chloramphenicol in the newborn infant. a physiologic explanation of its toxicity when given in excessive doses. N Engl J Med 262, 787–794.

WHO. (1977). Nitrates, nitrites and N-nitroso compounds. Environmental Health Criteria 5. Geneva: World Health Organization.

WHO (1981). Health care in the elderly: report of the technical group on use of medicaments by the elderly. Drugs 22, 279–294.

Williams RT (1974). Inter-species variations in the metabolism of xenobiotics. Biochem Soc Trans 2, 359–377.

Wong ZA, Wei Ching-I, Rice DW, et al. (1981). Effects of phenobarbital pretreatment on the metabolism and toxicokinetics of aflatoxin B1 in the rhesus monkey. Toxicol Appl Pharmacol 60, 387–397.

Appendix 1   Mechanisms[a] Underlying Certain Modifying Factors

Toxicant	Responsible Mechanism	Toxic Response
Bioactivation Differences		
2-Naphthylamine	2-Naphthyl hydroxylamine	Bladder tumor in dog, human, but not in rat, mouse
Acetylaminofluorene	N-Hydroxy metabolite	Carcinogenic in rat, mouse, and hamster, but not in guinea pigs
Toxicokinetic Characteristics		
Lead, cadmium	Greater absorption in the young	Greater toxic effects
Penicillin, tetracycline	Slower excretion in the young	Longer half-life
Morphine	Blood–brain barrier inefficient in the young	Greater CNS effect
Sulfur dioxide	Higher breathing rate in the young	Greater lung damage
Toxicodynamic Characteristics		
DDT	Susceptibility of receptor	Less susceptible in the young
Anatomic Characteristics		
Butylated hydroxyanisole, butylated hydroxytoluene	Presence of fore stomach in rat	Hyperplasia of forestomach
Physiological Characteristics		
Squill	Vomiting reflex	Absence in rat leading to toxic effect

[a]Other than detoxication.

Appendix 2   Strain-Related Differences in Drug-Induced Responses

Parameter	Tissue	Strain/stock	
		Resistant	Susceptible
Ciprofibrate-induced peroxisomal proliferation	Liver	Sprague-Dawley	Long-Evans
Acetaminophen-induced necrosis	Kidney	Sprague-Dawley	F344
Streptozotocin-induced autoimmune reactivity	Popliteal lymph node	F344	Sprague-Dawley or Wistar
Amiodarone-induced phospholipidosis	Lung	Sprague-Dawley	F344
Diethyl stilbesterol-induced carcinoma	Mammary tissue	COP	F344
Saccharin-induced histopathological changes	Urinary bladder	Sprague-Dawley	Wistar
Mepirizole-induced ulceration	Duodenum	DONYRU	Sprague-Dawley or F344
Azaserine-induced carcinoma	Pancreas	F344	Wistar
B-adrenoceptor suppression of lipolysis	Adipocyte	Wistar	Sprague-Dawley
Diethyl stilbesterol-induced prolactin secretion	Pituitary	Sprague-Dawley	F344

Resistant does not imply a lack of effect but a significantly lower responsiveness than susceptible.

6

Conventional toxicity studies

INTRODUCTION

Usefulness

As noted in prior chapters, toxicants vary greatly in their potency, target organ, and mode of action. To provide proper orientation for additional in-depth targeted studies, conventional toxicity studies are generally carried out first. These studies are designed to provide indications of the appropriate dosage range, the probable adverse effect, and the target organ (e.g., liver), system (e.g., respiratory), or special toxicity (e.g., carcinogenicity).

In addition to providing preliminary information for proper orientation of additional investigations, the conventional toxicity studies per se yield data that can be used to assess the nature of the adverse effects and the "no-observed-adverse-effect level" (NOAEL) of the toxicant, which are required in the safety assessment described in chapter 27. For example, approximately half of the pesticides evaluated by the WHO Expert Committee on Pesticide Residues in the past 30 years have been based on conventional toxicity studies, despite the extensive database that is also available (Lu, 1995).

Categories

In order to examine the different effects associated with various lengths of exposure, the conventional studies are generally divided into four categories: (*i*) *Acute toxicity studies* involve either a single administration of the chemical under test or several administrations within a 24-hour period. In this study, the lethal dose 50% (LD_{50}) and acute toxicities are determined within 14 days of treatment. (*ii*) *Short-term* (also known as subacute and subchronic) toxicity studies involve repeated administrations, usually on a daily or five times per week basis, over a period of about 10% of the life span, namely, three months in rats and one or two years in dogs. However, shorter durations such as 14- and 28-day treatments have also been used by some investigators. (*iii*) *Long-term* (also known as chronic) toxicity studies involve repeated administrations over the entire life span of the test animals or at least a major fraction of it, for example, 18 months in mice, 24 months in rats, and 7–10 years in dogs and monkeys. These types of studies are essential for assessment of the carcinogenic potential of chemicals. (*iv*) Generational studies involve the administration of compounds to the parent or first generation, and subsequently compounds are given to the offspring for a second generation. These types of studies are crucial for assessment of reproductive capability as well as for determination of developmental functions.

Importance of Selection of Rat Strains

In the search for compounds to enhance our living standards, there is a necessity for understanding normal human functions and mechanisms which underlie dysfunction in these processes. Utilization of a suitable animal model, which simulates humans, is necessary to develop new pharmaceutical agents to alleviate diseases or chemicals to enhance lifestyle. It is incumbent upon investigators to choose a species in which pharmacokinetic principles are established and resemble those of humans. The choice of rodent has specific advantages in that there are similar pharmacodynamic parameters resembling those in humans. Other advantages include availability, low cost, ease of breeding, and an extensive literature database to enable comparisons to present findings. Factors that need to be recognized as playing an important role in chemical-induced outcomes include strain, supplier, gender, and dietary intake. This is especially critical in the risk-assessment process.

In an effort to establish animal models to extrapolate to human responses, one must be apprised that choosing the rat strain can affect the responses observed under normal or chemically altered conditions. Even by limiting genetic variability by simply using the same strain, factors such as supplier and dietary intake can bring about differences in the responsiveness of one strain as well as between strains. Further, the rodent may be susceptible while the human is nonresponsive.

ACUTE TOXICITY STUDIES

These studies are designed either to determine the median lethal dose (LD_{50}) of the toxicant or a rough estimate of it. The LD_{50} has been defined as "a statistically derived expression of a single dose of a material that can be expected to kill 50% of the animals." In addition, such studies may also indicate the probable target organ of the chemical and its specific toxic effect and provide guidance on the doses to be used in the more prolonged studies.

In certain cases, especially those with low acute toxicities, it may not be necessary to determine the precise LD_{50}s. Simple lethality data can serve useful purposes. For example, synergistic and antagonistic effects can be demonstrated using some animals as shown by the data presented in Table 6.1. Furthermore, even the information that a sufficiently large dose produces few or no deaths may suffice. This *limit test* has been applied. For example, a number of food colors were given to rats at a dose of 2 g/kg. Since none of the rats died, it was considered sufficient

Table 6.1 Using Lethality in Demonstrating Chemical Interaction

	Lethality (Number of Deaths/Number on Test)		
KBrO$_3$ (mg/kg)	Control (Saline)	Cysteine[a] (400 mg/kg)	Diethyl maleate[b] (0.7 mL/kg)
169	5/5	0/5	
130	5/5	0/5	
49	0/5		4/5
29	0/5		4/5

With five animals per dose group, the interactions between KBrO$_3$ and the "antagonist" (cysteine) and a "synergist" (diethyl maleate) are evident.
[a]Antagonistic.
[b]Synergistic.
Source: From Kurakawa et al. (1987).

to rule out any serious acute toxicity and no LD$_{50}$ was determined (Lu and Lavallée, 1965). This view was accepted by the Joint FAO/WHO Expert Committee on Food Additives (WHO, 1966). EPA (1994) recommends the use of 5 g/kg.

When the route of exposure is inhalation, the end point is either the median lethal concentration (LC$_{50}$) with a given duration of exposure or the median lethal time (LT$_{50}$) with a given concentration of the chemical in the air.

Experimental Design

Selection of Species of Animal

In general, the rat, and sometimes the mouse, is selected for use in determining the LD$_{50}$. The preference stems from the fact that they are economical, readily available, and easy to handle. Further, there are more toxicological data on these species of animals, a fact that facilitates comparisons of toxicities to other chemicals.

Sometimes a non-rodent species is desirable. This is true, especially when the LD$_{50}$ values in rats and mice are markedly different or when the pattern or rate of biotransformation in humans is known to be significantly different from rats and mice.

The LD$_{50}$ determination is preferably done in animals of both genders, and also in adult and young animals, because of their differences in susceptibility. In recent years, the use of an LD$_{50}$ has been supplanted due to the unnecessary overuse of too many animals, and the data generated are not essential for determination of risk for humans. The beneficial value of LD$_{50}$ data does not outweigh the cost of animal welfare.

Route of Administration

Generally, the toxicant is administered by the route by which humans will be exposed. The oral route is most commonly used. The dermal and inhalation routes are used increasingly, not only for chemicals that are intended for human use by such routes but also for chemicals whose health hazards to personnel handling these chemicals are to be assessed (see chaps. 12 and 15). Parenteral routes are mainly used in assessing the acute toxicity of parenteral drugs. In addition, immediate or very prompt and complete or nearly complete absorption generally follow intravenous and intraperitoneal injection. The intravenous route is advantageous in the determination of the distribution of a compound in the organic system and given in the radioactive form.

Dosage and Number of Animals

To properly ascertain an LD_{50}, it is necessary to try to select a dose that will kill about half of the animals, another that will kill more than half (preferably less than 90%), and a third dose that will kill less than half (preferably more than 10%) of the animals. OECD (1992), among others, recommends a "Sighting" study to aid in the selection of the doses, which can be accomplished with no more than five animals. Dosing of the animals is done sequentially, with at least a 24-hour interval to allow adjustment of the dose that the next animal is to receive.

To determine a relatively precise LD_{50}, 40–50 animals are used, with a ratio of 1.2 between successive doses (Lu and Lavallée, 1965). For most chemicals, however, approximate LD_{50}s are adequate. These doses can be estimated using six to nine animals (Bruce, 1985). As indicated previously, this type of study is outdated and not necessary in light of the cost of animals in order to gain data of limited value.

Observations and Examinations

After administering the toxicant to the animals, they should be examined for the number and time of death in order to estimate the LD_{50}. More importantly, their signs of toxicity should be recorded. Table 6.2 provides a list of body organs and systems that might be affected, along with the specific signs of toxicity. The observation period should be sufficiently long so that delayed effects, including death, would not be missed. The period is usually 7–14 days but may be much longer.

Gross autopsies should be performed on all animals that have died, as well as on at least some of the survivors, especially those that are morbid at the termination of the experiment. Autopsy can provide useful information on the target organ, especially when death does not occur shortly after the dosing. Histopathological examination of selected organs and tissues may also be indicated.

Multiple Endpoint Evaluation

To derive additional information concerning the chemical on test, the toxic signs, such as those listed in Table 6.2, should be critically observed and recorded for evaluating nonlethal endpoints. These endpoints may assist in characterizing the nature of the toxicant.

Table 6.2 Relationship Between Toxic Signs and Body Organs or Systems

System	Toxic signs
Autonomic	Relaxed nictitating membrane, exophthalmos, nasal discharge, salivation, diarrhea, urination, piloerection
Behavioral	Sedation, restlessness, sitting position—head up, staring straight ahead, drooping head, severe depression, excessive preening, gnawing paws, panting, irritability, aggressive and defensive hostility, fear, confusion, bizarre activity
Sensory	Sensitivity to pain; righting, corneal, labyrinth, placing, and hind limb reflex; sensitivity to sound and touch; nystagmus, phonation
Neuromuscular	Decreased and increased activity, fasciculation, tremors, convulsions, ataxia, prostration, straub tail, hind limb weakness, pain and hind limb reflexes (absent or diminished), opisthotonos, muscle tone, death
Cardiovascular	Increased and decreased heart rate, cyanosis, vasoconstriction, vasodilation, hemorrhage
Respiratory	Hypopnea, dyspnea, gasping, apnea
Ocular	Mydriasis, miosis, lacrimation, ptosis, nystagmus, cycloplegia, pupillary light reflex
Gastrointestinal, gastrourinary	Salivation, retching, diarrhea, bloody stool and urine, constipation, rhinorrhea, emesis, involuntary urination and defecation
Cutaneous	Piloerection, wet dog shakes, erythema, edema, necrosis, swelling

Source: From McNamara (1976).

Evaluation of the Data

Dose–Response Relationship

When the mortality, or the frequency of other effects expressed in percentages, is plotted against the dose on a logarithmic scale, an S-shaped curve is obtained (Fig. 6.1, Curve B). The central portion of the curve (between 16% and 84% response) is sufficiently straight for estimating the LD_{50} or ED_{50}. However, a much wider range of the curve can be straightened by converting the percentages to probit units. This procedure is especially useful in estimating, for example, the LD_{01} or LD_{99}, when the extreme ends of this curve have to be used.

The probit units correspond to normal equivalent deviations around the mean, for example, +1, +2, +3... and −1, −2, −3... deviations, whereas the mean value itself has a zero deviation. However, to avoid negative numbers, the probit units are obtained by adding five to these deviations. The corresponding figures in these systems are as follows:

Detailed methods for estimating the LD_{50} and its standard errors are given in many papers and books on statistics, including those of Bliss (1957), Finney (1971), and Weil (1952).

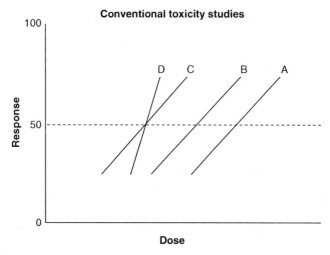

Figure 6.1   Median lethal doses and slopes of the dose–response (death) relationships of four chemicals. Chemical A is less toxic than the others. Chemical C is as toxic as D at the median lethal dose level but is more toxic at lower dose levels. Chemical B is less toxic than D at the median lethal dose level, but it may be more or less so at lower doses.

Deviations	Probit	% Response
−3	2	0.1
−2	3	2.3
−1	4	15.9
0	5	50
1	6	84.1
2	7	97.7
3	8	99.9

Relative Potency

The potency of toxicants varies significantly. Table 6.3 illustrates the range of LD_{50} values.

To render LD_{50} values more meaningful, it is advisable to also determine their standard errors (or the confidence limits) and the slopes of the dose–response curves. The importance of the slope can be readily appreciated when comparing two substances with similar LD_{50}s. The one with a flatter slope will likely produce more deaths than the other at doses smaller than the LD_{50}s (Fig. 6.1, chemicals C and D). The examples in Table 6.4 illustrate the marked differences in slopes.

Uses of LD50 Values and Signs of Toxicity

These values are useful in a number of ways.

Table 6.3   Acute LD_{50} Values for a Variety of Chemical Agents

Agent	Species	LD_{50} (mg/kg body weight)
Ethanol	Mouse	10,000
Sodium chloride	Mouse	4000
Ferrous sulfate	Rat	1500
Morphine sulfate	Rat	900
Phenobarbital, sodium	Rat	150
DDT	Rat	100
Picrotoxin	Rat	5
Strychnine sulfate	Rat	2
Nicotine	Rat	1
d-Tubocurarine	Rat	0.5
Hemicholinium-3	Rat	0.2
Tetrodotoxin	Rat	0.1
Dioxin (TCDD)	Guinea pig	0.001
Botulinum toxin	Rat	0.00001

Source: From Loomis (1978).

Table 6.4   Dose–Response Relationships[a]

Aflatoxin B_1 [b]		Botulinum toxin[c]			
Dose (ppb)	Response (tumor)	Dose (pg)	Response (death)	Dose (pg)	Response (death)
0	0/18	1	0/10	34	11/30
1	2/22	5	0/10	37	10/30
5	1/22	10	0/30	40	16/30
15	4/21	15	0/30	45	26/30
50	20/25	20	0/30	50	26/30
100	28/28	24	0/30	55	17/30
		27	0/30	60	22/30
		30	4/30	65	20/30

[a]Note relatively shallow dose–response relationship with aflatoxin B_1 wherein a 100-fold increase existed between the minimal and maximal effective doses, in contrast to the steep slope of botulinum toxin where there was a mere 50% increase.
[b]Data quoted from Food Safety Council (1978).
[c]Data supplied by E.J. Schantz (Food Research Institute, University of Wisconsin, Madison, Wisconsin, USA). Part of the data also appears in the Report of Food Safety Council (1978).

1. Classification of chemicals according to relative toxicity. A common classification is as follows:
2. Other uses include evaluation of the hazard from accidental overdosage; planning subacute and chronic toxicity studies in animals; providing information about (a) variations in response among different animal species and strains, (b) the susceptibility of a particular animal population, and (c) quality control of chemical products to detect toxic impurities, etc.

Category	LD_{50}
Supertoxic (mg/kg)	5 or less
Extremely toxic (mg/kg)	5–50
Highly toxic (mg/kg)	50–500
Moderately toxic (g/kg)	0.5–5
Slightly toxic (g/kg)	5–15
Practically nontoxic (g/kg)	>15

For toxicants with important health implications (e.g., TCDD), LD_{50}s are determined in several species of animals. The extent of variation of these values indicates the range of differences in the toxicokinetics and/or toxicodynamics among these species.

Guidelines for acute oral, dermal, and inhalation toxicity studies have been published by various national and international agencies (e.g., EPA, 1994). However, the prevailing advice is to estimate approximate LD_{50}s unless otherwise indicated.

SHORT-TERM AND LONG-TERM TOXICITY STUDIES

Humans are more often exposed to chemicals at levels much lower than those that are acutely fatal, but they are exposed over longer periods of time. To assess the nature of the toxic effects under these more realistic situations, short-term and long-term toxicity studies are conducted. These studies are also known as subacute (or subchronic) and chronic toxicity studies. The procedures involved in these two types are similar except their duration.

Experimental Design

Species and Number

Generally, two or more species of animals are used. Ideally, the animals chosen should biotransform the chemical in a manner essentially identical to humans. Since this is often unattainable, the rat and the dog are usually selected. This preference is based on their appropriate size, ready availability, and the great preponderance of toxicological information on chemicals in these animals. As noted in chapter 5, different strains of rats may respond markedly differently to toxicants.

Equal numbers of male and female animals should be used. Generally, 10–50 rats are used in each dose group as well as in the control group. As a rule, this procedure will provide data that are statistically analyzable. Smaller numbers of rats (10 animals/group/gender and thus totally 50 animals for four groups plus control) are used because of the greater number of examinations that can be made on each animal and because of their size and the expense involved.

Route of Administration

The chemical should be administered by the route of the intended use or exposure in humans. For most chemicals, the common route is oral. The preferred procedure is to incorporate the chemical in the diet, although the drinking water is sometimes used as the vehicle. The latter method is advisable when the chemical may react with a component in the diet. The chemical, especially if it is reactive, volatile, or unpalatable, is often administered by gavage or in gelatin capsules, a procedure more often used in dogs. The daily dose of the chemical may also be incorporated in a bolus of canned dog food.

Dermal application, exposure by inhalation, and parenteral routes are used for special purposes, such as industrial and agricultural products and drugs.

Dosage and Duration

As the aims of these studies are to determine the nature and site of the toxic effects, as well as the NOAEL, it is advisable to select three doses: a dose that is high enough to elicit definite signs of toxicity but not high enough to kill many of the animals, a low dose that is expected to induce no toxic effect, and an intermediate dose. Sometimes, one or more additional doses are included to ensure that the above objectives are achieved. As noted earlier, a control group must be included. These animals will not receive the chemical under test but must be given the vehicle used in the study.

The doses are generally selected on the basis of the information obtained in the acute toxicity studies, using both the LD_{50} and the slope of the dose–response curve. Any information on related chemicals and on their metabolism, especially the presence or absence of bioaccumulation, is also taken into account. Sometimes, a range-finding or dose range finding study is done. It consists of dosing five rats of each gender at each of the three or four dose levels for seven days. The criteria for assessing toxic effects are mortality, body weight gain, relative liver and kidney weight, and food consumption. The results from seven-day tests are generally better than the LD_{50} values in predicting the dose levels for the longer-term toxicity study.

In studies in rats, the dose levels may be constant concentrations and expressed in mg/kg diet (ppm) or constant dosage and expressed in mg/kg body weight of the animals. As the animal grows, there are changes in the body weight as well as in the food consumption. For the constant dose regimen, the concentration of the chemical must, therefore, be adjusted periodically to maintain a relatively constant dose in mg/kg body weight. This is usually done at weekly intervals during the period of rapid growth and biweekly thereafter.

In the short-term studies, the duration in rats is generally 90 days. In dog, the duration is often extended to six months or even one year. The duration of long-term studies in rats is generally 24 months, and seven or more years in dogs.

Observations and Examinations

Body Weight and Food Consumption

Body weight and food consumption should be determined weekly. Decreased body weight gain is a simple, yet sensitive, index of adverse effects. Food consumption is also a useful indicator. In addition, a marked decrease in food consumption can induce effects that mimic or aggravate the toxic manifestations of the chemical. In such cases, *paired feeding* or parenteral feeding may have to be instituted. Where the animals receiving the toxicant are affected more than those maintained on a reduced feed alone, the toxicant, apart from the undernutrition, is responsible for the effect.

General Observations

These should include appearance, behavior, and any abnormality. Dead and moribund animals should be removed from the cages for gross and possibly microscopic examination. Frequent observation is necessary to minimize cannibalism.

Laboratory Tests

Hematological examinations usually include hematocrit, hemoglobin, erythrocyte count, total leukocyte count, and differential leukocyte count. All dogs should be sampled before the initiation of treatment and at one week, one month, and at the end. Tests at other intervals may be warranted. Because of the small blood volume of rats, only half of them are sampled at various intervals, while the others are sampled only at the end. Special tests such as reticulocyte count, platelet count, methemoglobin, and glucose-6-phosphate dehydrogenase (G-6-PD) may be indicated.

Clinical laboratory tests usually include fasting blood glucose, serum aspartate aminotransferase (AST or SGOT), alanine aminotransferase (ALT or SGPT), alkaline phosphatase (AP), creatine kinase (CK), lactate dehydrogenase (LDH), total protein, albumin, globulin, blood urea nitrogen (BUN), triglycerides, cholesterol, creatinine, and such elements as sodium, potassium, calcium, and chloride. Other tests may be done where indicated. For example, cholinesterase activity is assessed when testing organophosphorus and carbamate pesticides.

Urinalysis usually includes color, specific gravity, pH, protein, glucose, creatinine, ketones, formed elements (red blood cells, etc.), and crystalline and amorphous materials.

Postmortem Examination

Whenever possible, all animals that are found dead or dying should be subjected to a gross pathological examination. If the state of the tissue permits, histological examinations should also be done. In addition, the weights of a number of organs, either in absolute values or in terms of the body weights, should be determined as they serve as useful indicators of toxicity.

The organs that are usually weighed are liver, kidneys, adrenals, heart, brain, thyroid, and testes or ovaries. Those that are histologically examined are the following: all gross lesions, brain (three levels), spinal cord, eye and optic nerve, a major salivary gland, thymus, thyroid, heart, aorta, lung with a bronchus, stomach, small intestine (three levels), large intestine (two levels), adrenal glands, pancreas, liver, gallbladder (if present), spleen, kidneys, urinary bladder, skeletal muscle, and bone and its marrow.

A list indicating the correlation between general observations, clinical laboratory tests, and postmortem examinations is produced as Appendix 1.

Guidelines for short-term and long-term studies have been published by WHO (1978, 1990), and the U.S. Environmental Protection Agency (EPA, 1994) among others.

Evaluation

Comprehensive short-term and long-term toxicity studies, using the various parameters of observations and examinations described earlier, usually yield information on the toxicity of the chemical under test, with respect to the target organs, the effects on these organs, and the dose–effect and dose–response relationships. Such information often provides indication on the additional specific types of studies that should be conducted. The quantitative data from the short-term and other studies have been suggested for use in the determination of the NOAEL. This suggestion, however, has not been widely accepted because it is considered more prudent to use the data from long-term studies. This is especially true for chemicals (e.g., food additives, pesticides, and environmental pollutants) to which humans may be subjected to lifetime exposure. On the other hand, short-term studies may suffice in testing such chemicals, as most pharmaceuticals are used for short durations. However, in the case of occupational exposure one needs to be cognizant that chemicals may cause delayed effects long after exposure as in the case of asbestos workers. It should also be borne in mind that confounding factors such as cigarette smoking or diet will also exert effects on the responses to chemical exposures.

The NOAEL from the long-term studies, along with data on their acute toxicity and metabolism as well as information from genetic, reproductive, and any other studies, is used in determining their "acceptable daily intakes" for humans. For further discussion on the procedure used for this purpose, see chapter 27.

GOOD LABORATORY PRACTICE

In 1975 and 1976, the U.S. Food and Drug Administration (FDA) raised questions about the integrity of toxicological data received from certain laboratories. On inspecting these facilities, FDA discovered a number of unacceptable laboratory practices, such as selective reporting, under-reporting, lack of adherence to a specified protocol, poor animal care procedures, poor record keeping, and inadequate supervision of personnel. In an attempt to improve the validity of the data, FDA proposed a set of regulations for good laboratory practice in 1978. These were later included in the Regulation for the Enforcement of the Federal Food, Drug, and Cosmetic Act.

These regulations (FDA, 1987) contain detailed guidance on provisions for the following:

1. Personnel, stipulating the responsibilities of the study director, testing facility management, and quality assurance unit
2. Facilities for animal care, animal supply, and handling test and control chemicals
3. Equipment, regarding its design, maintenance, and calibration
4. Testing facilities operation, including standard operating procedures, reagents and solutions, and animal care
5. Test and control chemicals, such as their characterization and handling
6. The protocol and conduct of a laboratory study
7. Records, their storage, retrieval, and retention, as well as the preparation and contents of reports
8. Disqualifications of testing facilities

The U.S. Environmental Protection Agency also proposed a set of good laboratory practice standards. They contain provisions similar to those of the FDA regulation regarding testing of health effects. However, the EPA standards also contain provisions for environmental effects testing. At an international level, OECD (1982) has also produced a set of similar guidelines. Good Manufacturing Practice and Good Clinical Practice are also needed to implement quality standards in drug research and development in pharmaceutical companies.

REFERENCES

Bliss CL (1957). Some principles of bioassay. Am Sci 45, 449–466.
Bruce RD (1985). An up-and-down procedure for acute toxicity testing. Fundam Appl Toxicol 5, 151–157.
EPA. (1994). Health Effects Test Guidelines. Hazard Evaluation. Code of Federal Regulations, Title 40, Parts 792, 798.
FDA. (1987). Good laboratory practice regulations; Final rule. Fed Reg 52, 33768–33782.
Finney DJ (1971). Probit Analysis. Cambridge, MA: Cambridge University Press.
Food Safety Council. (1978). Proposed system for food safety assessment. Food Cosmet Toxicol 16, 1–136.
Kurakawa Y, Takamura N, et al. (1987). Comparative studies on lipid peroxidation in the kidney of rats, mice and hamsters and the effect of cysteine, glutathione and diethyl maleate treatment on mortality and nephrotoxicity after administration of potassium bromate. J Am Coll Toxicol 6, 487–501.
Loomis T (1978). Essentials of Toxicology, 3rd edn. Philadelphia, PA: Lea & Febiger.
Lu FC (1995). A review of the acceptable daily intakes of pesticides assessed by WHO. Regul Toxicol Pharmacol 21, 352–364.
Lu FC, Lavallée A (1965). The acute toxicity of some synthetic colors used in drugs and foods. Can Pharm J 97, 30.

McNamara BP (1976). Concepts in health evaluation of commercial and industrial chemicals. In: Mehlman MA, Shapiro RE, Blumenthal H, eds. New Concepts in Safety Evaluation. Washington, DC: Hemisphere.

OECD. (1982). Good Laboratory Practice in the Testing of Chemicals. Organization of Economic Cooperation and Development. France.

OECD. (1992). OECD Guidelines for Testing Chemicals. Acute Oral Toxicity. Organization of Economic Cooperation and Development. France.

Weil CS (1952). Tables for convenient calculation of median effective dose (LD50 or ED50) and instructions for their use. Biometrics 8, 249–263.

WHO. (1966). Specifications for Identity and Purity and Toxicological Evaluation of Food Colors, WHO/Food Add./66.25. Geneva, Switzerland: World Health Organization.

WHO. (1978). Principles and Methods for Evaluating the Toxicity of Chemicals. Part I, Environmental Health Criteria 6. Geneva, Switzerland: World Health Organization.

WHO. (1990). Principles for toxicological assessment of pesticide residues in food. Environ Health Criteria 104. Geneva, Switzerland: World Health Organization.

Workshop on Subchronic Toxicity Testing. (1980). In: Page N, Sawbney D, Ryon MG, eds. Proceedings of the Workshop EPA-560/11–80-028. Springfield, VA: National Technical Information Service.

FURTHER READING

Ecobichon DJ (1992). The Basis of Toxicity Testing. Boca Raton, FL: CRC Press.

Appendix 1   General Observations, Clinical Laboratory Tests, and Pathology Examinations that may be Used in Short- and Long-term Toxicity Studies

Organ or Organ System	General Observations	Clinical Laboratory Tests on Blood	Pathology Examination[a]
Liver	Discoloration of mucus membranes, edema, ascites	ALT (SGPT), AP, AST (SGOT), LDH cholesterol, total protein, albumin, globulin	Liver
Urinary system	Urine volume, consistency, color	BUN, total protein, albumin, globulin, glucose	
Gastrointestinal (GI) system	Diarrhea, vomit, stool, appetite	Total protein, albumin, globulin, sodium, potassium	Stomach, GI tract, gallbladder (if present), salivary gland, pancreas
Nervous system	Posture, movements, responses, behavior		Brain, spinal cord, and sciatic nerve
Eye	Appearance, discharge, ophthalmological examination		Eye and optic nerves
Respiratory system	Rate, coughing, nasal discharge	Total protein, albumin, globulin	One lung with a major bronchus
Hematopoietic system	Discoloration of mucus membranes, lethargy, Weakness	Packed red cell volume, hemoglobin, erythrocyte count, total and differential leukocyte count, platelet count, prothrombin time, activated partial thromboplastin time	Spleen, thymus, mesenteric lymph nodes, bone marrow smear and section
Reproductive system	Appearance and palpation of external reproductive organs	FSH. LH, estrogen, testosterone	Testes and epididymis or ovaries. Uterus or prostate and seminal vesicles[b]
Endocrine system	Skin, hair coat, body weight, urine, and stool characteristics	Glucose, Na, K, AP (dog), cholesterol	Thyroid, adrenal, pancreas
Skeletal system	Growth, deformation, lameness	Calcium, phosphorus, AP	Bone and breakage strength
Cardiovascular system	Rate and characteristic of pulse, rhythm, edema, ascites	Creatine kinase, LDH	Heart, aorta, small arteries in other tissues
Skin	Color, appearance, odor, hair coat	Total protein, albumin, globulin	Only in dermal studies
Muscle	Size, weakness, wasting. decreased activity	AST creatine, phosphokinase	Only if indicated by observations, clinical chemistry, or gross lesions.
Bone	Deformity, weakness	Calcium, phosphorous, uric acid, AP	Spongy appearance

[a]All animals should undergo a thorough gross examination; organs or tissues listed should be examined microscopically.
[b]These organs should also be weighed.
Source: From Workshop on Subchronic Toxicity Testing (1980).

7

Carcinogenesis

INTRODUCTION

Historical Background

The relations between cancer and exposure to chemicals have long been noted. Thus, in 1761, Hill found that users of tobacco snuff had a high rate of nasal cancer, and Sir Percival Pott (1744–1788, English surgeon) observed, in 1775, that exposure to soot by chimney sweeps induced cancer of the scrotum (Pott, 1775). Twenty years later, Sommering noted that cancer of the lip was often associated with pipe smoking. Rehn discovered in 1895 that bladder tumors occurred among workers in aniline dye factories. In the twentieth century, cancers induced by a variety of chemicals under different exposure conditions have been observed. In 1915, Katsusaburo Yamagiwa and Koichi Ichikawa (1918) first succeeded in inducing experimental tumors in the skin of sensitive rabbit ears by applying coal tar (a complex mixture of chemicals) repeatedly to their skin every two or three days for a period of more than 100 days (Bishop, 1987). Later in 1930, Earnest Kennaway demonstrated that dibenzanthracene, a chemical constituent of coal tar was able to produce cancer in rats and in 1933, Cook et al. (1933) also showed that benzo(a)pyrene isolated from coal tar was carcinogenic in mouse skin.

In view of the seriousness of carcinogenesis, and the rapid development of new chemicals, many governmental agencies as well as academic and industrial laboratories have undertaken extensive research and testing in laboratory animals. These endeavors have provided leads for further epidemiological studies.

Definition and Identification

The term *chemical carcinogenesis* is generally defined to indicate the induction or enhancement of neoplasia by chemicals. Although in the strict etymologic sense this term means the induction of carcinomas, it is widely used to indicate tumorigenesis. In other words, it includes not only epithelial malignancies (carcinomas) but also mesenchymal malignant tumors (sarcomas). The cells tend to replicate, thereby invading surrounding tissues and metastasizing to remote parts of the body.

A chemical may be identified as a carcinogen based on observations in humans and supported by tests in laboratory animals. It should be emphasized that chemicals can induce tumors in rodents but that these types of tumors do not occur in humans; for example, solvent-induced renal tumors are dependent on proteins not present in humans. Thus this type of chemical-induced tumor is not relevant for humans. Human data may be derived from clinical observations as noted above. However, the relationship between the development of a cancer and the exposure to a chemical is complex. First, there is a long latency, generally in years or decades, between the time of exposure and the development of the cancer. Furthermore, humans are exposed to a multiplicity of potentially carcinogenic factors; in particular individuals are exposed to mixtures of chemicals where one compound alone may or may not induce carcinogenesis, but may be dependent upon each other in some cases to produce an effect. In addition, exposure of the female parent to chemicals during pregnancy can result in cancer development in offspring without any evidence of cancer in the mother. In view of these facts, very extensive epidemiological studies are needed. Further, exposure to a certain chemical may not induce cancer until the individual's immune system becomes compromised such as in AIDS.

In addition to human data, laboratory tests in animals can provide valuable supporting evidence. An important one involves chronic exposure of animals to the test chemical. However, animals, as humans, develop cancer even without being exposed to a known carcinogen. In view of this, it is generally agreed (e.g., WHO, 1969) that the presence of one or more of the following responses of the test animal be considered as positive for carcinogenesis:

1. An increase in the frequency of one or several types of tumors that also occur in the controls
2. The development of tumors not seen in the controls
3. The occurrence of tumors earlier than in the controls
4. An increase in the number of tumors in individual animals, compared to that in the controls

Weight of Evidence

Evidence of carcinogenicity consists of human and animal data. However, because of interspecies differences in response to chemicals, sound human data are given much greater weight. In fact, the earliest discoveries of chemical carcinogens were made in humans, as noted earlier. In view of the seriousness of cancer, however, it will be grossly imprudent to wait for relevant results to be generated from long-term human studies to assess each chemical for its carcinogenicity. Consequently, appropriate studies need to be carried out in animals. The significance of the results unfortunately varies greatly among different studies. For example, aflatoxin B_1 induced tumors in a variety of animals, with small doses (in ppb) and with a relatively short latent period. On the other hand, saccharin yielded positive results inconsistently, with very large doses (in tens of thousands of ppm) and only after very long periods of treatment. Atrazine induced mammary tumors in a

Table 7.1 Classification of Carcinogens Based on "Weight of Evidence"

Categories	IARC	EPA	Human Data	Animal Data
Human carcinogen	1	A	Sufficient	Sufficient or limited
Probable human carcinogen	2A	B1, B2[a]	Limited or inadequate[b]	Sufficient
Possible human carcinogen	2B	C	Absent or inadequate	Sufficient or limited[b]
Not classifiable	3	D	Absent or inadequate	Inadequate or absent
Not carcinogenic	4	E	Absent or extensive negative data	Negative evidence in at least two species

[a]EPA classifies carcinogens with sufficient animal data as "probable human carcinogen" and places them in category B1 or B2 depending on the weight of human data.
[b]IARC accepts positive genotoxicity in lieu of human data.

rat Sprague-Dawley strain, which does not resemble the human reproductive system in function; and thus findings were not of biological relevance to humans. Furthermore, the experimental design and conduct of the studies also differ in their adequacy.

To facilitate the evaluation of such diverse findings, a *weight of evidence* scheme has been adopted. This scheme must take into account the species used, as interspecies data cannot always be utilized as in the case of atrazine-induced mammary tumors in Sprague-Dawley rats. The findings may be considered "sufficient" when there are benign and malignant tumors in multiple species or strains or in multiple experiments, or there are large numbers of tumors or at an unusual site or being that of a special type.

"Limited" evidence means positive results in only one species, strain or experiment, or when the experimental design or conduct is inadequate. "Inadequate" evidence applies to results that are difficult to interpret. Similarly, data obtained in humans also vary greatly in their significance. Using these criteria, EPA (1996) and IARC (1987) classified chemical carcinogens in five categories (Table 7.1). In addition, the National Toxicology Program classified them into two categories: Group 1, Known to be human carcinogens (K); Group 2, Reasonably anticipated to be human carcinogens (R), and American Conference of Governmental Industrial Hygienists has three categories: Group A1, Confirmed human carcinogen; Group A2, Suspected human carcinogen; Group A3, Confirmed animal carcinogen with unknown relevance to humans; Group A4, Not Classifiable as a Human Carcinogen, and Group A5: Not Suspected as a Human Carcinogen.

MODE OF ACTION

Chemical carcinogenesis, as shown in Figure 7.1, is a multistage process. Carcinogenic chemicals act by initiating certain genetic changes in a cell (initiation),

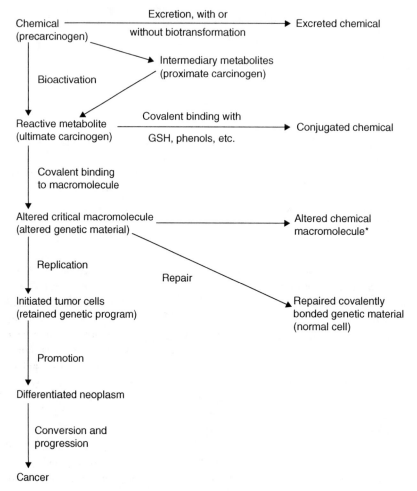

Figure 7.1   A schematic diagram depicting the fate of a genotoxic carcinogen and its relation with carcinogenesis. Events in the left-hand column lead to cancer formation, whereas those in the right-hand column are harmless. Asterisk (*) indicates that the step may be important during other stages of carcinogenesis.

promoting the formation of a benign neoplasm (promotion), converting the benign neoplasm to a malignant cancer (progression), or enhancing the activity of another chemical.

Bioactivation

Most carcinogenic chemicals per se are inactive. However, they undergo bioactivation in the body to yield reactive metabolites. A common type of reactive metabolite is epoxide. For example, aflatoxin B_1 is converted to aflatoxin-8,9-epoxide.

Benzene, vinyl chloride, and a number of polycyclic hydrocarbons also form epoxides. Other carcinogens, such as AAF and certain aminoazo dyes form *N*-hydroxy derivatives (see Appendix 1 of chap. 3). Certain chemicals are bioactivated to ultimate carcinogens via an intermediary step. An example of this is benzo (*a*)pyrene (BaP) which forms BaP-7,8-epoxide, the intermediary carcinogen. The latter then transforms to BaP-7,8-diol-9,10-epoxide, the ultimate carcinogen. Styrene undergoes oxidative metabolism to styrene 7,8-oxide, which is the intermediary carcinogen (Nestmann et al., 2005). Chromium undergoes reduction to a lower oxidation state to induce carcinogenesis (Shi et al., 1998). Arsenic requires transformation to induce cancer but this only occurs in populations possessing a certain phenotype, indicating that not only bioactivation is crucial but the presence of specific gene material needs to be present for an effect.

Interaction with Macromolecules

The reactive metabolites covalently bind to macromolecules such as DNA, RNA, proteins, and lipids to form DNA-, RNA-, proteins and lipid adducts, respectively (Poirier et al., 1977; Kwack and Lee, 2000). Some of them, such as proteins and lipids, may not play a critical role in carcinogenesis, but the biological role of protein adducts and lipid adducts needs to be fully investigated. When DNA is the target, the reaction may lead to point mutation, frame-shift mutation, and others. These changes may not persist: they may be reversed by an error-free DNA repair or disappear when the cell dies. However, some of them may persist, not be reversed by an error-prone DNA repair and lead to mutation and cancer.

Initiation

If the cell with an altered DNA undergoes mitosis, the alteration will be retained. The cell with the altered DNA is termed an "initiated" cell. The endpoint of initiation is "mutation," an alteration in genotype. Depending on the site of the alteration, the cell may be partially or fully preneoplastic. The process generally involves the conversion of proto-oncogenes to oncogenes.

Proto-oncogenes may be converted into *oncogenes* through translocation to a different chromosomal site, or other mechanisms such as genetic amplification, insertion, and gene mutation (Bishop, 1987). In addition, there are *oncosuppressor genes* or *antioncogenes*; a lack of their expression or an inactivation of their products may also lead to carcinogenesis (Weinberg, 1989). One of them, the p53 suppressor gene, is mutated in about half of human cancers (Greenblatt et al., 1994; Sugimura and Ushijima, 2000). In the case of silica, the generation of reactive oxygen species (ROS) results in the activation of nuclear transcription factors, induction of oncogene expression, redox regulation of p53 tumor suppressor gene, and induction of apoptosis (Shi et al., 1998, 1999). ROS generation as a step in the pathway of carcinogenesis is also involved in cigarette smoking, radon, and polycyclic aromatic hydrocarbons (Vallyathan et al., 1998).

Promotion

The initiated cell, with altered genotype, may remain dormant for a long period of time before it becomes a benign tumor through cell proliferation in the presence of *promoters* (Butterworth and Goldworthy, 1991). The dormancy is probably due to the suppressant influence of the surrounding normal cells exerted through certain intercellular communication (Trosko and Chang, 1988). The influence can be reduced by programmed cell death (apoptosis), cell killing (e.g., from cytotoxic chemicals), cell removal (e.g., partial hepatectomy), growth factors (e.g., hormones), and other factors.

While initiation is generally considered to be a permanent process, promotion is not. Furthermore, it is reversible. Therefore, for an initiated cell to continue to replicate, it must be exposed to a promoter more or less continuously. The endpoint of promotion is the formation of a benign tumor with altered genotype and phenotype.

Conversion and Progression

These are characterized by biochemical and/or morphological changes in the activity or structures of the genome. The mechanism of action is not fully understood, but may involve activation of the initiated cells by exposure to clastogenic agents or complete carcinogens (Pitot et al., 1988). During this period, the neoplasm may convert from benign to malignant tumor, which is invasive and metastatic.

Similar to initiation, progression is an irreversible process. Table 7.2 provides a list of the characteristics of initiation, promotion, and progression.

CATEGORIES OF CARCINOGENS

Carcinogens may also be classified according to their *mode of action* into genotoxic and nongenotoxic carcinogens.

Genotoxic Carcinogens

Genotoxic carcinogens initiate tumors by producing DNA damage (Fig. 7.1). These are of two types.

Direct-Acting Carcinogens

These chemicals are also known as ultimate carcinogens. They are electrophilic (electron-loving, electron-deficient) and can bind to DNA and other macromolecules (electron-rich molecules, nucleophiles). Examples are alkyl and aryl epoxides, lactones, sulfate esters, nitrosamides, nitrosoureas, ochratoxin A (Clark and Snedeker, 2006), arsenic (Bernstam and Nriagu, 2000), benzene (Pyatt et al., 2007), and platinum amine chelators. Because of their high reactivity, these direct-acting carcinogens are often more active in vitro but less so in vivo.

Table 7.2   Morphologic and Biologic Characteristics of the Stages of Initiation, Promotion, and Progression in Hepatocarcinogenesis in the Rat

Initiation	Promotion	Progression
Irreversible with constant "stem cell" potential. Initiated "stem cell" not morphologically identifiable. Genotoxic and rapid	Reversible, epigenetic, slow and long latency	Irreversible Measurable and/or morphologically discernible alteration in cell genome's structure
Efficacy sensitive to xenobiotic and other chemical factors	Promoted cell population existence dependent on continued administration of the promoting agent	
Spontaneous (fortuitous) occurrence of initiated cells can be quantitated	Efficiency sensitive to dietary and hormonal factors	Growth of altered cells sensitive to environmental factors during early phase
Requires cell division for "fixation" leading to mutation	Cellular proliferation and clonal expansion leading to benign tumor	Conversion of benign into malignant tumor
Dose–response does not exhibit a readily measurable threshold	Dose–response exhibits measurable threshold and maximal effect dependent on dose of initiating agent	Benign and/or malignant neoplasms characteristically seen
Relative effect of initiators depends on quantitation of focal lesions following defined period of promotion	Relative effectiveness of promoters depends on time and dose rate to reach maximal effect and dose rate	"Progressor" agents act to advance promoted cells into this stage but may not be initiating agents

Source: Adapted from Pitot et al. (1988).

Precarcinogens

They are also known as procarcinogens. They require conversion through bioactivation to become ultimate carcinogens, either directly or via an intermediary stage, the proximate carcinogens. Most of the presently known chemical carcinogens fall into this class. These include the polycyclic aromatic hydrocarbons (PAHs), diesel exhaust particles, aromatic amines, halogenated hydrocarbons, nitrosamines, cycasin, aflatoxin B, pyrrolizidine alkaloids, safrole, and thioamides. Different types of bioactivation (such as formation of epoxides, *N*-hydroxy derivatives) are involved in their conversion to the direct-acting agents, as discussed in chapter 3. These chemicals may also activate proto-oncogene to oncogene and inactivate oncosuppressor genes. Another type of activation involves the generation of ROS, which subsequently stimulates the multistep sequence resulting in carcinogenesis.

As noted above, timely and error-free DNA repair plays an important part in the prevention of neoplastic transformation. An interesting example is dimethyl nitrosamine. Its damage to hepatocyte DNA is rapidly repaired in the rat but only slowly in the hamster, and the latter is thus more susceptible than the rat to this carcinogen. Furthermore, in rat it induces tumors in the brain where the repair mechanism is deficient.

Nongenotoxic Carcinogens

These substances do not damage DNA but enhance the growth of tumors induced by genotoxic carcinogens or induce tumors through other mechanisms such as epigenetic regulation [e.g., DNA methylation, histone modification, nucleosome positioning (physical alteration), and posttranscriptional gene regulation by non-coding RNA (micro-RNAs)] (Ducasse and Brown, 2006; Kanwal and Gupta, 2010). These are briefly described subsequently.

Co-carcinogens

These substances that are not carcinogenic on their own enhance the effects of genotoxic carcinogens when given simultaneously. They may act by affecting an increase in the concentration of the initiator, the genotoxic carcinogen itself, or that of the reactive metabolite. This can be achieved either by an increase of the absorption of the carcinogen, via the gastrointestinal tract or the skin, or by an increase of the bioactivation. The same result can also be achieved through a decrease of the elimination of the initiator either by inhibiting the detoxification enzymes or by depleting the endogenous substrates involved in phase II reactions, such as glutathione.

Apart from increasing the concentration of the reactive species at the site of action, co-carcinogens may inhibit the rate or fidelity of DNA repair, or they may enhance conversion of DNA lesions to permanent alterations.

Tobacco smoke contains relatively small amounts of genotoxic carcinogens, such as PAH and tobacco-specific nitrosamines; its marked carcinogenic effects are perhaps attributed to catechols which act as co-carcinogens.

Promoters

These chemicals increase the effects of initiators when given subsequently. The classic example of this phenomenon was provided by studies demonstrating that an initial application on the mouse skin of a carcinogenic PAH did not induce skin cancer until after applying, at the same site, phorbol esters from croton oil (Berenblum and Shubik, 1947, 1949). The application of the promoters could be delayed for months or even a year without losing the effect. These studies clearly demonstrate the *two-stage* process of carcinogenesis as well as the persistence of the effect of the initiator.

Incidentally, croton oil is also co-carcinogenic since it is effective when applied at the same time as the initiator.

The possible mechanisms of action of promoters include the following:

1. Stimulation of cell proliferation through cytotoxicity leading to compensatory regeneration or hormonal effects
2. Inhibition of gap junction intercellular communication, thereby releasing the initiated cells from the restraint exercised by the surrounding normal cells
3. Immunosuppression
4. An increase in cell turnover rates and transformation

Cytotoxicants such as nitrilotriacetic acid, a non-eutrophying replacement for phosphate in household detergent, produce tumors through cell proliferation resulting from cell injury and death. Unleaded gasoline and a number of other chemicals have been shown to induce renal tubular necrosis resulting from the deposition of $\alpha 2u$-globulin in male rats. The cell death and subsequent regeneration are believed to produce kidney tumors in male rats (Swenberg et al., 1989).

Hormones such as estradiol and diethylstilbestrol have been shown to produce an increase in tumors in animals (e.g., breast cancer in mice) and in humans (e.g., endometrial cancer in menopausal females maintained on estrogen). These substances are not genotoxic but act as promoters. The actual initiators are not known. Androgens have little, if any, carcinogenic effect. The herbicide aminotriazole and certain fungicides induce thyroid tumors also through a hormonal mechanism (McClain, 1989).

Gap junction intercellular communication is an important mechanism in regulating cell growth. A number of chemicals interfere with this mechanism, thereby inducing hyperplasia and acting as promoters in carcinogenesis (Trosko and Chang, 1988). Klaunig (1991) listed, among others, a number of pesticides (e.g., chlordane, DDT, dieldrin, endosulfan, and lindane) and pharmaceuticals (phenobarbital and diazepam) as being able to inhibit hepatic gap junctional intercellular communication.

Immunosuppressive drugs such as cyclosporin A and azathioprine are increasingly being used in conjunction with organ transplantation. They have been shown to produce leukemias and sarcomas in some of these patients and in mice and rats. The genotoxic agents are likely to be viruses, and the immunosuppressive drugs promote the development of the tumors through nongenotoxic mechanisms (Ryffel, 1992).

Peroxisome proliferators consist of a variety of chemicals that have the common property of inducing rodent liver tumors and increasing peroxisomes in liver cells (Melnick, 2001). These chemicals have therefore been considered as a special class of carcinogen (Reddy and Lalwani, 1983). Examples are hypolipidemic drugs, such as clofibrate and fenofibrate, certain phthalate plasticizers, such as di(2-ethylhexyl) phthalate, and the solvent 1,1,2-tricholoroethylene. These chemicals are not genotoxic, but by increasing the number of peroxisomes, they may increase the formation of H_2O_2, leading to the formation of ROS and thereby enhancing cell replication (Lake, 1995).

Solid-State Carcinogens

These are exemplified by asbestos and implanted materials such as plastics, metal, and glass. These substances exert no genotoxic effects, but they produce tumors of mesenchymal origin. Although the precise mode of action is not known, the tumors they induce are preceded by an exuberant foreign-body reaction including hyperplastic fibrosis with a high frequency of chromosomal changes in the pre-neoplastic cells (Weisburger and Williams, 1993). In many cases there is concomitant exposure to the substances in cigarette smoke, and the frequency of lung cancer in individuals exposed to asbestos and cigarette smoke is markedly higher than those exposed to asbestos alone. The absence of tumors in subjects exposed to asbestos alone, but the presence of cancer in patients exposed to asbestos and cigarette smoke, is a strong indication that asbestos may be acting as an initiator rather than a direct carcinogen (Vallyathan et al., 1998).

Metals and Metalloids

Arsenic, cadmium, chromium, nickel, uranium, and their compounds are carcinogenic in humans. A number of others such as beryllium, cobalt, and lead are considered to be carcinogens in animals (IARC, 1987). Arsenic was thought to be an exception in that it is carcinogenic in humans but not in animals (Bernstam and Nriagu, 2000). Recent data, however, show that intratracheal instillation of As_2O_3 in Syrian hamsters resulted in an increase in pulmonary adenomas, and after intrauterine exposure, apparently induced lung tumors in mice. Radon and its daughters diffuse into the ambient air, become attached to particles in uranium mines, and upon inhalation produce lung cancer.

The mechanisms underlying metal-induced carcinogenesis are not fully understood, but may involve genotoxic and/or epigenetic activities. Sunderman (1984) has listed a number of promising avenues for research. Among them are the formation of cross-links between DNA and proteins or between adjacent DNA strands, and impairment of the fidelity of DNA replication by altering the conformation of DNA polymerases. Radon was shown to penetrate bronchial epithelial nuclei resulting in DNA mutation leading to malignant transformation of cells (Vallyathan et al., 1998). These substances may be classified as genotoxic carcinogens because they alter the gene expression in one way or the other. In addition, damages of cytoskeleton by certain metals may contribute to their carcinogenicity (Chou, 1989). A probable mechanism of metal carcinogenesis includes an increase in ROS and RNS formation through redox cycling reactions by disrupting metal homeostasis (e.g., Fe, Co, Cu, Cr), oxidative stress, and depletion of glutathione (e.g., As, Cd, and Pb) (Jomova and Valko, 2011). As epigenetic modes of action, perturbation of DNA methylation and global or gene specific histone modification are reported (Arita and Costa, 2009).

Secondary Carcinogens

This term has been used to refer to substances that are not directly carcinogenic but can induce cancer following a distinctly noncarcinogenic effect. For example, polyoxyethylene monostearate (Myrj 45), at very high doses, elicited bladder stones that in turn produced bladder tumors. No tumors were observed in any of the animals that had no bladder stones. On the other hand, this term has also been used in connection with those genotoxic carcinogens that require bioactivation.

SOME HUMAN CARCINOGENS/TARGET ORGANS

As noted above, the designation of a chemical, or mixture, as a human carcinogen is based on sufficient human data and, as a rule, some animal data. Human carcinogens induce cancers in different organs or systems. Table 7.3 lists the target organs of some human carcinogens, grouped by the "reason"/site of exposure.

In addition to the carcinogens related to diet and lifestyle, it is generally recognized that high intake of fat and/or calories and deficiencies in vitamins A and E pose risks of increasing certain cancers. However, these factors, in the strict sense, are not carcinogens, but they modify/promote carcinogenesis by certain indirect mechanisms. Caloric restriction reduces carcinogenesis and increases the survival time.

As noted above, certain biochemical changes take place in the body after exposure to a carcinogen. Some of these changes can be detected in biological samples. Clinically, they may serve to monitor such exposure or to assess the progress of cancer and progress of treatment. Appendix 1 describes a few examples to illustrate their uses.

TESTS FOR CARCINOGENICITY

Short-Term Tests for Mutagenesis/Carcinogenesis

In recent years, a number of relatively simple and much shorter tests have been devised and employed to detect the mutagenic activity of chemicals. These tests utilize a variety of systems, including microbes, insects, and mammalian cells, as well as a battery of parameters such as gene mutation, chromosomal aberration, and DNA repair. These mutagenesis tests and tests using cell transformation as endpoints will be described and discussed in the next chapter.

Although not all mutagens are carcinogenic, nor vice versa, the relationship between these two activities is nevertheless so close that mutagenesis tests are performed frequently as a rapid screening of chemicals for their potential carcinogenicity. To improve the reliability of the results, a battery of these tests is usually conducted (e.g., U.S. ISGC, 1986). Weisburger and Williams (1993) recommended the following short-term in-vitro tests:

1. Bacterial mutagenesis
2. Mammalian mutagenesis

Table 7.3   Some Human Carcinogens and Their Target Organs

Dietary and Lifestyle	
Aflatoxin	Liver
Alcoholic beverages	Pharynx, esophagus, liver, larynx, oral cavity
Betel chewing	Mouth, pharynx, larynx
Tobacco smoke	Lung, larynx, oral cavity, pharynx, esophagus, pancreas, kidney, urothelial
Industrial and environmental	
4-Aminobiphenyl	Bladder
Aromatic amines	Bladder
Azo dyes	Bladder
Arsenic	Skin, bronchus, liver
Asbestos	Lung, pleura, peritoneum
Benzene	Bone marrow
Benzidine	Bladder
Cadmium	Lung, prostate
Chromium (VI) compounds	Respiratory tract
2-Naphthylamine	Bladder
Nickel compounds	Nasal sinus, bronchus
Polynuclear aromatic hydrocarbons, from coke, coal, tar, etc.	Skin, bronchus, stomach
Vinyl chloride monomer	Liver, hemangiosarcoma
Wood dust	Nasal sinus
Manufacturing	
Anthraquinone dyes	Kidney, liver, urinary bladder
Aluminum production	Lung, bladder
Auramine manufacture	Bladder
Boot and shoe manufacture	Nasal cavity, hematopoietic system
Coke production	Skin, lung, kidney
Iron and steel founding	Nasal cavity
Magenta manufacture	Bladder
Painting	Lung
Rubber industry	Bladder, hematopoietic system
Medicinal	
Azathioprine	Lymph node, skin
Cyclophosphamide	Bladder, bone marrow
Estrogens	Cervix, uterus, breast
Methoxsalen (8-methoxypsoralen) with UV radiation	Skin
Phenacetin	Renal pelvis, bladder
Thorotrast (thorium-232)	Liver, bile duct

3. Mammalian cell DNA repair
4. Chromosome integrity
5. Cell transformation

   The results of these tests are also useful in defining the mechanism of action. Descriptions of these tests are provided in chapter 8.

Limited Carcinogenicity Tests

Limited carcinogenicity tests are superior to the mutagenesis tests in that the endpoint is tumor formation. Furthermore, the duration of these tests is much shorter than that of the long-term carcinogenicity studies.

Skin Tumors in Mice

Mouse skin responds to topical application of chemicals such as PAH and crude products such as tar from coal and petroleum, by the formation of papillomas and carcinomas. This procedure, introduced by Berenblum and Shubik (1947), has been widely used. Mouse skin responds positively apparently because it has the enzymes that convert the substances into active metabolites.

Some chemicals act as both initiators and promoters; they may, therefore, be referred to as complete carcinogens. Others act mainly or exclusively as initiators. Their carcinogenicity is revealed only after the application of a promoter, which is an incomplete carcinogen. Results obtained in the mouse skin test reported in the literature on the effects of chemicals as initiators and as promoters have been compiled by Pereira (1982).

Pulmonary Tumors in Mice

Strain A mice spontaneously have an essentially 100% lung tumor incidence by 24 months of age. Positive results from carcinogens can be obtained in about 24 weeks when few controls have tumors. With some chemicals, the test can be completed in 12 weeks.

Altered Foci in Rodent Liver

It has been demonstrated that distinct liver foci appear before the development of hepatocarcinoma. These foci are resistant to iron accumulation, a phenomenon that can be identified histochemically. There are also abnormalities in certain enzymes, which can be demonstrated histochemically. The latter alteration occurs in rats but not in mice. These foci can be detected within three weeks of exposure and occur in large numbers in 12–16 weeks (Goldfarb and Pugh, 1982).

Breast Cancer in Female Rats

Polycyclic hydrocarbons can induce breast cancers in young female Sprague-Dawley and Wistar rats. The tumors can develop in less than six months (Huggins et al., 1959). The Sprague-Dawley rat lacks progesterone but has very high estrogen levels.

Long-Term Carcinogenicity Studies

These studies are designed to provide definitive information on the carcinogenic effects of chemicals on the test animals. Because of the great expense and time required, they are undertaken usually after a review of other data, such as the chemical structure and results from short-term mutagenesis tests and long-term chronic toxicity studies, which are described, respectively, below and in chapter 6.

Guidelines on the long-term carcinogenicity studies are outlined in this section. More detailed descriptions and references to some comments are provided in a number of papers (WHO, 1969; OECD, 1981; U.S. ISGC, 1986).

Animals

Rats and mice are generally preferred because of their small size, short life span, ready availability, and an abundance of information on their response to other carcinogens. Hamsters are also used, especially in studies on cancers of the bladder, breast, gastrointestinal tract, and respiratory tract. Dogs and nonhuman primates are occasionally used for their positive response to 2-naphthylamine, the latter is also used for their higher phylogenetic order. But their use is limited because of their large size and relatively long life span, thereby requiring a 7- to 10-year exposure to the chemical on test.

The characteristics of a preferred strain are as follows:

1. Known sensitivity to substances of similar chemical structure
2. Low incidence of spontaneous tumors
3. Similarity of its rate and pattern of biotransformation and those of humans, if known.

Both genders should be included in these studies; differences in response to the carcinogenic activity of chemicals are well documented. To provide a sufficient number of animals surviving until the appearance of tumors for statistical analysis, it is a common practice to start the tests with at least 50 animals of each gender per dose group, including the controls.

Inception and Duration

The studies are generally started shortly after weaning the animals to allow maximum duration of exposure. The duration of the studies is generally 24 months in rats and 18 months in mice. If the animals are in good condition, the duration may be extended to 30 and 24 months, respectively.

Route of Administration

The chemical under test should be given to the animals by the route of human exposure and the usual route is oral. This principle readily applies to food additives and contaminants as well as most drugs. For industrial and environmental chemicals, the main route of entry is inhalation. Alternatively, the test chemical may be instilled intratracheally.

Doses and Treatment Groups

Usually two or three dose levels are included in such studies. In addition, control groups are also included for comparison. The doses are selected on the basis of the short-term studies and metabolism data, with the aim that the high dose would produce some minor signs of toxicity but not significantly reduce the life span of the animals. The two lower doses are generally some fractions of the high dose (e.g., one-half and one quarter) and are expected to permit the animals to survive in good health or until a tumor develops.

The "maximally tolerated dose" (MTD) is generally used as the high dose in long-term carcinogenicity study. It is estimated from 90-day studies and defined as one that would (i) not produce morphologic evidence of toxicity of a severity that interferes with the interpretation of the long-term study, and (ii) not comprise so large a fraction of the animal's diet that it might lead to nutritional imbalance (U.S. ISGC, 1986), and (iii) not produce toxic effects without causing death and to decrease body weight gain by no more than 10% relative to controls (OECD, 2002). Ideally, the MTD should provide some signs of toxicity without causing tissue necrosis or metabolic saturation, and without substantially altering normal life span due to effects other than tumors. However, the use of MTD has been criticized, especially when it is much higher than the expected human exposure; there is the possibility of alteration of metabolic pattern by "overloading" the animals (Mermelstein et al., 1994).

An untreated group consisting of the same number, or a larger number, of animals as each dose group is included. In addition to these negative controls, another group of animals is often incorporated that is given a known carcinogen at a dose level that has been shown to be carcinogenic. The positive controls provide more confidence in the results on the test chemical by serving as a check on the sensitivity of the particular lot of animals used, as well as the adequacy of the facilities and procedures in the specific laboratory. It will also provide some indication of the relative potency of the test chemical. If a vehicle, such as acetone or dimethyl sulfoxide, is to be used, its possible effect should also be tested in a group of animals as vehicle control.

Observations and Examinations

The animals should be examined daily for mortality and morbidity. Dead and moribund animals should be removed from the cage for gross and microscopic examinations whenever the condition of the tissues permits. The onset, location, size, and growth of any unusual tissue masses should be carefully examined and recorded. Signs of toxicity should also be noted. All animals found dead or dying should be subjected to gross autopsy. The survivals at the end of the study should be sacrificed and examined. In addition, a number of organs should be weighed, including the liver, kidneys, heart, testes, ovaries, and brain. Samples of all tissues should be preserved for histologic examination. Microscopic examinations should be done on all tumor growths and all tissues showing gross abnormalities.

Reporting of Tumors

As carcinogenesis can manifest in a variety of forms (see the section Definition and Identification), it is necessary to record the following:

1. The number of various types of tumors (both benign and malignant) and any unusual tumors
2. The number of tumor-bearing animals
3. The number of tumors in each animal
4. The onset of tumors whenever determinable

EVALUATION

Preliminary Assessment

Chemical Structure

A number of chemicals are known to be carcinogenic. A list of known human carcinogens is presented in Table 7.3. In addition, a large number of chemicals have been shown to be carcinogenic in animals (see the section Genotoxic Carcinogens). As chemicals that have structures similar to any of these or other carcinogens/mutagens are not necessarily carcinogens, they should be assigned high priority in carcinogenicity testing programs. In fact, certain chemical structures have been shown to be correlated with carcinogenicity (e.g., Ashby and Tennant, 1988). Doi et al. (2005) demonstrated that substitution of a functional group in the anthraquinone dye resulted in the presence of carcinogenicity, or the absence, or the development at a different site. Amino substitutions diminished while bromine substitutions enhanced the carcinogenicity and extended the target tissues to forestomach and lungs, as well as kidney and liver.

Mutagenicity

Mutagenic agents produce heritable genetic changes essentially through their effects on DNA. The mutagenicity tests also provide information on the mode of action as well as on the question as to whether metabolic activation is required for the mutagenicity. Although positive results from these tests do not constitute positive evidence that the chemical is carcinogenic, they do indicate that extensive testing is required. Furthermore, the mutagenesis data are useful in the risk assessment of the chemical in question. On the other hand, negative results do not establish the safety of the chemical.

Limited Carcinogenicity Tests

The endpoint in these tests is tumor formation. Therefore, certain chemicals, such as co-carcinogens that yield negative results in mutagenesis tests, may be positive in these tests. Positive results from more than one of these limited carcinogenicity tests may be considered unequivocal qualitative evidence of carcinogenicity.

Definitive Assessment

Data from well-designed and properly executed long-term carcinogenicity studies generally provide a sound basis for assessment of the carcinogenic potential.

General Considerations

Results from these studies are generally more reliable than those from the rapid screening tests. But the conclusiveness of the results depends on a number of factors. For example, too few animals surviving until tumor development may preclude statistical analysis of the data. This event may occur as a result of insufficient animals placed in each dosage group and/or excessive mortality resulting from improper husbandry or from competing toxicity of the chemical given at inordinately high dose levels. The thoroughness of the postmortem examination also plays an important role. This applies to the gross as well as the microscopic examinations.

Tumor Incidence

As noted at the beginning of the chapter, carcinogenesis may manifest in one of the four forms or any combination thereof. An appreciable increase in the tumor-bearing animals is the most common form. The occurrence of unusual tumors is an important phenomenon if there are a significant number of them; when one or only a few of them are detected, further critical examination is required. An increase in the number of tumors per animal without a concomitant increase in the tumor-bearing animals usually indicates co-carcinogenicity only. The tumors in the experimental animals may not be at the same stage of development. The stages may include, for example, atypical hyperplasia, benign tumors, carcinomas in situ, invasion of adjacent tissues, and metastasis to other parts of the body. Although tumors of the same type, but at different stages. should be separately tabulated, they should be combined for statistical analysis.

Dose–Response Relationship

As a rule, a positive dose–response relationship is apparent. However, there may be a lower tumor incidence in the high-dose group. This phenomenon usually results from poor survival among these animals, which succumb to competing toxic effects of the chemical.

Reproducibility of the Results

The confidence in a carcinogenicity study is enhanced if the results are produced in another strain of animals. Reproducibility in another species is even more significant. However, if negative results are obtained in another species, this fact may not nullify the positive findings but does justify further investigation.

Evaluation of Safety/Risks

The various approaches used in the evaluation of the safety/risk of carcinogens are discussed in chapter 25. The following points, however, are worthy of emphasizing.

First, while the tests enumerated above are a valuable basis for risk/safety assessment, other data relating to the mechanism of action and influences of modifying factors are also essential (U.S. ISGC, 1986). The significant differences between genotoxic and nongenotoxic carcinogens are also considered as valid reasons for assessing their risks differently: it is generally assumed that genotoxic carcinogens exhibit no threshold, whereas nongenotoxic carcinogens induce cancer secondary to other biological effects which are likely to show no-effect dose levels. However, a chemical, such as chloroform, may act as an epigenetic as well as a genotoxic carcinogen.

Furthermore, there are chemicals with carcinogenicity secondary to non-carcinogenic biologic or physical effects that are elicited only at dose levels that could never be approached in realistic human exposure situations. There was general consensus that there are threshold doses for such secondary carcinogens (Lu, 1976; Munro, 1988). The U.S. ISGC (1986) also cautions that extremely high doses of a toxicant may exhibit *qualitatively* different distribution, detoxication, and elimination of the toxicant. The response at such doses, therefore, may not be applicable to more realistic exposure conditions. Furthermore, evidence of extensive tissue damage, disruption of hormonal function, formation of urinary stones, and saturation of DNA repair function should be carefully reviewed.

Carcinogens also differ in the potency and latent periods. Some carcinogens are active in a particular species, whereas others affect several species and strains of animals. All these factors must be taken into account in evaluating the safety/risk of carcinogens. The type of tumor observed needs to be taken into account if one is comparing rodent to human data, especially if the tumor is species dependent and does not have relevance for humans.

Finally, it is important to bear in mind that chemicals differ tremendously in their value to humans. For example, the use of a food color can often be suspended on the basis of suggestive carcinogenicity data. On the other hand, life-saving drugs, even when there is evidence of their carcinogenicity in humans, may still be used clinically. There are also environmental carcinogens, including those in food, that cannot be eliminated with present technology (see also Ames, 1989). The concentration of chemical is crucial in the decision-making process if one is to ban a chemical due to its carcinogenic properties.

REFERENCES

Ames, BN (1989). What are the major carcinogens in the etiology of human cancer? Environmental pollution, natural carcinogens, and the causes of human cancer: six errors. In: De Vita VT Jr, et al., eds. Important Advances in Oncology, 1989, Philadelphia, PA: J. P. Lippincott.

Arita A, Costa M (2009). Epigenetics in metal carcinogenesis: nickel, arsenic, chromium and cadmium. Metallomics 1, 222–228.

Ashby J, Tennant RW (1988) Chemical structure, Salmonella mutagenicity and extent of carcinogenicity among 222 chemicals tested in rodents by the U.S. NCI/NTP. Mutat Res 204, 17–115.

Berenblum I, Shubik P (1947). A new quantitative approach to the study of the stages of chemical carcinogenesis in the mouse's skin. Br J Cancer 1, 383–391.

Berenblum I, Shubik P (1949). An experimental study of the initiating stage of carcinogenesis, and a re-examination of the somatic cell mutation theory of cancer. Br J Cancer 3, 109–118.

Bernstam L, Nriagu J (2000). Molecular aspects of arsenic stress. J Toxicol Environ Health B 3, 293–322.

Bishop JM (1987). The molecular genetics of cancer. Science 235, 305–311.

Butterworth BE, Goldworthy TL (1991). The role of cell proliferation in multistage carcinogenesis. Proc Soc Exp Biol Med 198, 683–687

Chou IN (1989). Distinct cytoskeletal injuries induced by As, Cd, Co, Cr, and Ni compounds. Biomed Environ Sci 2, 358–365.

Clark HA, Snedeker SM (2006). Ochratoxin A: its cancer risk and potential for exposure. J Toxicol Environ Health B 9: 265–296.

Cook JW, Hewett CL, Hieger I (1933). The isolation of a cancer-producing hydrocarbon from coal tar. Parts I, II and III. J Chem Soc 24, 395–405.

Doi AM, Irwin RD, Bucher JR(2005). Influence of functional group substitutions on the carcinogenicity of anthraquinone in rats and mice: analysis of long-term bioassays by the National Cancer Institute and the National toxicology Program. J Toxicol Environ Health B 8: 109–126.

Ducasse M, Brown MA (2006). Epigenetic aberrations and cancer. Mol Cancer 5, 60,

Environmental Protection Agency (EPA). (1996). Guidelines for carcinogen risk Assessment. Fed Reg 61, 17957–18010.

Goldfarb S, Pugh MB (1982). The origin and significance of hyperplastic hepatocellular islands and nodules in hepatic carcinogenesis. J Am Coll Toxicol 1, 119–144.

Greenblatt MS, Bennett NP, Hollstein M, et al. (1994). Mutations in the p53 tumor suppressor gene: Clues to cancer etiology and molecular pathogenesis. Cancer Res 55, 4855–5878.

Gu S-Y, Zhang Z-B, Wan J-X, et al. (2007). Genetic polymorphism in CYP1A1, CYP2D6, UGT1A6, UGT1A7 and SULT1A1 genes and correlation with benzene exposure in a Chinese occupational population. J Toxicol Environ Health A 70, 916–924.

Huggins C, Briziarelli G, Sutton H Jr. (1959). Rapid induction of mammary carcinoma in the rat and the influence of hormones on the tumors. J Exp Med 109, 25–41.

IARC. (1987). Monographs for Carcinogenic Chemicals: Overall Evaluation of Carcinogenicity: An Updating of IARC Monographs. vols. 1–42(suppl. 7). Lyon, France: International Agency for Research on Cancer.

Jomova K, Valko M (2011). Advances in metal-induced oxidative stress and human disease. Toxicology 283, 65–87.

Kadlubar FF, Butler MA, Kaderlick KR, et al. (1992). Polymorphisms for aromatic amine metabolism in humans: relevance for human carcinogenesis. Environ Health Perspect 98, 69–74.

Kanwal R, Gupta S (2010). Epigenetics and cancer. J Appl Physiol 109, 598–605.

Klaunig JE (1991). Alterations in intercellular communication during the stage of promotion. Proc Soc Exp Biol Med 198, 688–692.

Kwack SJ, Lee BM (2000). Correlation between DNA or protein adducts and benzo[a] pyrene diol epoxide I-triglyceride adduct detected in vitro and in vivo. Carcinogenesis 21, 629–632.

Lake BG (1995). Mechanisms of hepatocarcinogenicity of peroxisome-proliferating drugs and chemicals. Ann Rev Pharmacol Toxicol 35, 483–507.

Lu FC (1976). Threshold doses in chemical carcinogenesis: introductory remarks. Oncology 33, 50.

McClain, RM (1989). The significance of hepatic microsomal enzyme induction and altered thyroid function in rats: implications for thyroid gland neoplasia. Toxicol Pathol 17, 294–306.

Melnick RL (2001). Is peroxisome proliferation an obligatory precursor step in the carcinogenicity of di(2-ethylhexyl)phthalate (DEHP)? Environ Health Perspect 109, 437–442.

Mermelstein R, Marrow PE, Christian MS (1994). Organ or system overload and its regulatory implications. J Am Col Toxicol 13, 143–147.

Munro IC (1988). Risk assessment of carcinogens: present status and future directions. Biomed Environ Sci 1, 51–58.

Nestmann ER, Lynch BS, Ratpan F (2005). Perspectives on the genotoxic risk of styrene. J Toxicol Environ Health B 8, 95–107.

OECD. (1981). OECD Guidelines for Testing of Chemicals. Paris, France: Organization for Economic Cooperation and Development.

OECD. (2002). Guidance notes for analysis and evaluation of chronic toxicity and carcinogenicity studies. OECD series on testing and assessment no. 35, OECD, Paris. [online] Available from: http://www.olis.oecd.org/olis/2002doc.nsf/LinkTo/NT00002BE2/$FILE/JT00130828.PDF.

Pereira MA (1982). Mouse skin bioassay for chemical carcinogens. J Am Coll Toxicol 1, 47–82.

Pitot HC, Beer D, Hendrich S (1988). Multistage carcinogenesis: the phenomenon underlying the theories. In: Iversen OH, ed. Theories of Carcinogenesis. Washington, DC: Hemisphere.

Poirier MC, Yuspa SH, Weinstein IB et al. (1977). Detection of carcinogen-DNA adducts by radioimmunoassay. Nature 270, 186–188.

Pott P (1775). Cancer scroti. In: Chirurgical Observations Relative to the Cataract, the Polypus of the Nose, the Cancer of the Scrotum, the Different Kinds of Ruptures, and the Modification of the Toes and Feet. London: Hawes: Clarke, Collins, p. 63–68.

Pyatt DW, Aylward LL, Hays SM (2007). Is age an independent risk factor for chemically induced acute myelogenous leukemia in children? J Toxicol Environ Health B 10, 379–400.

Qian GS, Ross RK, Yu MC, et al. (1994). A follow-up study of urinary markers of aflatoxin exposure and liver cancer risk in Shanghai, China. Cancer Epidemiol Biomarkers Prev 3, 3–10.

Reddy JK, Lalwani ND (1983). Carcinogenesis by hepatic peroxisome proliferators: evaluation of the risk of hyperlipidemic drugs and industrial plasticizers to humans. CRC Crit Rev Toxicol 12, 1–58.

Ryffel B (1992). The carcinogenicity of cyclosporin. Toxicology 73, 1–22.

Seidegard J, Pero RW, Markowitz MM, et al. (1990). Isoenzyme(s) of glutathione transferase (class mu) as a marker for susceptibility to lung cancer: a follow-up study. Carcinogenesis 11, 33–36.

Shi X, Castranova V, Halliwell B, et al. (1998). Reactive oxygen species and silica-induced carcinogenesis. J Toxicol Environ Health B 1, 181–197.

Shi X, Chiu A, Chen CT, et al. (1999). Reduction of chromium (VI) and its relationship to carcinogenesis. J Toxicol Environ Health B 2, 87–104.

Steinmaus C, Moore LE, Shipp M, et al. (2007). Genetic polymorphism in MTHFR 677 and 1298, GSTM1 and T1 and metabolism of arsenic. J Toxicol Environ Health A 70, 159–170.

Sugimura T, Ushijima T (2000). Genetic and epigenetic alterations in carcinogenesis. Mutat Res 462, 235–246.

Sunderman FW Jr (1984). Recent advances in metal carcinogenesis. Am Clin Lab Sci 14, 93–122.

Swenberg JA, Short B, Borghoff S, et al. (1989). The comparative pathobiology of α2μ-globulin nephropathy. Toxicol Appl Pharmacol 97, 35–46.

Trosko JE, Chang CC (1988). Chemical and oncogene modulation of gap junctional inter-cellular communication. In: Langenbach R, et al. eds. Tumor Promoters: Biological Approaches for Mechanistic Studies and Assay Systems. New York, NY: Raven Press.

U.S. ISGC. (1986). Chemical carcinogens: a review of the science and its associated prin-ciples. U.S. Interagency Staff on Carcinogens. Environ Health Persp 67, 201–282.

Vallyathan V, Green F, Ducatman B, et al. (1998). Roles of epidemiology, pathology, molecular biology, and biomarkers in the investigation of occupational lung cancer. J Toxicol Environ Health B 1, 91–116.

WHO (1969). Principles for the testing and evaluation of drugs for carcinogenicity. WHO Tech Rep Ser 426, 5–26.

Weinberg RA (1989). Oncogenes, antioncogenes, and the molecular bases of multistep carcinogenesis. Cancer Res 49, 3713–3721.

Weisburger JH, Williams GM (1993) Chemical carcinogenesis. In: Amdur MO, Doull J, Klaassen CD, eds. Casarett and Doull's Toxicology. New York, NY: McGraw-Hill, 127–200.

Yamagiwa K, Ichikawa K (1918). Experimental study of the pathogenesis of carcinoma. J Cancer Res 3, 1–21.

Zhu Y-J, Li C-P, Tang W-Y, et al. (2007). Single nucleotide polymorphism of the JWA gene is associated with risk of leukemia: a case-control study in a Chinese population. J Toxicol Environ Health A 70, 895–900.

FURTHER READING

WHO. (1993). Biomarkers and Risk Assessment: Concepts and Principles. Environ Health Criteria 155. Geneva: World Health Organization.

Appendix 1   Biomarkers of Carcinogenesis/Human Cancers

Biomarkers of Exposure and Initiation

Initiation is associated with covalent binding of electrophilic carcinogens or their reactive metabolites to DNA. The carcinogen–DNA adduct can be demonstrated and quantified to indicate exposure and effect of the carcinogen. This procedure has been applied to situations wherein human exposure to a particular carcinogen is suspected, for example, in the determination of exposure to aflatoxin B_1 and its relationship to hepatocellular carcinoma (Qian et al., 1994).

Biomarker of Promotion

Promotion has been most extensively studied in skin carcinogenesis. A variety of biochemical changes have been noted in initiated as well as normal cells on treatment with promoters, the most active of which is TPA (12-o-tetradecanoyl phorbol-13-acetate). The changes include accumulation of plasminogen activator and increased prostaglandin synthesis. Growth factors, protein kinase C, TPA- and dioxin-responsive elements in genes, interaction of promoters with oncogenes, and/or suppressor genes are being studied to determine their role as markers of preneoplasia in the liver.

Tumor Markers

α-Fetoprotein (AFP) is a product of fetal liver and hepatocarcinoma. AFP had, therefore, been used to screen large populations for hepatocellular carcinomas, allowing early detection and treatment. However, it has been shown to be nonspecific. Human chorionic gonadotropin (HCG) is a sensitive marker and can be used to detect cancers of male and female sex organs at a subclinical phase. Carcinoembryonic antigen (CEA) is found in patients with carcinoma of the colon and rectum. Prostate-specific antigen (PSA) has been shown to be a useful biomarker of tumor and other lesions of the prostate. CA 125 is useful in diagnosing and monitoring treatment of ovarian cancer. Telomerase is a ribonucleoprotein enzyme that adds TTAGGG repeats onto telomeres to compensate for shortening and instability of desmosomes. Telomerase is detected in most cancers and immortal cell lines. Oncogene expression, tumor suppressor gene inactivation, formation of DNA and protein adducts, and endogenous production of paraneoplastic hormones by the tumor, all these are potential useful tools for the determination of which specific agents interact with cells to produce tumors.

Biomarkers of Susceptibility

Individuals with certain genetic disposition may be more susceptible to carcinogenesis. For example, those with xeroderma pigmentosa are prone to skin cancer. Polymorphism of x-oxidation has been linked to susceptibility to colon cancer (Kadlubar et al., 1992) and polymorphism in glutathione S-transferase to increased lung cancer (Seidegard et al., 1990). In the case of arsenic-induced carcinogenesis, polymorphism in the genes encoding the enzymes involved in the methylation of arsenic can lead to increased frequency of skin cancer (Steinmaus et al., 2007). A single nucleotide polymorphism in the JWA gene was found to be associated with a higher frequency of leukemia in the Chinese population (Zhu et al., 2007). Genetic polymorphisms in various metabolic enzymes were attributed to result in a higher frequency of benzene-induced carcinogenesis in China (Gu et al., 2007).

8

Mutagenesis

INTRODUCTION

Mutagenesis can occur as a result of interaction between mutagenic agents (mutagens) and the genetic materials of organisms. Although spontaneous mutations and natural selection are the major means of evolution, a number of toxicants, in recent decades, have been found to induce mutagenic effects in a variety of organisms. Mutations can be produced by external factors (e.g., high temperatures), toxic chemicals (most carcinogens, etc), radiation (ionizing and non-ionizing), and internal factors (e.g., cellular metabolism and respiration (reactive oxygen species and reactive nitrogen species), DNA replication/transcription error). Electromagnetic fields and free radicals generated from electronic equipments/devices, medical devices (e.g., X-ray, MRI, etc.), electricity, microwave, radar, and cellular phone could be the sources of mutations. Mutations are classified into microlesion (e.g., gene mutation: frame shift and base substitution) and macrolesion (e.g., chromosomal abnormalities: gap, fragments, deletion, ring, translocation, and numerical change). Some people have mutations in the skin cells or other tissues, termed somatic mutations. In contrast, germ mutations occur only in the sex cells and they are more threatening because germ mutations can be passed on to next generations.

Health Hazards

The hereditary effects of human exposure to these mutagenic substances cannot be ascertained at present. However, some spontaneous abortions, stillbirths, and heritable diseases have been shown to be related to changes in DNA molecules and to chromosomal aberrations. There are approximately 1000 dominant gene mutations responsible for various illnesses, including the hereditary neoplasms such as bilateral retinoblastoma, and about the same number of recessive gene disorders such as sickle-cell anemia, cystic fibrosis, and Tay–Sachs disease. In addition, abnormal chromosomal numbers are associated with diseases such as Down's syndrome, Klinefelter syndrome, and Edward's syndrome. These have been estimated to occur with an incidence of 0.5% among the live births in the United States.

Table 8.1 Examples of Chromosomal Abnormalities Associated with Human Cancers

Neoplasm	Abnormality of Chromosome
Chronic myelogenous leukemia	Translocation of chromosomes 9 and 22
Acute monocytic leukemia	Loss of long arm of chromosome 11
Small cell lung cancer	Loss of short arm of chromosome 6
Myeloproliferative diseases	Extra chromosome 1
Retinoblastoma	Deletion of chromosome 13

The true effects of any additional mutagen in the environment can only be manifested after a lapse of several generations. The seriousness of this matter, therefore, warrants extensive investigations in the various fields of mutagenesis.

A number of human diseases are the result of defects of the DNA repair systems. For example, patients with xeroderma pigmentosa are deficient in excision repair in the skin; they are susceptible to ultraviolet light and many chemical carcinogens and thus are prone to developing skin tumors. Those with ataxia telangiectasia have such deficiencies in the lymphoid system and are susceptible to X-rays and the carcinogen methyl nitro-nitrosoguanidine. Fanconi anemia is associated with defective DNA repair in the blood and skeleton. The afflicted persons are susceptible to mitomycin C and psoralens.

On the other hand, tests for mutagenicity in recent years have become more widely used because of their value as a rapid screening for carcinogenicity (see chap. 7). This development stems mainly from the fact that most mutagens have been found to be carcinogens. Furthermore, these tests, with a variety of endpoints, are useful in the elaboration of the mode of action of carcinogens. It is also worth noting that various gene mutations and chromosomal abnormalities have been detected in human tumors. Some examples are listed in Table 8.1. For a more extensive review on this topic, see Rabbitts' review (1994).

Categories of Mutagenesis and Their Tests

It is well known that DNA, consisting of nucleotide bases, plays a key role in genetics. First, it transmits the genetic information from one generation of cells to the next generation through self-replication. This is done by the separation of the double strands of the DNA molecule and the synthesis of new daughter strands. Second, the genetic information coded in the DNA molecule is expressed through the transcription of a complementary RNA strand from one strand of DNA, which serves as a template, and the subsequent translation of the information from the RNA to the amino acids in proteins. Every set of three nucleotide bases, a codon, specifies an amino acid. Derangement of the bases, therefore, alters the amino acid content of the protein synthesized.

Table 8.2   Basic Biochemical Characteristics of all Double-Stranded DNA

1. DNA consists of two different purines (guanine, adenine) and two different pyrimidines (thymine and cytosine).
2. A nucleotide pair consists of one purine and one pyrimidine [adenine/thymine (A–T) or guanine/cytosine (G–C)].
3. Nucleotide pairs are connected to a double helix molecule by sugar-phosphate backbone linkages and hydrogen bonding.
4. The A–T base pair is held by two hydrogen bonds, while the G–C is held by three.
5. The distance between each base pair in a molecule is 3.4 Å, producing 10 nucleotide pairs per turn of the DNA helix.
6. The number of adenine molecules must equal the number of thymine molecules in a DNA molecule. The same relationship exists for guanine and cytosine molecules. However, the ratio of A–T to G–C base pairs may vary in DNA from species to species.
7. The two strands of the double helix are complementary and antiparallel with respect to the polarity of the two sugar-phosphate backbones, one strand being 3′-5′ and the other being 5′-3′ with respect to the terminal OH group on the ribose sugar.
8. DNA replicates by a semiconservative method in which the two strands separate and each is used as a template for the synthesis of a new complementary strand.
9. The rate of DNA nucleotide polymerization during replication is approximately 600 nucleotides per second. The helix must unwind to form templates at a rate of 3600 rpm to accommodate this replication rate.
10. The DNA content of cells is variable (1.8×10^9 Da for *Escherichia coli* to 1.9×10^{11} Da for human cells).

Source: From Brusick (1987).

In earlier studies, mutagenic activity was demonstrated mainly in fruit flies and onion root tips because of the simpler techniques involved. More recently, many new test systems have been developed. They range in complexity from microorganisms to intact mammals. The use of such widely different organisms is based on the fact that all double-stranded DNA share the same biochemical characteristics, which are listed in Table 8.2.

At present, there are more than 100 test systems. A number of exemplary tests are outlined in this chapter under four major categories, namely, gene mutation, chromosomal effects, DNA repair and recombination, and others, which are designed to confirm carcinogenicity. Because of the brevity of their description, at least one reference is cited for each test. Additional references and more details are given elsewhere on these and other tests (EPA, 1994; OECD, 1987; Hoffmann, 1996).

It is worth noting that gene mutation may be detected in all organisms including bacteria. On the other hand, effects related to chromosomes (aberrations, aneuploidy, and DNA repair) can be detected only in higher organisms, that is, those with chromosomes.

GENE MUTATION

Gene mutations involve additions or deletions of base pairs or substitution of a wrong base pair in the DNA molecules. Substitutions consist of transitions and transversions. The former involve the replacement of a purine (adenine, guanine) by another or a pyrimidine (cytosine, thymine) by another. With transversion, a purine is replaced by a pyrimidine, or vice versa. When the number of base pairs added or deleted is not a multiple of three, the amino acid sequence of the protein coded distal to the addition or deletion will be altered. This phenomenon is called frame-shift mutation and is likely to affect the biological property of the protein.

Figure 8.1 clearly illustrates the effects of a deletion and an addition of a nucleotide base.

In addition, a mutagenic chemical, or a part of it, may be incorporated into the DNA molecule. For example, a number of electrophilic compounds react with DNA forming covalent addition products, known as "DNA adducts." Thus acetyl aminofluorene (AAF) binds specifically to the carbon at the 8th position of guanine. For a partial list of such chemicals, see discussions on procarcinogens in "Categories of Carcinogens" in chapter 7. Alkylating agents, such as ethylnitrosourea and diethyl sulfate, donate an alkyl group to DNA.

These various changes in the DNA molecule may cause the substitution of a new amino acid in the subsequently coded protein molecule or result in a different sequence of amino acids in the protein synthesized. Furthermore, a protein synthesis termination codon may be formed, giving rise to a shortened protein. While the first type of effect may or may not result in a modification of the biological property of the protein molecule, the latter two types almost invariably do.

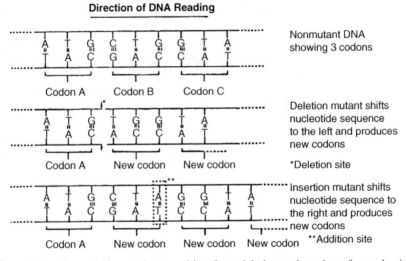

Figure 8.1 Frame-shift mutations resulting from deletion or insertion of a nucleotide base. A series of new codons is formed distal to the deletion or insertion, and hence new amino acids in the protein synthesized. *Source*: From Brusick (1987).

Microbial Tests In Vitro

These involve prokaryotic and eukaryotic microorganisms.

Prokaryotic Microorganisms

Such microorganisms consist of various strains of bacteria. For the detection of point mutations, the commonly used bacteria are *Salmonella typhimurium* and *Escherichia coli*. Most bacterial systems are intended to detect reverse mutation. For example, the Ames test (Ames, 1971) measures the reversion of histidine-dependent mutants (His–, auxotroph) of *S. typhimurium* to the histidine-independent wild type (His+, autotroph). The mutants are incubated in a medium that contains insufficient histidine to permit visible growth. If the toxicant added to the culture medium is capable of inducing reverse mutation, then the bacteria can become histidine-independent and grow appreciably in the histidine-deficient medium. It is customary to use several strains because of their specificity. Their mutation to histidine independency results from either frame-shift or base-pair substitution; different mutagens may affect one strain but not the other.

A number of strains of *S. typhimurium* have been rendered more sensitive to the effects of mutagens through alterations in the permeability of their cell walls (deficient in lipopolysaccharide) and in their DNA excision repair capabilities (through a specific deletion in the DNA molecule) and through the bearing of an ampicillin-resistance factor (Ames et al., 1975; McCann et al., 1975). These various tester strains (e.g., TA 98, 100, 1535, 1537, and 1538) may be susceptible to different mutagens.

As many mutagens are inactive before bioactivation, the test can be carried out with a bioactivating system included in the in-vitro procedure. The bioactivating system called S-9 usually consists of the microsomal fraction (containing the mixed-function oxidase system) of the liver of the rat or other animals, although the human liver is also used for special purposes. The activity of the microsomal enzyme is usually enhanced by pretreating the animal with an inducing agent, such as 3-methylcholanthrene, phenobarbital, or polychlorinated biphenyls. Appropriate cofactors are also added to the mixture prior to incubation.

Strains of *E. coli* that are tryptophan-dependent are also used to detect reverse mutation. Mutagenic changes will result in tryptophan-independent strain (Ames et al., 1975).

Eukaryotic Microorganisms

Certain strains of *Saccharomyces*, *Schizosaccharomyces*, *Neurospora*, and *Aspergillus* have been developed to detect mainly reverse mutations and, to a limited extent, forward mutations. Like the bacterial systems, these systems in general also include bioactivating enzymes and cofactors. For example, a type of mutant of *Saccharomyces cerevisiae* requires adenine and produces red-pigmented colonies, whereas the wild-type microorganisms are adenine-independent and produce white colonies. Thus the reverse mutation can be determined by the prevalence of white colonies (Brusick and Mayer, 1973).

Microbial Tests In Vivo (Host-Mediated Assay)

In this type of test, the microorganisms are injected into the peritoneal cavity of the host mammal (usually the mouse). They can also be injected into the circulatory system or the testes. The toxicant is injected into the host, usually prior to the introduction of the microorganisms. After an elapse of few hours, the host is sacrificed. The microorganisms are then collected and examined for manifestations of mutation. These assays have the advantage of incorporating the biotransformation of the toxicant in the host mammal, but at the same time have the drawback that the microorganisms can only be kept in the host for a relatively short time. Apart from microorganisms, cells from multicellular animals can also be used in the host-mediated assay (Gabridge and Legator, 1969). Despite its theoretical advantage, the procedure has been found to be insensitive to certain types of carcinogens and hence is unsuitable as a routine screening procedure (Simmons et al., 1979).

A modified procedure involves pretreatment of the host with a toxicant, collecting the urine from the host, and injecting the urine, which may contain a high concentration of the metabolite(s) of the toxicant, back into the host. This modified procedure demonstrates positive mutagenicity with 2-AAF, which yields negative results with the regular host-mediated assay (Durston and Ames, 1974).

Insects

The fruit fly *Drosophila melanogaster* is the most commonly used insect. It is characterized well genetically. It has an advantage over microorganisms in that it metabolizes toxicants in a manner that is similar to mammals. Furthermore, it is superior to mammals in two respects, namely, its generation time is only 12–14 days and it can be tested in sufficient numbers at a much lower cost.

The sex-linked recessive lethal test measures the lethal effect on the F_2 males after exposing the males of the parental generation. It is the preferred procedure because the X chromosome represents about 20% of the total genome, and it is capable of screening for point mutations and short deletions at about 800 loci on the X chromosome (Lee et al., 1983).

Mammalian Cells in Culture

The commonly used systems include cells from mouse lymphoma, human lymphoblasts, and cells from the lung, ovary, and other tissues of Chinese hamsters. These cells usually maintain a near-diploid chromosome number, grow actively, and have high cloning efficiency. Both forward and reverse mutations can occur, and the mutants respond selectively to nutritional, biochemical, serological, and drug-resistant growth manipulations. For example, cells from mouse lymphoma, which are heterozygous at the thymidine kinase locus (TK+/−), may undergo forward mutation, for example, via the action of a mutagen, and become TK−/−. Both genotype TK+/− and TK−/− can grow in a normal medium, but TK−/− can also grow in a medium containing 5-bromo-2′-deoxyuridine (BrdU). The mutagenicity of a toxicant can thus be determined by comparing the growth of the lymphoma cells in the presence and absence of the toxicant both in a medium containing BrdU and in a normal medium (DeMarini et al., 1989).

In Chinese hamsters, as in humans, the use of preformed hypoxanthine and guanine is controlled by an X-linked gene. Mutant cells at these loci are deficient in the enzyme, hypoxanthine-guanine phosphoribosyl transferase, and can be identified by their resistance to toxic purine analogs, such as 8-azaguanine or 6-thioguanine, which kill the cells that utilize these analogs (DeMarini et al., 1989).

These cell lines are generally deficient in metabolizing enzymes. Therefore, such enzyme systems are often added (*microsome mediated*). Alternatively, these cells can be co-cultivated with other cells that possess greater ability to biotransform toxicants. Such a *cell-mediated* system involves the use of freshly isolated hepatocytes as a feeder system (Williams, 1979). It offers an additional advantage of having capabilities to conjugate as well as to degrade toxicants.

Gene Mutation Tests in Mice

The Mouse Spot Test

This test is designed to detect gene mutation in somatic cells. Basically it involves treating the pregnant mouse whose embryos are heterozygous at specific coat color loci and examining the newborn for any mosaic patches in its fur. Such patches indicate the formation of clones of mutant cells that are responsible for the color of the fur. This test is relatively inexpensive and takes only a few weeks to complete. Although it may yield false-positive results, it has not yet yielded false-negative results. The spot test is, therefore, a useful prescreen for heritable germinal mutations in mammals (Russell, 1978).

The Specific Locus Test

The specific locus test was developed for determining the mutagenicity of ionizing radiation in the germ cells. This procedure was later adapted to assess the mutagenicity of chemicals (Searle, 1975). It has the advantage of directly detecting in intact mammals the mutagenic effects of toxicants in the germ cells, but it usually requires a very large number of animals.

It involves exposing non-mutant mice to the chemical and subsequently mating them to a multiple-recessive stock. The mutant offspring has an altered phenotype expressed in hair color, hair structure, eye color, ear length, and other traits. Some mutants are mosaic rather than the whole animal. Mutations can also be detected by the rejection or acceptance of skin grafts made between first-generation offspring. It can be further characterized immunogenetically (Russell and Shelby, 1985).

CHROMOSOMAL EFFECTS

The effect of a toxicant on chromosomes may be large enough to be visible micro-scopically, and may manifest as structural aberrations or as changes in number. The former, *aberrations*, include deletions, duplications, and translocations. The latter, *aneuploidy* (45 or 47 chromosomes), involve a decrease or an increase in the number of the chromosomes (euploid, 2n = 46 chromosomes) and another type of aneupolidy is triploid (3n = 69, three haploid sets of 23 chromosomes), or tet-rapolid (4n = 92, in plants), called *polyploidy*. Some of the effects are heritable.

The mode of action underlying these effects may involve molecular cross-linkage, which may cause an arrest of the synthesis of DNA, thereby leaving a gap in the chromosome. An unsuccessful repair of the DNA damage may also be responsible. Nondisjunction (failure of a pair of chromosomes to separate during mitotic division) can lead to mosaicism. A nondisjunction during gametogenesis (meiotic nondisjunction) gives rise to daughter cells that contain either one extra chromosome or one less than normal. The former is known as *trisomy* (e.g., Down syndrome associated with mental retardation and heart problems is caused by an extra copy of chromosome 21, also known as trisomy 21, and babies born with trisomy 18 have severe mental retardation/other birth defects and they do not sur-vive for more than the first few months of life) and the latter as *monosomy*. Babies with monosomy are most commonly fatal during prenatal development. Turner syndrome is caused by the absence of one sex chromosome, also known as 45, XO. About 99% of pregnancies affected with Turner syndrome are miscarried. The estimated chances for a woman to deliver a child with an aneuploidy are dramatically increasing as maternal age increases.

A number of test systems have been developed to determine the chromo-somal effects. The following are the major systems:

Insects

Drosophila melanogaster has the advantage in that the chromosomes of some of its cells are superior in size and morphology. In addition, the chromosomal effects can be readily confirmed genetically, such as the sex-linked recessive lethality. The chromosomal effects include loss of X and Y chromosomes and translocations of fragments between second and third chromosomes.

Effects on the sex chromosome can also be detected by phenotypic changes, such as body color eye color, and shape of the eye (National Research Council, 1983).

Cytogenetic Studies with Mammalian Cells

In-Vitro Tests

For cytogenetic tests, the commonly used cells are derived from Chinese hamster ovaries and human lymphocytes. These cells are cultured in a suitable medium. They are then exposed to different concentrations of the test chemical in the presence or absence of a bioactivator system (usually the microsomal fraction of the rat liver homogenate). The test generally includes two positive control mutagens, namely, ethylmethane sulfonate, which is direct acting, and dimethyl nitrosamine , which requires bioactivation. After an appropriate incubation period, the cell division is arrested by the addition of colchicine. The cells are then mounted, stained, and scored (Preston et al., 1981).

An example of scoring of *aberrations* is shown below: chromatid gap, chromatid break, chromosome gap, chromosome break, chromatid deletion, fragment, acentric fragment, translocation, triradial chromosome, quadriradial chromosome, pulverized chromosome, pulverized cells, ring chromosome, dicentric chromosome, minute chromosome, greater than 10 aberrations, polyploid, and hyperploid (Brusick, 1987).

Fluorescent in situ hybridization, a sensitive cytogenetic technique, was also introduced to analyze the presence or absence of specific DNA sequences on chromosomes by fluorescence microscopy.

In-Vivo Tests

Mammalian cells used in the in-vivo study of chromosomal effects include germ cells and somatic tissues. The chemical to be tested is administered to intact animals, such as rodents and humans. The somatic tissues commonly used are bone marrow and peripheral lymphocytes. A classic protocol using bone marrow from mice, rats, or hamsters has been provided by the Ad Hoc Committee of the Environmental Mutagen Society and the Institute for Medical Research (1972). The scoring is the same as in the in-vitro test.

The *micronucleus* test is a somewhat simpler in-vivo procedure. It involves the use of polychromatic erythrocyte stem cells of CD-1 mice. Six hours after two treatments with the test chemical, given 24 hours apart, the animals are killed and the bone marrow is collected from the femur of the mice that have undergone the two treatments. An increase in the number of micronucleated cells over the controls (about 0.5%) is considered positive (Schmid, 1976). Many other types of cells may also be used. These micronuclei represent fragments of chromosome and chromatid resulting from spindle/centromere dysfunction.

For tests on *germ cells*, the male animal is usually used. In order to allow cells of different stages of spermatogenesis to be exposed, the chemical is given daily for five days and the animals sacrificed one, three, and five weeks following the last dose. The sperm is collected surgically from the cauda epididymides. After mounting and staining, the incidence of abnormal sperm heads is determined, and it is compared with the negative and positive controls (Wyrobek and Bruce, 1975).

Sister Chromatid Exchange

This test measures a reciprocal exchange of DNA between two sister chromatids of a duplicating chromosome. The exchange takes place because of a breakage and reunion of DNA during its replication. The test can be done with mouse lymphoma cells, Chinese hamster ovary cells, and human lymphocytes. It may also be done in vivo by collecting cells from treated animals. The procedure involves labeling of cells with 5-BrdU (5-bromo-deoxyuridine), and after two cycles of replication, the cells are stained with a fluorescent-plus-Giemsa technique. The frequency of sister chromatid exchange per cell and per chromosome is scored and compared. The exchange is visible because, in one chromatid, the semiconservative replication of DNA results in a substitution of BrdU in *one* polynucleotide strand; in the other chromatid, the BrdU is substituted in *both* polynucleotide strands (Wolff, 1977).

Although the mechanism underlying the sister chromatid exchange is not fully understood, it shows that a chemical has attacked the chromosomes or impaired their replication. The test has the advantage of being simple to perform. Furthermore, its endpoint is often observed at concentrations much lower than those required for other tests (NRC, 1983).

Dominant Lethal Test in Rodents

This test is designed to demonstrate toxic effects on germ cells in the intact male animal, usually the mouse or rat. The effects can manifest in the mated females as dead implantations and/or preimplantation losses (the difference between the number of corpora lutea and the number of implantations). These effects are generally due to chromosomal damages, which lead to developmental errors that are fatal to the zygote. However, other cytotoxic effects can also cause early fetal death (see also chap. 18).

Heritable Translocation Test in Mice

This test is intended to detect the heritability of chromosomal damages. The damages, consisting of reciprocal translocation in the germ line cells of the treated male mice, are transmitted to the offspring. By mating the male F_1 progeny with untreated female mice, the chromosomal effects are revealed by a reduction of viable fetuses. The presence of these reciprocal translocations can be verified by the presence of translocation figures among the double tetrads at meiosis (Adler, 1980).

DNA REPAIR AND RECOMBINATION

These biological processes are not mutations per se, but they occur after DNA damage. These phenomena, therefore, indicate the existence of DNA damages, which are caused essentially by mutagens. There are three main types of DNA damages that can be repaired: missing, incorrect, or altered bases; interstrand crosslinks; and strand breaks.

Bacteria

Among *E. coli* there are those with normal DNA polymerase I enzyme, which is capable of repairing DNA damage, and those deficient in this enzyme. Mutagens induce DNA damage and thereby impair the growth of the *E. coli* that is deficient in the repair enzyme, whereas the growth of those with this enzyme is not affected. The DNA repair-efficient strain is included to rule out the effect of cytotoxicity (Rosenkranz et al., 1976).

Similarly, there are also recombination efficient and deficient strains of *Bacillus subtilis*. Damage to DNA is repaired in the former strain through recombination but not in the latter. Mutagens will thus inhibit the growth of the latter but not the former.

Yeasts

Various eukaryotic microorganisms, such as *Saccharomyces cerevisiae*, have been used to test the mutagenicity of chemicals by the induced mitotic crossing-over and mitotic gene conversion. These effects on DNA result in the growth of colonies with different colors (Zimmermann et al., 1984).

Mammalian Cells/UDS

Unscheduled DNA synthesis is an indication of DNA repair. It can be detected in human cells in culture. The synthesis is determined by the amount of radioactive thymidine incorporated per unit weight of DNA over the control value. This is done both in the presence and absence of an added activator system (Stich and Laishes, 1973). Such synthesis can also be determined in primary rat hepatocytes. The extent of DNA synthesis is determined using an autoradiographic method. Since these cells have sufficient metabolic activity, there is no need to add an activator system (Williams, 1979).

Because of their greater relevance to genetic risk, germ cells have also been used in unscheduled DNA synthesis tests: male mice are treated with a suspected mutagen, and $[^3H]$-thymidine ($[^3H]$-dT) is injected intratesticularly. Any incorporation of $[^3H]$-dT into the DNA of meiotic and postmeiotic germ cells indicates the production of repairable damage to the DNA (Russell and Shelby, 1985).

OTHER TESTS

As noted in chapter 7, a number of related mutagenesis tests are used to determine carcinogenicity.

In-Vitro Transformation of Mammalian Cells

Cells from the BALB/3T3 mouse are commonly used in this test. Others include Syrian hamster embryo cells, mouse 10T1/2 cells, and human cells. Normally these cells will grow in the culture medium to form a monolayer. Those treated with a carcinogen, however, will reproduce without being attached to a solid surface and grow over the monolayer. The appearance of such multilayered colonies indicates malignant transformation. This endpoint can be confirmed by injecting these cells into syngeneic animals. In general, malignant tumors will develop if the cells have undergone transformation (Kakunaga, 1973). Therefore, in general, positive results from this test are especially significant.

Nuclear Enlargement Test

HeLa cells are grown in culture medium and treated with different concentrations of the chemical on test. After an appropriate duration, the cells are harvested and counted. They are then stripped of their cytoplasmic material and the size of the nucleus is determined with a particle counter. An increase in the nuclear size indicates the carcinogenicity of the chemical (Finch et al., 1980).

EVALUATION

Selection of Test Systems

Since mutagens affect the genetic material in different ways, they may yield negative results in one test but positive in others. To rule out false negatives (and false positives), it is advisable to conduct several tests, preferably of different categories. OECD (1987) recommended a series of tests for screening, confirmation, and risk assessment (Table 8.3). Ideally, test systems with both high sensitivity and specificity will be the best choice.

The Committee on Chemical Environmental Mutagens of the National Research Council has recommended a mutagen assessment program (National Research Council, 1983). It suggests that the mutagenesis tests be placed in three tiers. Tier I consists of (i) the *Salmonella*/microsome gene-mutation test, (ii) a mammalian cell gene-mutation test, and (iii) a mammalian cell chromsomal breakage test. If all tests are negative, the chemical is considered a presumed mammalian non-mutagen. If two of these tests are positive, it is classified as a presumed mammalian mutagen. If only one is positive, then the Tier II test (*Drosophila* sex-linked lethal mutation) is conducted. For further screening of the most crucial chemicals, supplemental tests are done. A specific-locus test is recommended for chemicals with a potential mutagenicity in mammalian germ cells, and a dominant lethal test should be done for those having chromosomal effects [see also WHO (1990)].

Many chemicals have been tested for genotoxicity (mutagenicity, carcinogenicity, and developmental toxicity) using a multiplicity of tests. To facilitate the task of a "weight-of-evidence" analysis of the genotoxicity of the chemicals and an analysis of the merit of the tests used in generating the data, a method has been proposed by the International Commission for Protection Against Environmental Mutagens and Carcinogens (ICPEMC, 1992).

Table 8.3   Utility and Application of Assays

A. Assays that may be used for mutagen and carcinogen screening
   Salmonella typhimurium reverse mutation assay
   Escherichia coli reverse mutation assay
   Gene mutation in mammalian cells in culture
   Gene mutation in *Saccharomyces cerevisiae*
   In-vitro cytogenetics assay
   Unscheduled DNA synthesis in vitro
   In-vitro sister chromatid exchange assay
   Mitotic recombination in *S. cerevisiae*
   In-vivo cytogenetics assay
   Micronucleus test
   Drosophila sex-linked recessive lethal test
B. Assays that confirm in-vitro activity
   In-vivo cytogenetics assay
   Micronucleus test
   Mouse spot test
   Drosophila sex-linked recessive lethal test
C. Assays that assess effects on germ cells and that are applicable
      for estimating genetic risk
   Dominant lethal assay
   Heritable translocation assay
   Mammalian germ cell cytogenetic assay

Source: From OECD (1987).

Significance of Results

Relation Between Mutagenicity and Carcinogenicity

A number of investigators have shown the association between carcinogens and mutagens. For example, McCann et al. (1975) reported in their study of 300 substances for mutagenicity in the *Salmonella*/microsome test. The results were compared with the reported carcinogenicity or noncarcinogenicity of these substances. The authors demonstrated a high correlation between these toxic effects: 90% (156/175) of carcinogens are mutagenic in the test. Few noncarcinogens showed any degree of mutagenicity.

More recently, Mason et al. (1990) compiled information on the correlation between carcinogenicity in rodents and mutagenicity as determined by *S. typhimurium*. The correlations varied between 55% and 93%.

It is of interest to note that many recent studies have demonstrated that certain human leukemias, lymphomas, and solid tumors are associated with specific chromosomal alterations, some of which are listed in Table 8.1. Furthermore, gene mutations and chromosomal damages can convert proto-oncogenes to active oncogenes (Bishop, 1991; Barrett, 1993). For further discussions on the effects of such conversion, see the section on "Mode of Action" of carcinogenesis in chapter 7.

Heritable Effects

At present there is no direct correlation between laboratory tests for heritable mutations induced by chemical toxicants and human experience. Nevertheless, if a substance has been shown to be mutagenic in a variety of test systems including heritable mutations in intact mammals, it must be considered as a mutagen in humans unless there is convincing evidence to the contrary. Fortunately, for many chemicals, such as food additives, pesticides, cosmetics, and most drugs, where human exposure can be avoided, any incidence of mutagenicity will be sufficient to warrant suspension of their use (Flamm, 1977). For environmental pollutants and occupational toxicants that are mutagenic, all efforts should be made to reduce human exposure to them.

REFERENCES

Ad Hoc Committee of the Environmental Mutagen Society and the Institute of Medical Research (1972). Chromosome methodologies in mutagen testing. Toxicol Appl Pharmacol 22, 269–275.

Adler ID (1980). New approaches to mutagenicity studies in animals for carcinogenic and mutagenic agents. I. modification of heritable translocation test. Teratogen Carcinogen Mutagen 1, 75–86.

Ames BN (1971). The detection of chemical mutagens with enteric bacteria. In: Hollander A, ed. Chemical Mutagens: Principles and Methods for Their Detection, vol. 1. New York, NY: Plenum Press, 267–282.

Ames BN, McCann J, Yamasaki E (1975). Methods for detecting carcinogens and mutagens with the Salmonella/mammalian-microsome mutagenicity test. Mutat Res 31, 347–364.

Barrett JC (1993). Mechanisms of multistep carcinogenesis and carcinogen risk assessment. Environ Health Perspect 100, 9–20.

Bishop JM (1991). Molecular themes in oncogenesis. Cell 64, 235–248.

Brusick DJ, Mayer VW (1973). New developments in mutagenicity screening techniques with yeast. Environ Health Perspect 6, 83–96.

Brusick DJ (1987). Principles of Genetic Toxicology, 2nd edn. New York, NY: Plenum Press.

DeMarini DM, Brockman HE, deSerres FJ, et al. (1989). Specific-locus induced in eukaryotes (especially mammalian cells) by radiation and chemicals: a perspective. Mutat Res 220, 11–29.

Durston WE, Ames BN (1974). Simple method for the detection of mutagens in urine: studies with the carcinogen 2-acetylaminofluorene. Proc Natl Acad Sci USA 71, 737–741.

EPA (1994). Health Effects Test Guidelines, Title 40, Part 798. Washington, DC: U.S. Environmental Protection Agency.

Finch RA, Evans IM, Bosmann HB (1980). Chemical carcinogen in vitro testing: a method for sizing cell nuclei in the nuclear enlargement assay. Toxicology 15, 145–154.

Flamm WG (Chairman, DHEW Working Group on Mutagenicity Testing) (1977). Approaches to determining the mutagenic properties of chemicals: risk to future generations. J Environ Pathol Toxicol 1, 301–352.

Gabridge MG, Legator MS (1969). A host-mediated microbial assay for the detection of mutagenic compounds. Proc Soc Exp Biol Med 130, 831–834.

Hoffmann GR (1996). Genetic toxicology. In: Klaassen CD, ed. Casarett and Doull's Toxicology. New York, NY: McGraw-Hill.

ICPEMC. (1992). A method for combining and comparing short-term genotoxicity test data. The basic system. Mutat Res 266, 7–25.

Kakunaga T (1973). A quantitative system for assay of malignant transformation by chemical carcinogens using a clone derived from BALB/3T3. Int J Cancer 12, 463–473.

Lee WR, Abrahamson S, Valencia R, et al. (1983). The sex-linked recessive lethal test for mutagenesis in Drosophila melanogaster: a report of the U.S. EPA Gene-Tox Program. Mutat Res 123, 183–279.

Mason JM, Langenbach R, Sheldby MD, et al. (1990). Ability of short term tests to predict carcinogenesis in rodents. Annu Rev Pharmacol Toxicol 30, 149–268.

McCann J, Choi E, Yamasaki E, et al. (1975). Detection of carcinogens as mutagens in the Salmonella/microsome tests assay of 300 chemicals. Proc Natl Acad Sci USA 72, 5135–5139.

National Research Council (NRC) (1983). Identifying and Estimating the Genetic Impact of Chemical Mutagens. A Report of the Committee on Chemical Environmental Mutagens, National Research Council. Washington, DC: National Academy Press.

OECD (Organization for Economic Cooperation and Development) (1987). OECD Guidelines for Testing Chemicals. Washington, DC: OECD Publications and Information Center.

Preston RJ, Au W, Bender MA, et al. (1981). Mammalian in vivo and in vitro cytogenetic assays: a report of the U.S. EPA Gene-Tox Program. Mutat Res 87, 143–188.

Rabbitts TH (1994). Translocations in human cancer. Nature 372, 143–149.

Rosenkranz HS, Gutter G, Spek WJ (1976). Mutagenicity and DNA-modifying activity: a comparison of two microbial assays. Mutat Res 41, 61–70.

Russell LB (1978). Somatic cells as indictors of germinal mutations in the mouse. Environ Health Perspect 24, 113–116.

Russell LB, Shelby MD (1985). Tests for heritable genetic damage and for evidence of gonadal exposure in mammals. Mutat Res 154, 69–84.

Schmid W (1976). The micronucleus test. Mutat Res 31, 9–15.

Searle AG (1975). The specific locus test in the mouse. Mutat Res 31, 277–290.

Simmons VF, Rozenkranz HS, Zeiger E, et al. (1979). Mutagenic activity of chemical carcinogens and related compounds in the intraperitoneal host-mediated assay. J Natl Cancer Inst 62, 911–918.

Stich HF, Laishes BA (1973). DNA repair and chemical carcinogens. Pathobiol Annu 3, 341–376.

WHO. (1990). Summary Report on the Evaluation of Short-term Tests for Carcinogenesis. WHO Environ Health Criteria 109.

Williams GM (1979). The status of in vitro test systems utilizing DNA damage and repair for the screening of chemical carcinogens. J Assoc Anal Chem 63, 857–863.

Wolff S (1977). Sister chromatid exchange. Annu Rev Genet 11, 183–201.

Wyrobek AJ, Bruce WR (1975). Chemical induction of sperm abnormalities in mice. Proc Natl Acad Sci USA 72, 4425–4429.

Zimmermann FK, von Borstel RC, von Halle ES, et al. (1984). Testing of chemicals for genetic activity with Saccharomyces cerevisiae: a report of the U.S. EPA Gene-Tox Program. Mutat Res 133, 199–244.

9

Developmental toxicology

INTRODUCTION

Historical Background

Congenital malformations (structural or functional malformations) have been observed for centuries without knowing their etiology. It was only early last century that a variety of malformations were reported among the offspring of mothers who had been exposed to radiation, nutritional deficiencies, or certain viral infections. There was no connection suspected to exist between congenital malformation and chemicals because there was a tendency among toxicologists to assume that the natural protective mechanisms, such as detoxication, elimination, and placental barrier, were sufficient to shield the embryo from maternal exposure to chemicals. On the other hand, it was not unexpected that the natural protective mechanisms were ineffective against ionizing radiation, viruses, and nutritional deficiencies. In general, the time of exposure to developmental toxicants especially at the trimester in humans is critical for congenital malformations.

A new era in teratology was initiated as a result of the clinical use of thalidomide, a sedative hypnotic. This drug, first introduced in the late 1950s in Germany, was found to be relatively nontoxic in experimental animals such as rodents, but toxic in New Zealand White rabbits and chicken, showing species differences. It was used, among other indications, for the relief of morning sickness during pregnancy. In 1960, few cases of phocomelia and amelia were reported. In the following year, there were many more cases. Phocomelia is a very rare type of congenital malformation, with shortening or absence of limbs. The causative agent in these cases was soon traced to the ingestion of thalidomide by the mothers, mainly between the third and eighth week of pregnancy. The use of the drug was promptly prohibited. In spite of that action, more than 10,000 such malformed babies were born in a number of countries (Lenz and Knapp, 1962). The profound, tragic effect on the malformed individuals and the traumatic impact on the families and society were so great that all feasible steps were instituted in an attempt to prevent the occurrence of such a chemically man-made teratogenesis. One of these steps was to subject numerous drugs, food additives, pesticides, environmental contaminants, and other chemicals to various types of testing to determine their potential teratogenicity. An approach to evaluate reproductive and developmental toxicity was compiled by the National Academy of Sciences (Mitchell et al., 2004).

Some toxic effects on the fetus are not observable at birth. They may manifest as delayed developmental toxicity. An outstanding example is diethylstilbestrol. The offspring of mothers who had taken this drug to prevent premature birth showed adverse effects in their sex organs, only many years later. To embrace such delayed effects, the science "teratology" is now more commonly referred to as "developmental toxicology."

Embryology

After fertilization, the ovum undergoes a precise sequence of cell proliferation, differentiation, migration, and organogenesis. The embryo then passes through a set of metamorphoses and a period of fetal development before birth.

Predifferentiation Stage

During this stage, the embryo is not susceptible to teratogenic agents. These agents either cause death of the embryo by killing all or most of the cells or have no apparent effect on the embryo. Even when some mildly harmful effects have been produced, the surviving cells can compensate and form a normal embryo. This resistant stage varies from five to nine days depending on the species.

Embryonic Stage

This is the period when cells undergo intensive differentiation, mobilization, and organization. It is during this period that most of the organogenesis takes place. As a result, the embryo is most susceptible to the effects of teratogens. This period generally ends some time from the 10th to the 14th day in rodents and in the 14th week of the gestation period in humans. Furthermore, not all organs are susceptible at the same time of the pregnancy. Figure 9.1 shows that the rat embryo is most susceptible between days 8 and 12 for most organs, but the palate and urogenital organs are more susceptible at a later stage.

Fetal Stage

This stage is characterized by growth and functional maturation. Teratogens are thus unlikely to produce morphological defects during this stage, but they may induce functional abnormalities. Although morphological defects are in general readily detected at birth or shortly thereafter, functional abnormalities, such as CNS deficiencies, may not be diagnosed for some time after birth.

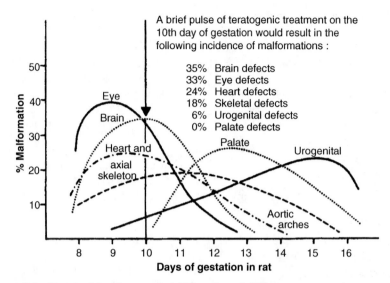

Figure 9.1 Expected incidences of malformation of different organs and systems the susceptibilities of which vary according to the days of gestation. A brief exposure to a teratogen on the 10th day of gestation is expected to induce a variety of malformations, with their incidences is shown here. *Source*: Reprinted from *Teratology: Principles and Techniques* by J. G. Wilson; courtesy of University of Chicago Press.

The effects of developmental toxicants may precede the fertilization as well as after the delivery. A summary of the relationship between the stage of exposure and its effects on development is summarized in Table 9.1.

TERATOGENS (DEVELOPMENTAL TOXICANTS) AND THEIR EFFECTS

Many chemical and physical agents may affect the conceptus. The effect may result in one or more of the following manifestations: death and/or various types of malformations. In addition, growth retardation, functional disorders, and certain other effects are observed shortly or much later after birth. They are generally referred to as developmental toxicity (Appendix 1).

A variety of agents are known to be teratogenic in humans. These include radiation, certain infections, nutritional imbalance, and certain drugs, metals and chemicals. The more important agents and their effects are outlined in this chapter. Additional information may be found in Shepard (1992), Beckman et al. (1997) and Golub et al. (1998).

Radiation for diagnostic or therapeutic purposes may cause embryonic death, leukemia, microcephaly, and skeletal and genital anomalies.

Infections that can cause congenital anomalies include German measles, herpes simplex, syphilis, and toxoplasmosis. A variety of congenital anomalies

Table 9.1   Relationship Between Developmental Stage and Fetal Outcome

Development Stage	Target System	Observed Effect
Spermatozoa	Whole body	Decreased birth weight
		Neonatal mortality
Oocyte	Whole organism	Cell death congenital anomalies
Placenta	Cardiovascular	Interference with active transport
		Alterations in maternal-fetal circulation
	Metabolism	Changes in biosynthesis of nutrients
		Changes in biotransformation of xenobiotics
Embryo	Whole organism	Intrauterine growth retardation
		Congenital anomalies
Fetus	Whole body	Growth retardation
	Reproductive and kidney	Genitourinary abnormalities
	Bone	Skeletal anomalies
Neonate	CNS	Neurobehavioral abnormalities
		Withdrawal symptoms
		Altered mental ability
	Reproductive	Altered fertility
	Respiratory	Respiratory depression
	Musculature	Hypotonia
	Whole organism	Neonatal death

Sources: From Lock and Kacew (1988), Kacew and Lock (1990), and Kacew (1995).

have been reported, for example, microcephaly, glaucoma, cataract, and hemolytic anemia.

Metabolic imbalance such as folic acid deficiency, diabetes, alcoholism, hyperthermia, rheumatic disease, congenital heart block, virilizing tumors, and phenylketonuria may cause spina bifida, anencephaly, mental retardation, etc.

Drugs and other chemicals that are known for their developmental toxicity are listed below with their major effects:

Acetozolamide: supernumerary ribs

Actinomycin D: supernumerary ribs

Alcohol: fetal alcohol syndrome; growth restriction (e.g., height, weight; bottom 10%), facial abnormalities (e.g., microcephaly, short palpebral fissures, thin upper lip, upturned nose, and microphthalmia) mental retardation, developmental delay, and hypotonia

Androgens: masculinization of female offsprings

Arsenic: neural tube defects, renal and gonadal agenesis, and eye defects

Cocaine: fetal loss; microcephaly; neurobehavioral, cranial-spinal, cardiovascular and ocular abnormalities

Diethylstilbestrol:

1. At birth: clitoromegaly in female newborns (Bongiovanni et al., 1959)
2. Years later: adenocarcinoma of the vagina and cervix of the female offspring (Poskanzer and Herbst, 1977); abnormal structural and functional disorders of the genital organs of the male offspring (Bibbo et al., 1977)

Dinoseb: supernumerary ribs
Diphenylhydantoin: microcephaly, mental retardation, and cleft plate
2-Methoxyethanol: supernumerary ribs
Methyl mercury: cerebral palsy, microcephaly, blindness, and cerebellar hypoplasia
Organophosphate pesticides: congenital anomolies, ear anomalies, and club foot (Weselak et al., 2007)
Phthalates: testicular damage
Retinoids (including vitamin A): malformations of the face, limbs, CNS, heart, and skeletal system
Thalidomide: phocomelia (short or absent limbs)
Valproic acid: spina bifida and supernumerary ribs

MODE OF ACTION

A variety of chemicals have been shown to be teratogenic in humans and/or animals. In view of the great diversity of the properties of these agents, it is not surprising that different mechanisms are involved in their teratogenic effects.

Interference with Nucleic Acids

Many agents interfere with nucleic acid replication, transcription, or RNA translation. Their effects may result in cell death or somatic mutation in the embryo. Structural or functional defects may occur where enough cells are so affected. Ionizing radiation and genotoxic carcinogens are likely to act through this mechanism. Although some chemicals, such as carbon tetrachloride and nitrosamines, also yield metabolites that react with nucleic acids, their reactive metabolites are too unstable to reach the embryo. Therefore, these toxicants are carcinogenic but not potent teratogens.

Deficiency of Energy Supply and Osmolarity

Certain teratogens can affect the energy supply for the metabolism of the organism by restricting the availability of substrates either directly (e.g., dietary deficiencies) or through the presence of analogs or antagonists of vitamins, essential amino acids, and others such as 6-amino-nicotinamide, which also interfere with glycolysis. In addition, hypoxia and agents inducing hypoxia (CO, CO_2) can be teratogenic by depriving the metabolic process of the required oxygen and probably also by the production of osmolar imbalances. These can induce edema and hematomas, which in turn can cause mechanical distortion and tissue ischemia.

Inhibition of Enzymes

Inhibitors of enzymes, such as 5-fluorouracil, can induce malformation through interference with differentiation or growth, by inhibiting thymidylate synthetase. 6-Aminonicotinamide, which inhibits glucose-6-phosphate dehydrogenase, is also a potent teratogen.

Oxidative Stress

Teratogens such as phenytoin undergo bioactivation and induce lipid peroxidation, protein oxidation, and protein degradation in both maternal and embryonic tissues. These biochemical changes may be responsible for the teratogenesis (Liu and Wells, 1995).

Others

It should be noted that the mode of action of many teratogens is as yet unknown. Furthermore, a potential teratogen may or may not exert teratogenic effects depending on factors like bioactivating mechanism, stability of the reactive metabolites, ability to cross the placental barrier, and detoxifying capability of the embryonic tissues. These and other factors are listed in Table 9.2.

TERATOGENS OF SPECIAL INTEREST

Thalidomide, as noted earlier, is otherwise a relatively safe drug but induced an episode of unprecedented tragic congenital malformation. This episode broadened the scope of teratology. Unfortunately, after some 25 years of intensive study, the mechanism underlying its teratogenicity remains to be confirmed. The proposed mechanisms include interference with folic acid or glutamic acid metabolism, depurination of DNA, and acylation of polyamines. In addition to these biochemical investigations, a number of target tissues have been studied without any definitive answer. These are limb mesenchyme tissue, mesonephric-limb tissue, and the developing neural crest tissue (Manson and Wise, 1993). A detailed account of the 24 different approaches that have been explored is provided by Stephens (1988).

One of proposed mechanisms of thalidomide teratogenicity is oxidative stress through ROS generation (Parman et al., 1999; Hansen and Harris, 2004). For the species specificity, rabbits are more sensitive to thalidomide-induced teratogenicity because rabbit limb bud cells and embryos have insufficient amounts of reduced glutathione to counteract ROS produced by thalidomide, whereas rodents are resistant to thalidomide because they have a higher glutathione detoxication

Table 9.2   Factors Associated with the Ability of Chemicals to Reach Target Fetus Site

Physicochemical properties	The ability of chemicals to reach the fetus depends on water solubility, lipid solubility, and molecular weight
Pharmacokinetics	Fetus effects observed are dependent on chemical concentration in maternal circulation in fetal blood supply, metabolism of chemicals in the placenta and fetus, and changing volume distribution and elimination (fetal renal function)
Chemical structure	Two chemicals of similar structure will cross the placenta, yet only the one with a specific structural form will affect
Duration of exposure	A single administration of a high dose can produce damage to the same extent as chronic, low-dose treatment
Implantation site	Improper implantation can result in malformation
Mechanical	Deformations in structures of uterine tissue affect circulation to placenta and fetus
Nutrition	Nutritional deficiency in the mother can influence placental transfer of essential nutrients to fetus. Excess nutrients can also cause adverse fetal effects
Physiological status	The absence of maternal hormones can alter the ability of fetus to cope with chemicals
Developmental state	Teratogenic agents act selectively on developing cells
Infection (disease)	Change in maternal body temperature can prolong half-life of drugs, predisposing the fetus to enhanced toxicity
Genetic	Inborn errors of metabolism can predispose a fetus to enhanced toxicity
Drug interactions	The presence of more than one drug and/or chemical can increase the susceptibility of the fetus
Environment	Various factors in outdoor or indoor environment can modify toxicokinetics and thereby affect placental transfer
Multifactorial (gene–environment interactions)	Various factors in environment in specific, susceptible population can modify toxicokinetics and placental transfer

Sources: From Lock and Kacew (1988), Kacew and Lock (1990), and Kacew (1995, 1997).

potential. On a molecular basis, Knobloch and coworkers (2007) demonstrated that thalidomide-induced limb defects and microphthalmia (small eyes) are caused by an oxidative stress–mediated upregulation of bone morphogenetic protein signaling, leading to Dkk1 (Wnt antagonist Dickkopf1) induction, inhibiting canonical Wnt (Notch and Wingless) signaling and increasing the programmed cell death. A thalidomide-binding protein, cereblon (CRBN) was also proposed as a primary target for thalidomide teratogenicity, which may be initiated by thalidomide-binding to CRBN and inhibiting its ubiquitin ligase activity (Ito et al., 2011). *Diethylstilbestrol* , a synthetic estrogen was used in the late 1930s to 1970s to prevent threatened abortion. Unfortunately, few of the young adult female off-spring (usually at age 19–22 years) of these mothers developed clear cell adenocarcinoma of the vagina and cervix; more of them developed other disorders of the vagina and cervix (Poskanzer and Herbst, 1977). Daughters of women who took diethylstilbestrol during pregnancy may also have a slightly higher risk of breast cancer (1.9 times) after age 40 than unexposed women of the same ages (Palmer et al., 2006). In addition, abnormal structural and functional disorders of the genital organs were observed in some male offspring (Bibbo et al., 1977).

TESTING PROCEDURES

Animals

Rats, rabbits, mice, and hamsters are the commonly used animals, because of their ready availability, easy handling, larger litter size, and short gestational period. The use of nonhuman primates has also been suggested because of their phylogenetic proximity to humans. There are advantages and disadvantages of various species of animals for use in teratology. On balance, it appears that rabbits and nonhuman primates offer more advantages.

Administration of the Chemical

At least three dosage levels are used. The higher dosage should include some maternal (and/or fetal) toxicity, such as reduction in body weight. The lowest dosage should induce no observable ill effect. One or more doses should be appropriately interspersed between the two extremes. Two control groups are included. One of these is given the vehicle or physiological saline, and the other receives a substance of known teratogenic activity. These groups will provide information on the incidence of spontaneous malformations and the sensitivity of the specific lot of animals under the existing experimental conditions. In addition to these contemporary controls, data from historical controls are also useful. The test substances should be administered by the route that simulates the human exposure situations. The timing of administering the chemical is important. For routine teratological studies, it is customary to administer the chemical during the entire period of organogenesis when the embryo is most susceptible.

Observations

The pregnant animals are examined daily for gross signs of maternal toxicity which may adversely affect the fetus. Fetuses are usually surgically removed from the mother about one day prior to the expected delivery to avoid cannibalism and permit counting of resorption sites and dead fetuses. The following observations are to be made and recorded: number of corpora lutea, implantations, resorptions, dead fetuses, and live fetuses. Other observations include gender, weight, length (crown rump), and abnormalities of each fetus (Chernoff and Rogers, 2004).

Detailed examinations are performed to determine the different types of abnormalities. Each fetus is examined for external defects. In addition, about two-thirds of the fetuses are examined for skeletal abnormalities after staining with alizarin red. The remaining one-third of the fetuses are examined for visceral defects after fixation in Bouin's fluid and sectioned with a razor blade.

Delayed effects of toxicants are generally observed on the fetal central nervous, genitourinary, or respiratory system. In testing toxicants suspected of having such potentials, a sufficient number of pregnant females are allowed to deliver their pups. These pups are nursed by either their biological mothers or by foster mothers. In the latter case, the potential effects of postnatal exposure are eliminated.

Neuromotor and behavioral tests may be used to detect CNS effects. In evaluating two known teratogens, Goldey et al. (1994) measured motor activity, acoustic startle, T-maze delayed alternation, and measurement of total and regional brain weight as well as glial fibrillary acidic protein. Male rats exposed to 2,3,7,8-tetrachlorodibenzo-*p*-dioxin in utero and lactationally may exhibit altered androgenic status, including reduced sperm count and testosterone levels (Mably et al. (1992). You et al. (1998) observed impaired male sexual development in rats exposed in utero and lactationally to p,p'-dichlorodiphenyldichloroethylene. Gestational exposure to phthalates resulted in abnormal fetal development of the male reproductive system.

More detailed information may be found in EPA (1994).

EVALUATION OF TERATOGENIC EFFECTS

Categories and Relative Significance

Resorption is a manifestation of death of the conceptus and is determined by the difference in the number of corpora lutea and implantations.

Fetal toxicity may manifest as reduced body weight on the nonviable fetus. This type of data is often useful as corroborating evidence in assessing the teratogenicity of the toxicant in question.

Malformations may involve external and/or internal structures. Minor abnormalities, or deviations, generally do not affect the survival of the fetus. Examples are supernumerary ribs and decreased or abnormal sternal ossification.

Major malformations, such as spina bifida or hydrocephalus, are incompatible with survival, growth, and fertility.

Minor anomalies are of doubtful significance. Examples are curly tail, straight legs, malrotated limbs and paws, wrist drop, protruding tongue, enlarged atria and/or ventricles, abnormal pelvic development, and translucent skin.

Extrapolation to Humans

The results obtained in teratogenesis studies in animals cannot be readily extrapolated to humans. However, the value of animal teratogenicity studies to the assessment of human health hazards was shown by Frankos (1985). Analyzing the

134 LU'S BASIC TOXICOLOGY

FDA data, he noted that 37 of the 38 known human teratogens were positive in at least one laboratory animal test species, and that 130 of the 165 chemicals showing no teratological findings were negative in at least one laboratory animal test species. In view of the above, it is prudent to carry out appropriate animal tests on all chemicals to which women of childbearing age may be exposed. If positive results are obtained with a substance, especially when this is so in more than one species of animal, exposure of women of childbearing age to this substance should be avoided, if possible.

REFERENCES

Beckman DA, Fawcett LB, Brent RL (1997). Developmental toxicity. In: Massaro EJ, ed. Handbook of Human Toxicology. Boca Raton, FL: CRC Press, 1022–1029.

Bibbo M, Gill W, Azizi F, et al. (1977). Follow-up study of male and female offspring of DES-exposed mothers. Obstet Gynacol 49, 1–8.

Bongiovanni AM, DiGeorge AM, Grumbach MM (1959). Masculinization of the female infant associated with estrogenic therapy alone during gestation: Four cases. J Clin Endocrinal Metab 19, 1004–1011.

Chernoff N, Rogers JM (2004). Supernumerary ribs in developmental toxicity bioassays and in human populations: Incidence and biological significance. J Toxicol Environ Health B 7, 437–449.

EPA (1994). Health Effects Test Guidelines/Code of Federal Regulations, Title 40, Part 789. Washington, DC: Environmental Protection Agency.

Frankos VH (1985). FDA perspectives on the use of teratology data for human risk assessment. Fundam Appl Toxicol 5, 615–625.

Goldey ES, O'Callaghan JP, Stanton ME, et al. (1994). Developmental neurotoxicity: Evaluation of testing procedures with methylagomethanol and methylmercury. Fundam Appl Toxicol 23, 447–464.

Golub MS, Macintosh MS, Baumrind N (1998). Developmental and reproductive toxicity of inorganic arsenic: Animal studies and human concerns. J Toxicol Environ Health B 1, 199–241.

Hansen J M, Harris C (2004). A novel hypothesis for thalidomide-induced limb teratogenesis: redox misregulation of the NF-kappaB pathway. Antioxid Redox Signal 6, 1–14.

Ito T, Ando H, Handa H. (2011). Teratogenic effects of thalidomide: molecular mechanisms. Cell Mol Life Sci 68, 1569–1579.

Kacew S (1995). Neonatal toxicology. In: Ballantyne GB, Marrs T, Turner P, eds. General and Applied Toxicology. London, UK: Macmillan.

Kacew S (1997). General principles in pediatric pharmacology and toxicology. In: Kacew S Lambert GH, eds. Environmental Toxicology and Pharmacology of Human Development. Washington, DC: Taylor and Francis.

Kacew S, Lock S (1990). Developmental aspects of pediatric pharmacology and toxicology. In: Kacew S, ed. Drug Toxicity and Metabolism in Pediatrics. Boca Raton, FL: CRC Press.

Knobloch J, Shaughnessy JD Jr, Rüther U (2007). Thalidomide induces limb deformities by perturbing the Bmp/Dkk1/Wnt signaling pathway. FASEB J 21, 1410–1421.

Lenz W, Knapp K (1962). Thalidomide embryopathy. Arch Environ Health 5, 100–105.

Liu L, Wells PG (1995). Potential molecular targets mediating chemical teratogenesis: in vitro peroxidase-catalyzed phenytoin metabolism and oxidative damage to proteins and lipids in marine maternal hepatic microsomes and embryonic 9000 g supernatant. Toxicol Appl Pharmacol 34, 71–80.

Lock S, Kacew S (1988). General principles in pediatric pharmacology and toxicology. In: Kacew S, Lock S, eds. Toxicologic and Pharmacologic Principles in Pediatrics. Washington, DC: Hemisphere Publishing.

Mably TA, Moore RW, Peterson RE (1992). In utero and lactational exposure of male rats to 2,3,7,8-tetrachlorodibenzo-p-dioxin: 1. Effects on androgenic status. Toxicol Appl Pharmacol 114, 97–107.

Manson JM, Wise LD (1993). Teratogens. In: Amdur MO, Doull J, Klaassen CD, eds. Casarett and Doull's Toxicology. New York, NY: McGraw-Hill, 226–254.

Mitchell AE, Bakshi KS, Kimmel CA (2004). Evaluating chemical and other agent exposures for reproductive and developmental toxicity. J Toxicol Environ Health 67, 1159–1314.

Palmer JR, Wise LA, Hatch EE, et al. (2006). Prenatal diethylstilbestrol exposure and risk of breast cancer. Cancer Epidemiol Biomarkers Prev 15, 1509–1514.

Parman T, Wiley MJ, Wells PG (1999). Free radical-mediated oxidative DNA damage in the mechanism of thalidomide teratogenicity. Nat Med 5, 582–585.

Poskanzer D, Herbst A (1977). Epidemiology of vaginal adenosis and adenocarcinoma associated with exposure to stilbestrol in utero. Cancer 39, 1892–1895.

Shepard TH (1992). Catalog of Teratogenic Agents, 7th edn. Baltimore, MD: Johns Hopkins University Press.

Stephens TD (1988). Proposed mechanisms of action in thalidomide embryopathy. Teratology 38, 229–239.

Weselak M, Arbuckle TE, Foster W (2007). Pesticide exposure and developmental outcomes: The epidemiological evidence. J Toxicol Environ Health B 10, 41–80.

You L, Casanova M, Archibeque-Engle S, et al. (1998). Impaired male sexual development in perinatal Sprague-Dawley and Long-Evans hooded rats exposed in utero and lactationally to p,p'-DDE. Toxicol Sci 45, 162–173.

Appendix 1   Teratogens in Animal Models

1. Physical agents: hypothermia and hyperthermia, hypoxia, radiation
2. Agents producing hypoxia: carbon monoxide, carbon dioxide
3. Infections: rubella viruses, syphilis
4. Dietary deficiency or excess: vitamins A, D, and E; ascorbic acid; nicotinamide; trace metals (Zn, Mn, Mg, and Co)
5. Vitamin antagonists: antifolate drugs, 6-aminonicotinamide
6. Hormone deficiency or excess: cortisone, hydrocortisone, thyroxine, vasopressin, insulin, androgens, estrogens
7. Natural toxins: aflatoxin B_1, ochratoxin A, ergotamine, nicotine
8. Heavy metals: arsenic, methyl mercury, phenyl mercuric acetate, lead, thallium, strontium, selenium
9. Solvents: benzene, carbon tetrachloride, 1,1-dichloroethane, dimethyl sulfoxide, propylene glycol, xylene
10. Insecticides, herbicides, fungicides
11. Azo dyes: trypan blue, Evans blue, Niagara blue
12. Antibiotics: dactinomycin, penicillin, streptomycin, tetracyclines
13. Sulfonamides: sulfanilamide, hypoglycemic sulfonamides
14. Drugs and chemicals: caffeine, carbutamide, chlorcyclizine, chlorpromazine and derivatives, diphenylhydantoin, hydroxyurea, imipramine, meclizine, nitrosamines, phthalates, pilocarpine, quinine, rauwolfia, thalidomide, triparanol, veratrum alkaloids, vinca alkaloids

10

Lactation

GENERAL REMARKS

Following birth, the fetal stage develops into the neonate or infant stage. Exposure to drugs and environmental agents can be either direct through inhalation, ingestion, etc. or indirectly via the mother's milk. The importance and necessity of breast milk in the developing neonate have been clearly shown (Kacew, 1994; Berlin and Kacew, 1997). Box 10.1 lists some of the disease conditions where the frequency of occurrences of these disorders was clearly diminished in breast-fed infants. Breast-feeding has distinct advantages nutritionally, immunologically, and psychologically, and despite the presence of environmental toxins, should be encouraged. At present, it should be stressed that human milk remains the best nutrient source for the healthy term infant (Redel and Shulman, 1994). This is clearly evident from the emphasis both professionals and laypersons place on the promotion of breast-feeding. The incidence of breast-feeding in North America has varied over the years from 25% (1970) to 56% (1981), and some studies show that about 54% of women discharged from hospital to home are breast-feeding (Berlin, 1989; Lawrence, 1989; Buttar, 1994). The resurgence in the number of women breast-feeding will increase even further as the educational awareness of benefits of lactation is promoted amongst men of expectant mothers. Wilson et al. (1986) estimated that a figure of 70% of breast-feeding mothers in the United States was equivalent to approximately 2.5 million women. Even at 50%, in 1994, there were 4 million new mothers in the United States, so more than 2 million infants went home receiving breast milk. A health goal established by a workshop sponsored by Human Health Services was that, by the year 2000, 75% of newborns would be breast-fed and 50% would still be breast-fed by six months of age. Meta-analyses of long-term effects of breast-feeding also demonstrated that the prevalence of overweight/obesity/type-2 diabetes is lower in breast-fed subjects (Horta et al., 2007). In addition, women who had breastfed for a lifetime total of at least two years are associated with a 23% lower risk of coronary heart disease than those who had never breastfed (Stuebe et al., 2009). However, the breast-feeding mother is subjected to exposure from environmental contaminants

---

Box 10.1   Adverse Infant Conditions Protected by Breast-Feeding

Infant mortality
Sudden infant death syndrome
Respiratory tract disease
Food allergies
Atopic dermatitis
Otitis media
Asthma
Immune system disorders
   Lymphomas
   Celiac disease
   Insulin-dependent diabetes mellitus
   Inflammatory bowel disease
   Crohn's disease
   HIV-related mortality
Cholera
Giardia lamblia diarrhea
Rotavirus diarrhea
Shigellosis
Bacteremia and meningitis
Chronic liver disease

Source: From Kacew (1994, 2000).

(e.g., heavy metals, xenoestrogens, pesticides, and solvents), and these pollutants may be present in human milk (Massart et al., 2005). In the majority of cases, it is still more beneficial to breast-feed despite the presence of such contaminants. Recently, the use of plastic baby bottles containing a chemical, bisphenol A (BPA), was linked to the development of abnormal endocrine functions in animals. Although excessive concentrations of BPA produced these changes in non-human organisms, regulatory agencies in some countries banned the use of this chemical in baby bottles. In the case of breast feeding there was no exposure of lactating infants to BPA again pointing out an advantage for breast versus bottle feeding.

BENEFITS OF BREAST-FEEDING

Breast-feeding confers certain benefits on infants, which are summarized in Table 10.1 and discussed in the following sections.

Immune System

The beneficial effects of breast-feeding against immune system disorders are well established (Davis et al., 1988; Mayer et al., 1988; Kramer, 1988). The finding that lead interferes with the immune system indicates that the presence of this metal in milk may not yield protection in lead-exposed mothers. It should also be noted that in the presence of environmental toxicants and a condition of malnourishment, the immune system is further compromised as there is an increased sensitivity to viral infection. The transmission of human immunodeficiency virus (HIV) during breast-feeding from infected mothers to suckling infants is well documented (Oxtoby, 1988). Based on this knowledge the question arises as to the advantages of bottle-feeding in HIV-infected mothers. In an extensive study, Lederman (1992) demonstrated that exclusive breast-feeding even in situations where mothers were HIV infected, there was a decrease in the estimated infant mortality rate, especially in population areas where HIV prevalence was low. Although lactation does not protect against HIV transmission, breast-feeding is clearly beneficial in reducing infant mortality. In a population where HIV infection is exceedingly high, bottle-feeding is preferable. Bearing this in mind the benefits of breast-feeding substantially outweigh HIV transmission, as one must consider infant mortality. In general, once a mother is infected, antibodies and numerous protective factors are produced in the mother's body and these are secreted in milk to protect babies (Jackson and Nazar, 2006). Clearly, breast-feeding protects against infant mortality regardless of the cause and this physiological process should not be discontinued.

Cancer

The beneficial effects of protecting breast-fed infants against lymphoid hypertrophy and lymphomas have been documented (Davis et al., 1988). This protective antineoplastic effect was found to extend to the mother where lactation for prolonged periods was correlated with a reduction in breast cancer (McTiernan and Thomas, 1986). Although Kvale and Heuch (1988) failed to demonstrate any association in a large cohort study, in the more extensive finding of Newcomb et al. (1994), a positive inverse correlation between lactation and risk of breast cancer was noted in premenopausal women. However, no reduction in the risk of breast cancer was found in postmenopausal women with a history of lactation. Regardless of the fact that breast cancer occurs in less than one quarter of all cases reported and that lactation provides a slight protective effect, it was concluded that any factor which reduces the incidence of breast cancer should be encouraged.

Avoidance of Food Allergies

In the case of food allergies or atopic dermatitis, it is generally accepted that breast-feeding delays the development of these disorders (Lucas et al., 1990). Although Kramer (1988) suggested that breast-feeding provided protection against allergic diseases, these manifestations occurred in exclusively breast-fed infants. However, it should be noted that the incidence of food allergies decreased dramatically in exclusive breast-fed infants. In recent studies the maternal diet was found to be a critical factor in the development of allergic manifestations in lactating infants. Ingestion of a maternal hypoallergenic diet devoid of cow's milk, eggs, and fish during lactation decreased the cumulative incidence and current prevalence of atopic dermatitis during the first six months of age with continuation to the age of four (Chandra et al., 1989; Sigurs et al., 1992). Breast-feeding per se is effective in protecting against allergic disorders provided the offending stimulus is not ingested by the mother for transmission to the infant via the milk.

Psychological Bonding

Breast-feeding is known to create a special psychological bond between an infant and a mother that ultimately leads to a socially healthier child. In addition, lactation enhances maternal postpartum recovery and body weight returns to prepartum levels more rapidly. The physiological process of breast-feeding plays a critical role in human growth and development. The use of bottles to feed nursing infants with milk formula in developing countries was found to enhance morbidity and mortality. In addition, with the knowledge that bottles contain BPA, the potential for endocrine disruption was eliminated through breast-feeding. In affluent nations, inadequate knowledge on growth patterns between breast-fed and bottle-fed infants resulted in inappropriate counseling against lactation. In an extensive study, Dewey et al. (1992) demonstrated that the growth pattern was equivalent between breast-fed and formula-fed infants from birth to the first three months. However, breast-fed infants gained significantly less weight from 3 to 12 months without any deleterious effects on nutrition, morbidity, motor activity level, or behavioral development. It is evident that breast-fed infants are leaner and do not display a faltering growth pattern; women should be encouraged to continue the lactational process beyond three months. With the knowledge that growth in breast-fed infants is generally less than in formula-fed, growth per se as an index of toxicity in the first year of life is not appropriate.

Maternal nutrient intake is an important factor in the growth pattern of the infant. If a deficiency of zinc exists, there may be a delay in infant growth. Thus, in conditions of adequate maternal zinc concentrations, lactation should be encouraged despite a decreased infant growth pattern. A maternal diet deficient in essential nutrients such as iron or calcium results in a greater bioavailability of mammary lead, with consequent developmental delay.

BIOMARKERS OF EXPOSURE

It is clear that chemicals are present in milk and that these agents may affect the suckling infant. However, limited data are available to determine whether the presence of the chemical is sufficient to exert an adverse effect. Diehl-Jones and Bols (2000), using dioxin, established the criteria or biomarkers of exposure. In essence, alterations in certain milk constituents provided evidence for a dioxin-like effect. Examples of biomarkers in milk include lysosyme, cathepsin; vitamins A to K; cytokines interleukin 1 or tumor necrosis factor; and hormones including estrogen, thyroxine, or prolactin. The determination of these biomarkers could then be used to ascertain the degree of exposure. The cellular modifications that one will measure are cytochrome P-450 induction, DNA adducts, apoptosis, and chemokinesis. This can prove crucial as in terms of therapeutic intervention following an exposure.

TOXICANTS

The nursing mother can serve as a source of neonatal exposure to drugs or chemicals (Wang and Needham, 2007). No matter whether the agent is an over-the-counter medication or prescribed by a physician, most drugs are detectable in breast milk. The presence of a drug in maternal milk may be construed as a potential hazard to the infant even though only 1–2% of total intake is likely to be found there. The basis for this observation is the fact that drug metabolizing enzymes involved in degrading and eliminating the drugs are not fully developed in the lactating neonate resulting in excess amounts of chemical present in the infant. Hence the primary consideration in maternal drug therapy is the risk to the nursing infant rather than the mere presence of xenobiotic in the milk. Based on the numerous advantages of breast-feeding, the benefit of this physiological process in the majority of cases far exceeds the potential risk. Although it may be inadvertent, the suckling infant also derives environmental chemicals from the mother. These chemicals are excreted in breast milk and pose a serious potential hazard to the infant (Berlin et al., 2002; Table 10.1). Unlike drug therapy, which can be voluntarily terminated, environmental exposure may be chronic and, consequently, more toxic. In addition, both environmental chemicals and drugs present in milk can enter the infant to exert a synergistic adverse effect. Some of these are discussed in the following sections:

Table 10.1   Toxicants Identified in Human Breast Milk and Their Adverse Infant Effects

Chemical	Effect
Silicone	Esophageal dysfunction
Hexachlorobenzene	Porphyria cutanea tarda
Polychlorinated biphenyls	Abnormal skin pigmentation, bone defects, growth retardation, hypotonia
Perchloroethylene	Obstructive jaundice
Methyl mercury	Developmental delay, abnormal muscle tone, mental retardation, decreased suckling response
Lead	Poor mental performance, central nervous system toxicosis
Nicotine	Decreased weight gain
Cadmium	Low birth weight

Source: From Kacew (1994), Berlin and Kacew (1997).

Silicone

Silicone is a polymeric substance, which is inert and is unlikely to produce a toxic manifestation. Based on these properties the use of silicone for breast implantation was considered ideal; however, retrospective studies revealed an increased incidence of rheumatological disorders, in particular, scleroderma and arthritis. Levin and Ilowite (1994) reported that in infants of breast-fed mothers with silicone implants, there was a decreased lower sphincter pressure and abnormal esophageal wave propagation. Clearly the inert material silicone was associated with infant esophageal disease as a result of lactational exposure. It has been suggested that leakage from the implant produces immunological substances that lead to scleroderma development. However, it should be noted that silicon concentrations in cows' milk exceed those in human breast milk by a factor of 10 and are even higher in infant formula (Semple et al., 1998). Normally human milk contains immunological components, which provide protection against diseases. In the presence of silicone the breast milk would contain components that may immunologically compromise the infant not only with esophageal dysfunction but also with increased susceptibility to other immune-related diseases.

Mercury

Lactational exposure of human infants to metals is a concern and raises the issue of risks versus benefits in the maintenance of the breast-feeding process. Mercury levels in milk are usually low (<1 ng/mL), but in environmental disasters as in Minamata, Japan, the levels reached 50 ng/mL. Numerous studies exist on the effects of either prenatal or during both pregnancy and postnatal exposure to metals on developing infants, but few reports are available on the consequences of the presence of metals exclusively in breast milk on children. Bearing in mind the consequences of methyl mercury poisoning, especially in Minamata, Japan, consideration should be given to the contribution of lactational exposure to the observed neuronal disturbances where nursing mothers ingesting mercury-contaminated fish resulted in severe neurological disorders in human infants (Matsumoto et al., 1965). Takeuchi (1968) clearly demonstrated the effects of epidemic methyl mercury exposure on fetal and newborn development. Industrial release of methyl mercury into Minamata Bay followed by accumulation in edible fish and ingestion by lactating females resulted in the transfer of metal to the suckling human infant. Similarly, Amin-Zaki et al. (1974) demonstrated that ingestion of homemade bread prepared from wheat treated with the fungicide methyl mercury by lactating mothers produced a significant rise in human infant metal levels. In fish-eating populations in Canada, maternal ingestion of mercury-contaminated food during pregnancy and lactation resulted in abnormal muscle tone and reflexes in boys but not in girls (McKeown-Eyssen et al., 1983). In a New Zealand study, Kjellstrom et al. (1989) reported developmental retardation in four-year-old children of mothers eating mercury-contaminated fish during pregnancy and lactation. Although emphasis was placed on the consequences of prenatal exposure in the Canadian and New Zealand studies, the contribution of milk mercury to toxic outcome was neglected. It should be noted that in some patients with Minamata disease, the neurological symptoms developed not at the time of exposure but years later. Further, the reported number of cases where children born in a mercury-contaminated area in Japan were healthy yet developed neuropathy in childhood. The contribution of breast milk mercury to late-onset Minamata disease remains to be resolved. Mammary transfer of methyl mercury to suckling infants has been reported to produce neurological lesions. This finding clearly indicates a positive correlation between exposure to high concentrations of metal in mammary tissue and toxicity in suckling infants.

Although the precise contribution of mammary-derived methyl mercury to the observed adverse effects on neurological and behavioral changes in suckling pups is not known, it was found that postnatal exposure directly to newborns of this metal produced ocular defects. In contrast, there was a lack of an ocular effect in fetuses of prenatal exposed dams, suggesting that lactation methyl mercury may in part contribute to the observed toxicity. It is well known that methyl mercury is secreted more readily in the maternal colostrum, the period at which eye defects are reported, and crosses into the suckling infant. Mercury itself decreases the suckling response in human infants. Because milk contains essential nutrients for neurological and behavioral development, it is conceivable that less suckling and feeding would contribute to the mercury-induced nervous disorders as there is less nutritional supply and this is associated with delayed growth processes.

Lead

In a number of studies conducted in the United States and Europe, the content of lead in human milk ranged from 5 ng/mL to 68 ng/mL (Rabinowitz et al., 1985). Levels in Boston averaged 1.7 ng/mL in 1979. Dillon (1974) found lead levels of approximately 26 ng/mL in seven different U.S. cities. In Mexico city, milk lead levels reached 45 ng/mL (Berlin and Kacew, 1997; Berlin et al., 2002). It is not surprising that upon examination of the source of infant lead intoxication, breast milk contained far less lead than either formula or environmental sources such as ceramic-leachable kitchenware, paint chips, etc. (Rabinowitz et al., 1985). There is evidence to suggest a correlation between poor mental performance, as evidenced by the Bayley Infant Assessment Test, and increased lead level (Needleman et al., 1983). These findings prompted Newman (1993) to recommend the promotion of breast-feeding, as human milk was a less suitable transmission vehicle for lead contamination compared with formula feeding. Further it should be stressed that the best source for daily nutrition among infants is human milk.

Although the contribution of exclusive mammary lead exposure to the observed central nervous system (CNS) toxic consequences remains undefined, there is evidence to suggest that the presence of lactational metal results in newborn toxicity. Direct application of topical lead ointment on the breast was reported to produce CNS toxicosis in the human infant (Dillon, 1974). The presence of lead in mammary tissue alters the nutritional value of milk as reflected by decreases in the essential elements copper, zinc, and iron, which are required for mammalian metabolism and CNS function. The absorption of calcium, iron, and vitamin D is affected by lead. In conditions of diets deficient in essential elements, lead absorption and toxicity is enhanced in infants. Because breast milk is a source of lead for suckling infants, it is conceivable that during iron-deficiency anemia or calcium-deficient dietary intake in mothers, the bioavailability of milk lead is increased, resulting in greater toxicity. Evidence suggests that lead exposure may interfere with maternal metabolic pathways resulting in decreased utilization of nutrients in the diet, and thus an absence of nutritional components present in milk. This altered milk composition will consequently adversely affect newborn development.

Halogenated Hydrocarbons

Chemical exposure via accidents and hazardous waste sites has resulted in toxicant accumulation in breast milk. The human maternal ingestion of a fungicide, hexachlorobenzene-treated wheat resulted in chemical accumulation in breast milk. Suckling infants subsequently developed symptoms of a disease, pembe yara, and a condition of prophyria cutanea tarda (Peters et al., 1982). Exposure to organophosphate pesticides such as chlorpyrifos and malathion is worthy of mention, as these compounds have been identified in breast milk (Berlin and Kacew, 1997). Ingestion of chlorpyrifos by a three-year-old infant resulted in delayed polyneuropathy with transient bilateral vocal paralysis (Aiuto et al., 1993). Although lactation per se was not involved in this specific case, the importance lies in the fact that the manifestations of exposure did not occur until one to three weeks later. One should be aware that the consequences of lactational exposure to toxicants can also be delayed. This is supported by the findings where a mother was exposed to 2,4-diphenoxyacetic acid (2,4-D) spray during pregnancy and lactation. Examination of the infant at 5 and 24 months of age revealed multiple malformations and severe mental retardation. Although the mammary tissue content of 2,4-D was not determined, prolonged maternal exposure with consequent transmission to the infant was suggested to result in the observed toxicity. The fact that lactational-derived organophosphate pesticides alter suckling infant metabolism and that toxicity may be delayed suggests that breast-feeding in severe exposure conditions should be minimized.

Ingestion of polychlorinated biphenyl–contaminated rice oil by nursing mothers was attributed to produce low–birth weight human infants, growth retardation, abnormal skin pigmentation as well as bone and tooth defects (Yamaguchi et al., 1971). In extensive studies in North Carolina, Rogan et al. (1986) measured the levels of polychlorinated biphenyls in human milk and found an associated hypotonicity and hyporeflexia in nursing infants. Organochlorine pesticides including, DDT, aldrin, and dieldrin have been identified in human milk (Berlin and Kacew, 1997; Wang and Needham, 2007). However, it is surprising that manifestations of toxicity in suckling infants following maternal organochlorine exposure have not been reported. This should not be deemed that the presence of organochlorine contaminants in breast milk fails to affect the infant, as these environmental toxicants induce mammary carcinoma and may act as co-carcinogens. It is well known that suckling infants of cigarette smoking mothers are more prone to respiratory irritation and infections. However, cigarette smoking in the presence of atmospheric pollutants exerted an additive toxic effect on the mother. Conceivably, the presence of organochlorine compounds and nicotine in breast milk will increase infant toxicity with the hydrocarbons acting as co-carcinogens. Hence in susceptible suckling infants these compounds may precipitate autoimmune diseases, lymphomas, etc.

Ethanol (Alcohol)

Alcohol ingestion during pregnancy is known to result in congenital anomalies termed "fetal alcohol syndrome" (FAS). FAS is characterized by mental deficiency, microcephaly, irritability, and poor muscle coordination in the affected subjects. This syndrome is associated with alcoholic women who drank heavily and chronically during pregnancy. Although the contribution of alcohol during lactation to FAS has not been established, it is known that the severity of manifestations in infants is correlated with the amount consumed. Hence, alcohol in breast milk could worsen adverse infant development that was initiated during pregnancy. There are some studies inferring that alcohol exposure during lactation may increase the susceptibility of the infant to develop cancer (Infante-Rivard and El-Zein, 2007).

Solvents

The aromatic hydrocarbon toluene is utilized as a solvent or thinner in numerous industrial products including paints, glue, and resins. The lipophilic property of toluene is of interest in light of the physicochemical properties of breast tissue. Hersh et al. (1985) demonstrated that in infants of approximately four years of age, maternal exposure to toluene throughout pregnancy via glue sniffing produced embryopathy, mental deficiency, and postnatal growth delay. There is no doubt that in-utero exposure to toluene was manifested in teratogenesis. However, as there was evidence of postnatal growth deficiency and that toluene has a high affinity for fat, it is also possible that these infants were exposed to this solvent via the mother's milk. This is supported by the finding that obstructive jaundice developed in lactating infants of mothers exposed to the dry-cleaning solvent, perchloroethylene (Bagnell and Ellenberg, 1977). It is well established that exposure to the organic solvents during pregnancy results in toxemia and anemia. Unfortunately, infants born to these mothers were not followed clinically during lactation. However, as these environmental chemicals accumulate in breast milk and produce metabolic maternal alterations, it is conceivable that solvents may alter infant development. The release of organic solvents from breast milk fat needs to be considered among solvent abusers in light of adverse consequent effects reported in children (Schreiber, 1997).

REFERENCES

Aiuto LA, Pavlakis SG, Boxer RA (1993). Life-threatening organophosphate-induced delayed polyneuropathy in a child after accidental chlorpyrifos. J Pediatr 122, 658– 660.

Amin-Zaki L, Elhassini S, Majeed MA, et al. (1974). Studies of infants postnatally exposed to methylmercury. J Pediatr 85, 81–84.

Bagnell PC, Ellenberg HA (1977). Obstructive jaundice due to a chlorinated hydrocarbon in breast milk. Can Med Assoc J 117, 1047–1048.

Berlin CM Jr, Kacew S, Lawrence R, et al. (2002). Criteria for chemical selection for progranms on human milk surveillance and research for environmental chemicals. J Toxicol Environ Health A 65, 1839–1851.

Berlin CM Jr (1989). Drugs and chemicals: Exposure of the nursing mother. Pediatr Clin North Am 36, 1089–1097.

Berlin CM Jr, Kacew S (1997). Environmental contamination human milk. In: Kacew S, Lambert GH, eds. Environmental Toxicology and Pharmacology of Human Development. Washington, D.C.: Taylor & Francis.

Buttar HS (1994). Neonatal risks of drugs excreted in breast milk. Can Pharm J 127, 14–19.

Chandra RK, Puri S, Hamed A (1989). Influence of maternal diet during lactation and use of formula feeds on development of atopic eczema in high risk infants. Br Med J 299, 228–230.

Davis MK, Savitz DA, Graubard BI (1988). Infant feeding and childhood cancer. Lancet 2, 365–368.

Dewey KG, Heining MJ, Nommsen LA, et al. (1992). Growth of breast-fed and formula-fed infants from 0 to 18 months: The DARLING study. Pediatrics 89, 1035–1041.

Diehl-Jones WL, Bols NC (2000). Use of response biomarkers in milk for assessing exposure to environmental contaminants: The case for dioxin-like compounds. J Toxicol Environ Health B 3, 79–107.

Dillon HK (1974). Lead concentration in human milk. Am J Dis Child 128, 491–492.

Hersh JH, Podruch PE, Rogers G, et al. (1985). Toluene embryopathy. J Pediatr 106, 922–927.

Horta BL, Bahl R, Martines JC, Victora CG (2007). Evidence on the long-term effects of breastfeeding: systematic reviews and meta-analyses. Geneva, Switzerland: World Health Organization. ISBN 9789241595230. http://whqlibdoc.who.int/publications/2007/9789241595230_eng.pdf. Retrieved 2011-09-18.

Infante-Rivard C, El-Zein M (2007). Parental alcohol consumption and childhood cancers: A review. J Toxicol Environ Health B 10, 101–129.

Jackson KM, Nazar AM (2006). Breastfeeding, the immune response, and long-term health. J Am Osteopath Assoc 106, 203–207.

Kacew S (1994). Current issues in lactation: Advantages, environment, silicone. Biomed Environ Sci 7, 307–319.

Kacew S (2000). Neonatal toxicology. In: Ballantyne B, Marrs T, Syversen T, eds. General and Applied Toxicology. New York, NY: Macmillan.

Kjellstrom T, Kennedy P, Wallis S, et al. (1989). Physical and mental development of children with prenatal exposure to mercury from fish. Stage 2. Interviews and psychological tests at age 6, Solna, National Swedish Environmental Board, 112 (Report no. 3642).

Kramer MS (1988). Does breast feeding help protect against atopic disease? Biology, methodology and a golden jubilee of controversy. J Pediatr 112, 181–190.

Kvale G, Heuch I (1988). Lactation and cancer risk: Is there a relation specific to breast cancer? J Epidemiol Community Health 42, 30–37.

Lawrence RA (1989). Breastfeeding and medical disease. Med Clin North Am 73, 583–603.

Lederman SA (1992). Estimating infant mortality from human immunodeficiency virus and other causes in breast-feeding and bottle-feeding populations. Pediatrics 89, 290–296.

Levine JJ, Ilowite NT (1994). Scleroderma like esophageal disease in children breast-fed by mothers with silicone breast implants. J Am Med Assoc 271, 213–216.

Lucas A, Brooke OG, Morley R, et al. (1990). Early diet of preterm infants and development of allergic or atopic disease: Randomized prospective study. Br Med J 300, 837–840.

Massart F, Harrell JC, Federico G et al. (2005). Human breast milk and xenoestrogen exposure: A possible impact on human health. J Perinatol 25, 282–288.

Matsumoto M, Koya G, Takeuchi T (1965). Fetal minamata disease. J Neuropathol Exp Neurol 24, 563–574.

Mayer EJ, Hamman RF, Gay EC, et al. (1988). Reduced risk of IDDM among breast-fed children. Diabetes 37, 1625–1632.

McKeown-Eyssen GE, Ruedy J, Neims A (1983). Methyl mercury exposure in northern Quebec. II. Neurological finding in children. Am J Epidemiol 118, 470–479.

McTiernan A, Thomas DB (1986). Evidence for a protective effect of lactation on risk of breast cancer in young women: Results from a case-control study. Am J Epidemiol 124, 353–358.

Needleman H, Bellinger D, Leviton A, et al. (1983). Umbilical cord blood lead levels and neuropsychological performance at 12 months of age. Pediatr Res 17, 179A.

Newcomb PA, Storer BF, Longnecker MP, et al. (1994). Lactation and reduced risk of premenopausal breast cancer. N Engl J Med 330, 81–87.

Newman J (1993). Would breast-feeding decrease risks of lead intoxication? Pediatrics 90, 131.

Oxtoby MJ (1988). Human immunodeficiency virus and other viruses in human milk: Placing the issues in broader perspective. Pediatr Infect Dis J 7, 825–835.

Peters HA, Gocmen A, Gripps DJ, et al. (1982). Epidemiology of hexachlorobenzene-induced porphyria in Turkey. Arch Neurol 39, 744–749.

Rabinowitz M, Leviton A, Needleman H (1985). Lead in milk and infant blood: A dose–response mode. Arch Environ Health 40, 283–286.

Redel CA, Shulman RG (1994). Controversies in the composition of infant formulas. Pediatr Clin N A 41, 909–924.

Rogan WJ, Gladen BC, McKinney JD, et al. (1986). Neonatal effects of transplacental exposure to PCBs and DDE. J Pediatr 109, 335–341.

Schreiber JS (1997). Transport of organic chemicals to breast milk: Tetra-chlorothene case study. In: Kacew S, Lambert GH, eds. Environmental Toxicology and Pharmacology of Human Development. Washington, D.C.: Taylor & Francis.

Semple JL, Lugowski SJ, Baines CJ, et al. (1998).. Breast milk contamination and silicone implants: Preliminary results using silicon as a proxy measurement for silicone. Plast Reconstr Surg 102, 528–533.

Sigurs N, Hattevig G, Kjellman B (1992). Maternal avoidance of eggs, cow's milk and fish during lactation: Effect on allergic manifestation, skin-prick test, specific 1gE antibodies in children at age 4 years. Pediatrics 89, 735–739.

Stuebe AM, Michels KB, Willett WC, et al. (2009). Duration of lactation and incidence of myocardial infarction in middle to late adulthood. Am J Obstet Gynecol 200, 138. e1–138.e8.

Takeuchi T (1968). Pathology of Minamata Disease. In: Kutsune M, ed. Minamata Disease. Japan: Kunamoto University.

Wang RY, Needham LL (2007). Environmental chemicals: From the environment to food, to breast milk, to the infant. J Toxicol Environ Health B 10, 597–609.

Wilson JT, Hinson JL, Brown RD, et al. (1986). A comprehensive assessment of drugs and chemical toxins excreted in breast milk. In: Hamosh M, Goldman AD, eds. Human Lactation, vol. 2. New York, NY: Plenum Publishing Corporation.

Yamaguchi A, Yoshimura T, Kuratsune M (1971). A survey of pregnant women having consumed rice oil contaminated with chlorobiphenyls and their babies. Fukuoka Acta Med 62, 117–122.

11

Toxicology of the immune system

GENERAL CONSIDERATIONS

The function of the immune system is to protect the host against foreign organisms (virus, bacterium, fungus), "foreign cells" (neoplasm), and other foreign substances. Its importance is evidenced by the seriousness of immunodeficiency: patients with this disorder are prone to be affected by infection and tumors. Immunodeficiency can be congenital or acquired; the latter is also known as acquired immunodeficiency syndrome (AIDS).

The immune system is composed of several types of organs, cells, and noncellular components. The functions of the individual components are, in general, interrelated. Thus, upon encountering a foreign substance, a cascade of reactions usually appears between different types of cellular and humoral components. These reactions involve the recognition, memory, and response to the foreign substance, and are designed for its elimination or control.

A variety of toxicants are known to suppress immune function. This effect will lead to lowered host resistance to bacterial and viral infections, and to parasitic infestation, as well as lowered control of neoplasm. In addition, certain toxicants may provoke exaggerated immune reactions leading to local or systemic reactions. Furthermore, it may even result in "autoimmune reactions."

This chapter briefly describes the components of the immune system and their functions and major immunotoxicants.

COMPONENTS OF THE SYSTEM

The immune system consists of a network of organs including the bone marrow, thymus, spleen, and lymph nodes. From these organs, various lymphocytes and other cells with different immune functions are derived.

Some of the components are involved in specific immune responses and others in nonspecific responses. Both types of cells are derived from the pluripotent cells in the bone marrow. From these cells the lymphoid stem cells are generated. Some of these cells are processed through the thymus and become

Table 11.1   Cells and Primary Soluble Mediators: Innate Vs. Acquired Immunity

Characteristic	Innate Immunity	Acquired Immunity
Cells involved	Polymorphonuclear cells	T cells
		B cells
	Monocyte/macrophage	Macrophages
	NK cells	NK cells
Primary soluble mediators	Complement	Antibody
	Lysozyme	Cytokines
	Acute phase proteins	
	Interferon α/β	
	Cytokines	

Source: From Burns et al. (1996).

T cells (T lymphocytes); others go through the "bursal equivalent" tissues (including bone marrow, lymph nodes, and lymphoid tissues in the gut such as appendix, cecum, and Peyer patches) to become B cells (B lymphocytes). Still others are released from the bone marrow without further processing. These are known as natural killer (NK) cells. Unlike the T cells and B cells, NK cells are also involved in nonspecific defense against neoplasms, and certain other foreign substances (Table 11.1).

Other pluripotent stem cells give rise to myeloid stem cells, from which monocytes, mast cells, and polymorphonuclear (PMN) cells are derived. Monocytes then become macrophages, which are involved in specific (acquired) and nonspecific (innate) immune reactions. In addition, there are three types of PMN cells, namely, neutrophils, eosinophils, and basophils. These cells are involved in nonspecific defense mechanisms.

T Cells

As noted above, the T cells, after passing through the thymus, enter the blood and constitute 70% of the circulating lymphocytes. Some settle in thymus-dependent areas of the spleen and lymph nodes. On contact with antigens processed by antigen-presenting cells (APCs; such as macrophages and B cells), the T cells undergo proliferation and differentiation. Some of these cells become "activated" and are responsible for mediating cellular immunity. Others become T memory cells, which can be activated by combining with antigens; still others by becoming *helper* cells. Once activated, helper T cells will proliferate and secrete lymphokines. The lymphokines will cause the B cells to become plasma cells.

The activated T cells react either directly with cell membrane–associated antigens or by releasing various soluble factors known as lymphokines. There are a large number of lymphokines (see the section "Other Types of Cells").

B Cells

Other stem cells undergo changes in certain tissues as noted above to become B cells (B lymphocytes). They enter the blood to constitute 30% of the lymphocytes. The primary immune response is initiated by the contact of antigen with B cells, which then differentiate and proliferate. Some of these become *memory* cells, which retain the surface immunoglobulin receptors, whereas others become *plasma* cells. The latter type bears IgM and IgD immunoglobulins on cell surface. Exposure of the memory cells to the same antigen at a later time results in the secondary immune response.

Other Types of Cells

Other lymphocytes lack the characteristic surface markers of the T cells and the B cells, but they participate in the nonspecific immune system functions. These are the null cells. Some of these, the *natural killer* cells, have spontaneous (without prior sensitization) cytolytic activity against other cells, especially leukemia and carcinoma cells.

   Macrophages are also derived from the stem-cell pool in the bone marrow. After their release, they appear in the bloodstream as monocytes and in the tissues as histiocytes. On contact with a foreign body, they engulf the foreign body and become activated macrophages. These cells are rich in cytoplasmic hydrolytic enzymes. Most bacterial cells are readily digested by these enzymes. Macrophages can also be activated to become APCs.

   Langerhans cells, located in the skin, are also derived from bone marrow and act as APCs. They serve to process dermal antigens and initiate contact allergy and rejection of skin graft.

   Among the *PMN cells*, neutrophil PMNs exert phagocytic activity. The eosinophils possess cytotoxic function, and basophils (which become mast cells in tissues) release histamine and other substances, thereby initiating local reactions to a foreign substance inducing immediate hypersensitivity.

Soluble Mediators

Immunoglobins (Ig family) are proteins produced by plasma cells (derived from B cells). They have specific antibody activities. Their specificity is determined by the amino acid sequence and the tertiary surface configuration. There are five major types of immunoglobins. Their characteristics and functions are outlined in Table 11.2.

   Interleukins (cytokines) are proteins produced by activated T cells (lymphokines) or monocytes/macrophages (monokines) in response to antigenic or mitogenic stimulation. They promote the proliferation of T cells, B cells, and hematopoietic stem cells.

Table 11.2 Characteristics of Immunoglobulins

Class	Mol. Weight	Mean Survival, $t_{1/2}$ (days)	Mean Serum Concentration (mg/dL)	Major Function
IgG	150,000	20	720–1500	Most prevalent; major antibody for toxins, viruses, and bacteria
IgA	170,000	6	90–325	In secretions from mucosa; for early antibacterial and antiviral defense
IgM	900,000	10	45–150	Major antibody after exposure to most antigens
IgD	180,000	3	3	Present on B cell surface, function as an antigen receptor
IgE	200,000	2	0.03	Fixed on mast cells, responsible for immediate type hypersensitivity

The complement system consists of more than 30 plasma and body fluid proteins. These proteins complement a variety of immune functions, such as adherence of antibody-coated bacteria to macrophages, modulation of immune response, and lysis of cells. Immunotoxicants can activate or inhibit the complements. Macrophages and certain lymphocytes are capable of synthesizing certain important cytokines, such as tumor necrosis factor (Ruddle, 1994), and growth factors; the latter play a central role in the fibrotic lung lesions in humans exposed to asbestos and silica (see chap. 12).

IMMUNOTOXICANTS

Major Immunotoxicants

A variety of substances have been found to affect the immune system. They may be placed in six categories as follows:

1. Medicinal products: among these, the antineoplastic drugs cyclophosphamide, nitrogen mustards, 6-mercaptopurine, azathioprine, methotrexate, 5-fluorouracil, actinomycin, doxorubicin, and diazepam are more frequently implicated. A number of other drugs that induced autoimmune reactions are listed in Table 11.3.
2. Heavy metals, organometals: beryllium, nickel, chromium, lead, gold, methyl mercury, platinum, organic tin compounds, sodium arsenite and arsenate, and arsenic trioxide.
3. Pesticides: pyrethroids, chlordane, DDT, dieldrin, methyl parathion, carbofuran, maneb, hexachlorobenzene, carbaryl, 2,4-D, paraquat, and diquat.
4. Halogenated hydrocarbons: 2,3,7,8-tetrachlorodibenzo-*p*-dioxin, PCB, polybrominated biphenyls, trichloroethylene, chloroform, pentachlorophenol, perfluorooctanoic acid, and perfluorooctane sulfonate.

Table 11.3   Examples of Drugs that Induce Autoimmune Syndromes

Autoimmune Syndrome	Examples of Drugs
Hepatitis	Erythromycin, floxacillin, halothane, methyldopa
Hemolytic anemia	Amoxicillin, nomifensine, probenecid, tolbutamide
Lupus erythematosus	Hydralazine, procainamide
Nephritis	Captopril
Neutropenia	Methyldopa, penicillamine
Oculocutaneous syndrome	Practolol
Thrombocytopenia	Acetaminophen, quinine

Source: From Pohl et al. (1988) and Behan et al. (1976).

5. Air pollutants: diesel exhaust particles, ambient particulate matter, asbestos fibers, and nanoparticles.
6. Miscellaneous compounds: aflatoxins, benzo[*a*]pyrene, methylcholanthrene, diethylstilbestrol, 2-methoxyethanol, benzene, corticosteroids, deoxynivalenol, 12-*o*-tetradecanoylphorbol-13-*o*-acetate, ochratoxin, penicillin, sulfites, subtilisin, formaldehyde, and toluene diisocyanates.

The effects of toxicants on the immune system are complex; some suppress the cell-mediated immunity, others the humoral immunity, and still others may even stimulate certain immune functions (Table 11.4).

Effects on Immune Functions

The function of the immune system is, as noted earlier, to protect the host against foreign organisms (viruses, bacteria, etc.), "foreign" cells (tumors), and other foreign substances. When the system functions properly, the foreign agents are eliminated promptly and efficiently. However, with certain agents, in some individuals, the immune system may respond in adverse manners. These may manifest as (i) immunosuppression and immunodeficiency, (ii) hypersensitivity and allergy, and (iii) autoimmunity. These are outlined next.

Hypersensitivity and Allergy

There are four types of such reactions. With Type I, the reactions are immediate (usually within 15 minutes), resulting from a second or subsequent exposure to an antigen. The first exposure to that antigen induces the production of IgE antibodies. Subsequent exposure to the same antigen triggers the release of existing histamine, heparin, serotonin, prostaglandins, chemokines, etc. These substances induce a variety of clinical manifestations, such as asthma, rhinitis, urticaria, and anaphylaxis. Allergenic agents are diverse in nature. Notable examples are metals (nickel, beryllium, platinum compounds), therapeutic agents (penicillin), food additives (sulfites, monosodium glutamate, tartrazine, and benzoates), food (chocolate, peanuts), pesticides (pyrethrum), and industrial chemicals such as TDI.

Table 11.4   Effects of In Vivo Exposure to Chemicals on Immune Functions and Host Resistance

Parameters	DES	BaP	TPA
Resistance to [A8] *Listeria* [A7] challenge	D	NE	1
Resistance to tumor challenge	D	NE	D
Trichinella expulsion	D	D	NE
Thymus weight	D	NE	D
Delayed hypersensitivity	D	NE	NE
Lymphocyte responses[a]	D	D[b]	D
T-cell quantification	D	–	D
Spontaneous lymphocyte cytotoxicity	NE	NE	D
Antibody plaque response	D	D	D
Immunoglobulins, M, G, and A levels	NE	NE	D
Macrophage phagocytosis	1	NE	1
Macrophage cytostasis	1	NE	1
RES clearance time	1	NE	1
Bone marrow cellularity[c]	D	D	NE

[a]Lymphocyte responses to phytohemagglutinin, concanavalin A, lipopolysaccharide, and mixed lymphocyte culture.
[b]Decreased, except the response to mixed lymphocyte culture.
[c]Colony-forming units, multipotent cells, and granulocyte/macrophage progenitors.*Abbreviations*: BaP, benzo[*a*]pyrene; D, decreased; DES, diethylstilbestrol; I, increased; NE, no effect; –, not tested; TPA, 12-*o*-tetradecanoylphorbol-13-*o*-acetate; .
Source: From Dean et al. (1982).

Type II and Type III hypersensitivity reactions are less common. Type II is characterized by cytolysis through IgG and/or IgM. The targets are usually erythrocytes, leucocytes, platelets, and their progenitors. The result of the cytolysis is hemolytic anemia, leucopenia, or thrombocytopenia. The offending agents include gold salts, chlorpromazine, phenytoin, sulfonamides, and TDI. Type III, also known as Arthus reactions, is mediated mainly by IgG. The antigen–antibody complexes are deposited in the vascular endothelium. Depending on the site, the damaged blood vessels may produce lupus erythematosus (e.g., procainamide) and glomerular nephritis (e.g., gold).

Type IV is a delayed hypersensitivity reaction. The latent period is usually between 12 and 48 hours. The reaction is mediated by T cells (rather than antibodies) and characterized by perivascular infiltration of monocytes, lymphocytes, and lymphoblasts (resulting from local transformation of lymphocytes). Clinically, this is seen with contact dermatitis and granulomatous reactions. A commonly encountered hypersensitivity inducer is nickel, which also induces immediate immune reaction. Others include beryllium, chromium, formaldehyde, thimerosal (a mercurial compound that was widely used as a vaccine), and TDI.

Autoimmunity

With autoimmune diseases, the immune system produces antibodies to endo-genous antigens, thus damaging normal tissues. Hemolytic anemia is an example of such disorders with phagocytosis of antibody-sensitized erythrocytes leading to hemolysis and anemia. Certain chemicals and metals have been reported to induce such diseases. For example, the pesticide dieldrin was found to produce hemolytic anemia. Exposure to gold and mercury has been associated with a type of glomerular nephritis that is considered an autoimmune disease (Dean et al., 1982). Trichloroethene, an industrial solvent, was shown to induce an autoimmune dis-order resembling systemic lupus erythematosus (Wang et al., 2007).

In addition, a number of drugs are known to exert toxicity through their effects on the cellular or humoral immunity, inducing autoimmune diseases. Clin-ically these conditions manifest as hepatitis, nephritis, hemolytic anemia, neutro-penia, thrombocytopenia, etc. (see also chaps. 12–15). Table 11.3 is a compilation of such drugs.

The mode of action of these drugs appears to be mediated through covalent binding of the drug or its metabolite to tissue macromolecules. The target specific-ity may be related to differences in tissue distribution of the conjugates. In general, the incidence of these side effects is low. The low incidence might be due to complex genetic makeup, which determines the levels of activating and detoxi-cating enzymes (Pohl et al., 1988; Park and Kiteringham, 1990).

Immunosuppression and Immunodeficiencies

Many immunotoxicants suppress immune functions (Bondy and Pestka, 2000). An extensively studied immunotoxicant is 2,3,7,8-tetrachlorodibenzo-p-dioxin. Its effect on the immune system is one of the most sensitive targets for toxicity. It suppresses all the specific immune functions tested, while sparing the nonspecific functions, such as the NK-cell activity and macrophage functions. Its immuno-toxicity is apparently mediated through binding to the *Ah* receptors on lymphoid cells (Luster et al., 1989). Cigarette smoke components are also effective immuno-suppressants. Alcohol depresses immune system, resulting in a depletion and loss of function of CD4(+) T lymphocytes, and subsequent suppression of IL-2 pro-duction, which regulates both innate and adaptive immunity. (Ghare et al., 2011). When the immune system is suppressed, people are more susceptible to infections and many diseases such as cancers, aging, diabetes, etc.

Other immunosuppressants have more restricted activities. For example, antineoplastic drugs such as cyclosporin adversely affect B cells; T cells that have undergone antigenic differentiation may also be affected. Metals such as lead and mercury impair both humoral and cell-mediated host resistance (Luebke et al. 2006). In addition, gold may also induce glomerular nephritis through an auto-immune mechanism resulting in deposits in the glomeruli. Nickel may suppress immune functions through a variety of mechanisms; however, its major clinical effect is hypersensitivity. Organochlorine pesticides impair immune functions mainly in neonatal animals (Loose, 1982). Carbaryl depresses antibody response and phagocytosis by granulocytes. Corticosteroids depress immune functions as well as inflammatory responses.

IMMUNOTOXICITY

As noted above, the immune system is composed of a variety of cellular and humoral components and has numerous activities. An immunotoxicant can affect any one or more of these components and activities.

Immunocompetence Tests in Intact Animals

These tests are designed to study the effects of chemicals on host resistance/ susceptibility to bacterial, viral, and parasitic diseases as well as to bacterial endotoxins and tumor cells. In general, mice are used because of the large number of animals required.

The test chemical is given to the animals by an appropriate route, preferably mimicking the human exposure. Usually three dose groups and a control group are included in the test. The duration of the dosing is generally 14 or 90 days. After this pretreatment, the animals are given a suitable quantity of the challenging agent. The quantity of the agent is selected on the basis that 10–20% of the mortality or morbidity is induced in the control animals. Increased mortality or morbidity indicates decreased host resistance. A list of various infectious agents has been compiled by Bradley and Morahan (1982).

Cell-Mediated Immunity

This can be studied in intact animals or with cells in vitro. In the intact animals, usually mice, the commonly used procedure is to determine the *delayed hypersensitivity* response to a specific antigen. The antigen, such as sheep erythrocytes or keyhole limpet hemocyanin, is injected into a footpad or an ear of the animal. Four days later, a challenging dose of the antigen is given at the sensitized site. The extent of the swelling or the amount of localized radioactivity is measured from a radiolabeled substance, such as ^{125}I-labeled human serum albumin or tritiated thymidine (Luster et al., 1982; Munson et al., 1982; Sanders et al., 1982).

In-vitro tests are conducted on cells collected from animals pretreated with the test chemical. Such tests include lymphocyte proliferation and lymphocyte subpopulation. The *lymphocyte proliferation* assay is done by culturing, in the presence of mitogens, lymphocytes collected from the spleen of pretreated animals. Mitogens such as phytohemagglutinin and concanavalin A are capable of inducing proliferation of normal T lymphocytes, whereas lipopolysaccharides, such as the cell membrane of Gram-negative bacteria, affect B lymphocytes. Immunosuppressive agents inhibit lymphocyte proliferation. The extent of proliferation can be determined by the incorporation of tritiated thymidine into DNA (Luster et al., 1982).

Lymphocytes, as noted above, consist of T cells, B cells, and null cells, and the T-cell population is composed of T-memory, T-helper, and T-killer cells. Techniques for their enumeration include the use of immunofluorescence, rosette formation, histochemistry, cell electrophoresis, cytolysis, and fluorescence-activated cell sorting (Norbury, 1982).

Humoral Immunity

A commonly used procedure, the plaque assay, involves quantitative determination of plaque-forming cells of the IgM class: four days after the mouse has been sensitized to an antigen (e.g., sheep erythrocytes), the spleen is removed and a cell suspension is made. A quantity of the antigen, along with a suitable complement, is added to the suspension. The mixture is then spread on a slide and the number of plaques is counted. This represents the primary humoral immune response. To determine the secondary immune response, the mouse is given on day 10 a second dose of the antigen. On day 15 the spleen is removed and the above procedure is repeated with an additional step of incubation with rabbit anti-mouse IgG to develop the IgG-producing plaques. Reduced plaques indicate immunosuppression (Spyker-Cranmer et al., 1982). Instead of sheep erythrocytes, which are T-dependent antigens, lipopolysaccharides, which are T-independent antigens, may be used.

The levels of various immunoglobulins (IgG, IgM, and IgA) in the serum may be directly measured. The techniques for their measurement have been reviewed by Davis and Ho (1976). The number of B cells in the spleen also provides information on the status of humoral immunity (Dean et al., 1982). The procedures and advantages of the enzyme-linked immunosorbent assay (ELISA) in testing chemicals for immunotoxicity have been elaborated by Vos et al. (1982).

Macrophage and Bone Marrow

The functions of macrophages can be tested in a number of ways: (i) the number of resident peritoneal cells, (ii) phagocytosis, (iii) lysosomal enzymes, (iv) cytostasis of tumor target cells, and (v) reticuloendothelial system uptake of ^{132}I-triolein. Parameters of bone marrow activity include (i) cellularity, (ii) colony-forming units of pluripotent cells, (iii) colony-forming units of granulocyte/macrophage progenitors, and (iv) iron incorporation in the bone marrow and spleen (Dean et al., 1982).

Others

A variety of pathotoxicological data are also useful indicators of immune function; (i) hematology profile: erythrocyte count, leukocyte count, and differential cell count; (ii) serum proteins: albumin, globulin, and albumin/globulin ratio; (iii) weights: body, spleen, thymus, and adrenals; and (iv) histology: thymus, adrenal, lung, kidney, heart, spleen, and cellularity of spleen and bone marrow. For example, thymic atrophy appears to be a very sensitive indicator of immunotoxicity. A paucity of lymphoid follicles and germinal centers in the spleen is indicative of B-cell deficiency, whereas T-cell deficiency is characterized by lymphoid hypoplasia in the paracortical areas (Dean et al., 1982).

REFERENCES

Behan PO, Behan WMH, Zacharias FJ, et al. (1976). Immunological abnormalities in patients who had the oculomueocutaneous syndrome associated with practol therapy. Lancer ii, 984–987.

Bondy GS, Pestka JJ. (2000) Immunomodulation by fungal toxins. J Toxicol Environ Health B 3, 109–143.

Bradley SG, Morahan PS (1982). Approaches to assessing host resistance. Environ Health Persp 43, 65–71.

Burns LA, Meade BJ, Munson AE (1996). Toxic responses of the immune system. In: Klaassen CD, ed. Casarett and Doull's Toxicology. New York, NY: McGraw-Hill, 335–402.

Davis NC, Ho M (1976). Quantitation of immunoglobulins. In: Rose NR, Friedman H, eds. Manual of Clinical Immunology. Washington, DC.: American Society of Microbiology.

Dean JH, Luster MI, Boorman GA, et al. (1982). Procedure available to examine the immunotoxicity of chemicals and drugs. Pharmacol Rev 34, 137–148.

Ghare S, Patil M, Hote P, et al. (2011). Ethanol inhibits lipid raft-mediated TCR signaling and IL-2 expression: potential mechanism of alcohol-induced immune suppression. Alcohol Clin Exp Res 35, 1435–1444.

Loose LD (1982). Macrophage induction of T-suppressor cells in pesticide exposed and protozoan-infected mice. Environ Health Persp 43, 89–97.

Luster MI, Ackermann MF, Germolec DR, et al. (1989). Perturbations of the immune system by xenobiotics. Environ Health Persp 81, 157–162.

Luster MI, Dean JH, Boorman GA (1982). Cell-mediated immunity and its application in toxicology. Environ Health Persp 43, 31–36.

Luebke RW, Chen DH, Dietert R, et al. (2006). The comparative immunotoxicity of five selected compounds following developmental or adult exposure. J Toxicol Environ Health B 9, 1–26.

Munson AE, Sanders VM, Douglas KA, et al. (1982). In vivo assessment of immunotoxicity. Environ Health Persp 43, 41–52.

Norbury KC (1982). Immunotoxicology in the pharmaceutical industry. Environ Health Persp 43, 53–59.

Park BK, Kiteringham N (1990). Drug–protein conjugation and its immunological consequences. Drug Metab Rev 22, 87–144.

Pohl LR, Satoh H, Christ DD, et al. (1988). The immunologic and metabolic basis of drug hypersensitivities. Annu Rev Pharmacol 28, 367–387.

Ruddle NH (1994). Tumor necrosis factor (TNFα) and lymphotoxin (TNFβ). Curr Opin Immunol 4, 327–332.

Sanders VM, Tucker AN, White KL Jr. et al. (1982). Humoral and cell-mediated immune status in mice exposed to trichloroethylene in the drinking water. Toxicol Appl Pharmacol 62, 358–368.

Spyker-Cranmer JM, Barnett JB, Avery DL, et al. (1982). Immunoteratology of chlor-dane: cell-mediated and humoral immune responses in adult mice exposed in utero. Toxicol Appl Pharmacol 62, 402–408.

Vos JG, Krajnac EI, Beekhof P (1982). Use of the enzyme-linked immunosorbent assay (ELISA) in immunotoxicity testing. Environ Health Persp 43, 115–121.

Wang G, Ansari GAS, Khan MF (2007). Involvement of lipid peroxidation-derived alde-hyde–protein adducts in autoimmunity mediated by trichloroethene. J Toxicol Environ Health A 70, 1977–1985.

FURTHER READING

Descates J (1999). An Introduction to Immunotoxicology. Philadelphia, PA: Taylor & Francis.

WHO (1996). Principles and methods for assessing direct immunotoxicity associated with exposure to chemicals. Environ Health Criteria 180. Geneva, Switzerland: World Health Organization.

12

Respiratory system inhalation toxicology

INTRODUCTION

With industrialization, the respiratory system of humans is increasingly exposed to airborne toxicants. Effects of these toxicants on human health and a number of testing procedures are briefly described in this chapter.

Structure

The respiratory tract is a complex system, both in structure and function. It consists of the nasopharynx, the tracheal and bronchial tract, and the pulmonary acini, which are composed of respiratory bronchioles, alveolar ducts, and alveoli. The nasopharynx serves to remove large particles from the inhaled air, add moisture, and moderate the temperature. The tracheal and bronchial tract serves as the conducting airway to the alveoli.

Functions

The pulmonary acini are the sites where oxygen and carbon dioxide are exchanged between the blood and the air, and are the main sites of absorption of toxicants that exist in the form of gases and vapors. The alveoli are lined with epithelial cells, especially those of type I. These cells have a very thin cytoplasm ($0.1–0.2\,\mu m$), but each covers a relatively large surface ($2290\,\mu m^2$). The cuboidal ($63\,\mu m^2$) type II cells can undergo mitosis and, in time, mature to type I cells. In addition, there are endothelial cells, macrophages, and fibroblasts.

Apart from its vital function in the exchange of oxygen and carbon dioxide, the respiratory system also regulates the blood concentrations of angiotensins, biogenic amines, and prostaglandins. Furthermore, it can excrete toxicants that have been absorbed from the lungs or via other routes. Although liver is the primary site of blood detoxification, pulmonary tissue possesses cytochrome P-450 (CYP-450) enzymes involved in xenobiotic detoxication.

Defense Mechanisms

The trachea and bronchi are lined with ciliated epithelium and covered with a thin layer of mucus secreted by certain cells in the epithelial lining. This lining, with the cilia and mucus, can move particles deposited on the surface up to the mouth. The particle-containing mucus can then be eliminated from the respiratory tract by spitting or swallowing.

The respiratory tract has various CYP-450 enzyme systems, which may detoxify certain toxicants. However, many toxicants may be activated by these enzyme systems. They are concentrated in the Clara cells and, to a lesser extent, in the type II cells (Dormans and Van Bree, 1995). The Clara cells are located at the boundary where alveolar ducts branch out from bronchioles.

Apart from clearance and detoxication, the respiratory tract also possesses mechanisms to phagocytize and engulf toxicants, notably solid particles. The main effector is the macrophage. Similar to the enzyme systems, the macrophage may also aggravate the toxic effects (Brain, 1992).

TOXICANTS AND THEIR EFFECTS

Many toxicants are known to adversely affect the respiratory system in humans and animals. Those that pose serious occupational hazards are listed in Appendix 1.

Inhalable toxicants exist in the form of gases, vapors, liquid droplets, and solid particulate matters. Gases and vapors are readily absorbed. The droplets and particulate matters may also be absorbed. However, they vary in size, and their sizes have marked effects on the extent of absorption. In general, large particles ($>10\,\mu m$) do not enter the respiratory tract. Very small particles ($<0.01\,\mu m$) are likely to be exhaled. The optimal size of particle for retention is between 1 and $3\,\mu m$ (see also chap. 2).

A toxicant may exert systemic effects after its absorption from the respiratory tract and distribution to other tissues or it may induce local effects on the respiratory tract, or both. A toxicant may also affect the respiratory tract after exposure from other routes.

Systemic Effects

Many chemicals can be absorbed from the inspired air. After absorption, they are carried by the circulating blood to various parts of the body and exert their effects, such as general anesthesia.

Toxic gases can be absorbed from various parts of the respiratory tract including the nasopharynx. The main site of absorption, however, is the alveoli, and the principal mechanism of absorption is simple diffusion. In addition, liquid aerosols and solid particulate matter can also be absorbed via different mechanisms. Further details regarding the uptake of toxicants are given in chapter 2.

Pulmonary Effects

A variety of pulmonary effects have been observed. These are briefly described under five categories. Additional details and references have been provided by Gordon and Amdur (1994).

Local Irritation

Ammonia and chlorine are classic examples of irritant gases. They produce bronchial constriction and edema, which result in dyspnea, but chronic effects are rare. Arsenicals induce irritation on acute exposure; after prolonged exposure they might induce development of lung cancer. Similarly, chronic exposure to cigarette smoke results in irritation in lung airways and ultimately in lung cancer. Residing in highly industrialized cities or in the vicinity of traffic has been shown to produce lung dysfunction and subsequently development of diseases such as asthma due to ambient particulate matter or diesel exhaust particles. Dust generated during storms was reported to produce lung irritation and increase the frequency of hospital visits with patients complaining of respiratory distress.

Cellular Damage and Edema

Toxic *gases*, such as ozone and oxides of nitrogen, produce cellular damage, perhaps through generation of reactive oxygen species and reactive nitrogen species followed by peroxidation of cellular membranes. Edema ensues as a result of the increased permeability through the damaged membrane. The edematous fluid, however, accumulates in the airway instead of in the interstitial space, as is the case with other tissues. Such effects are also observed after inhalation of toxicants that exist in small particles, such as diesel exhaust, nickel carbonyl, and certain beryllium and boron compounds.

Cellular damage usually affects type I cells in the alveoli. Death of these cells leads to proliferation of type II cells, which then flatten and become type I cells. However, more extensive damage will result in the exudation of fibrin-rich protein, neutrophils, and debris into the alveoli. These eventually become fibrous tissue. Asbestos fibers are known to produce fibrotic reactions and mesothelioma.

Certain organic *solvents*, such as perchloroethylene and xylene, are rapidly absorbed after inhalation and distributed to various parts of the body including the liver, which is the major site of biotransformation. Part of the solvent reenters the lungs through circulation and may form reactive metabolites, leading to covalent binding to macromolecules there. This process in turn produces pulmonary cellular damage and edema. It is also noteworthy that the lungs serve as a conduit for chemicals into the circulation followed by activation in other tissues and development of diseases in different organs. An example is benzene that enters via the lungs, forms reactive intermediates in the liver. These intermediates react with bone macromolecules subsequently, resulting in leukemia.

Ipomeanol is a toxin produced by the mold *Fusarium solani*, which grows on sweet potatoes. This toxin is interesting in that it produces necrosis of one type of cell only, namely, the Clara cells. These cells bioactivate the toxin to a reactive metabolite, which binds to the macromolecules and produces cellular necrosis. This is followed by edema, congestion, and hemorrhage in the lungs. Death may ensue (Timbrell, 1991).

Glucans are polyglucose compounds, which are constituents of fungi and bacteria that produce inflammatory lung diseases characterized by hypersensitivity and pneumonitis (Schuyler et al., 1998). Monocrotaline, a pyrrolizidine alkaloid, was reported to produce lung injury and pulmonary hypertension. In fact, monocrotaline is used as a model to study causes of pulmonary hypertension in humans (Schultze and Roth, 1998).

Fibrosis (Pneumoconiosis)

Pulmonary fibrosis is a serious, debilitating lung disease which results from the inhalation of "inorganic dust." *Silicosis*, with a history that goes back to thousands of years, is produced by crystalline forms of silica (silicon dioxide). Of the crystalline forms, quartz is the most stable. On heating, such as in volcanic eruption and mining, quartz may become tridymite or cristobalite. Both of these forms are more fibrogenic than quartz. The toxic effect stems from the rupture of the lysosomal membrane in a macrophage. The released lysosomal enzymes digest the macrophage, and this process, in turn, releases the silica from the lysed macrophage. This is a continuous process that is repeated. It was suggested that the damaged macrophage releases factors that stimulate the fibroblasts and the formation of collagen (Brain, 1980). Other cells, such as fibroblasts and epithelial cells, in response to macrophage inflammatory proteins, may also play a role in the fibrotic changes (Driscoll et al., 1993). Kuhn et al. (1995) suggest that cytokine is involved in the fibrosis and its increase precedes deterioration of pulmonary function, hence may serve as a biomarker for initiating intervention in exposed workers.

Another major cause of pulmonary fibrosis is *asbestos*. Asbestos refers to a large number of fibrous hydrated silicates of magnesium, calcium, and others. In addition, some of these mineral fibers, such as the blue asbestos (crocidolites), produce bronchogenic carcinoma and mesothelioma. The white variety (chrysotile) appears to have no effect on the incidence of mesothelioma. The potency of asbestos seems related to the chemical and physical properties. Fibers measuring $5\,\mu m$ in length and $0.3\,\mu m$ in diameter appear to be most potent. Various types of man-made refractory ceramic fibers have been used in the place of asbestos. In the rat, they also induce fibrosis and carcinoma, but appear to be less carcinogenic than asbestos (Mast et al., 1995). However, the incidence of carcinoma is markedly increased in smokers exposed to asbestos indicating that the presence of asbestos creates a more susceptible individual to lung cancer development.

Other fibrogenic substances include coal dust, kaolin, talc, aluminum, beryllium, and carbides of tungsten, titanium, and tantalum (Appendix 1). Coal worker's pneumoconiosis (also known as black lung disease) is produced by long exposure to coal dust, graphite, or man-made carbon.

Emphysema is also a debilitating disease. It may be induced by cigarette smoking or exposure to aluminum, cadmium oxide, or oxides of nitrogen, ozone, and others. It was suggested that the elastic fibers surrounding and supporting the alveoli and bronchi may be damaged by the elastase released from polymorpho-nuclear granulocytes under certain conditions (Spitznagel et al., 1980).

Allergic Response

This type of response is usually induced by pollens, spores of molds, bacterial contaminants, cotton dust, cement dust, and so on. Detergents containing enzymes derived from *Bacillus subtilis* were reported to produce asthma among workers. A common chemical used in plastic industry, toluene diisocyanate, as other isocya-nates, also produces hypersensitivity reactions. It is probable that this reactive chemical binds to proteins in the blood or lungs to form antigens, which stimulate antibody formation. The major response is bronchoconstriction triggered by the reaction between the antigens and circulating or fixed antibodies (Karol and Jin, 1991). Long-term exposure may result in other pulmonary effects such as chronic bronchitis and fibrosis.

Lung Cancer

Cigarette smoke contains a number of carcinogens, co-carcinogens, and irritants (Hoffmann and Hoffmann, 1997). These substances initiate and promote carcino-genesis. Furthermore, many other substances may induce oxidative stress, thereby adversely affecting health (Appendix 2). Some details of this topic have been out-lined by Halliwell and Cross (1994). It is well established that cigarette smoking is the leading cause of lung cancer in many countries and that it greatly increases the incidence of lung cancers among asbestos workers (chap. 5). Other causes of lung cancer include arsenic, chromates, nickel, uranium, and coke oven emissions.

Asbestos has been well known for its carcinogenicity in the respiratory tract in humans and animals. Man-made refractory ceramic fibers appear to be carcinogenic also, but only at maximum tolerated doses. Much investigation is in progress to determine their health hazards, if any, in humans. One important approach is to assess their persistence, which is a determinant of their toxicity (Bignon et al., 1994).

Effects on Upper Respiratory Tract

Large airborne particles in the inhaled air are mainly deposited in the nasal pas-sages. They may produce hyperemia, squamous- or transitional-cell metaplasia, hyperplasia, ulceration, and, in certain cases, carcinoma. For example, nickel sub-sulfide, nickel oxide, and nickel usually exist in large particles during their pro-duction and mining; therefore, their effects are mainly on the nasal passage (NAS, 1975). Inhalation of diesel exhaust particles was found to produce immediate nasal hyperresponsiveness, antioxidant responses, marked epithelial inflammation, and specific humoral responses (Nikasinovic et al., 2004). The larynx is also a site of chemical carcinogenesis, for example, with asbestos and chromium. Inhalation of gases and vapors such as sulfur dioxide and toluene may produce irritation of trachea and bronchi. Other toxic effects include deciliation, goblet-cell hyperplasia, and squamous metaplasia.

Effects of Exposure from Routes Other Than Inhalation

Paraquat, a herbicide, produces lung damage not only after exposure by inhalation but also after ingestion (Clark et al., 1966). Its storage in the lungs and its inherent toxicity are apparently the reasons for its pulmonary effects after noninhalation routes. It is of interest that ingestion of paraquat was used as a means of suicide. The mechanism of paraquat toxicity is the generation of reactive oxygen species, which is dependent on the mitochondrial inner transmembrane potential (Castello et al., 2007). In contrast, a closely related herbicide, diquat, although also toxic to cultured lung cells, is not toxic to the lungs either after inhalation or after ingestion. It is interesting that diquat is not retained by the lungs.

A number of drugs are known to induce pulmonary fibrosis in humans. These include bleomycin, busulfan, cyclophosphamide, gold salts, melphalan, methotrexate, BCNU, chlorambucil, and mitomycin. In these cases, there is an increase in interstitial collagen and in the number of type II cells. Methotrexate and streptomycin were found to induce pulmonary eosinophilia. Phenylbutazone, oxyphenylbutazone, aspirin, retinoic acid, and sulfonamides may produce pulmonary edema.

In addition, a number of amphiphilic drugs, such as chlorphentermine, chloroquine, amiodarone, and triparanol, are known to interact with the phospholipids in certain cells to form myeloid bodies and pulmonary foam cells in humans and animals. These bodies and cells were suggested to lead to alterations in cell activities and later to impairment of respiratory functions (Hruban, 1984). However, there is no evidence that drug-induced pulmonary phospholipidosis results in any functional changes in lung activity. It would seem that this is a morphological alteration but not a functional disturbance and can be termed adaptive. This adaptive change disappears upon drug cessation and pulmonary function remains normal.

REFERENCES

Bignon J, Saracci R, Touray JC (1994). Biopersistence of respirable synthetic fibers and minerals. Environ Health Persp 102(Suppl 5), 3–5.

Brain JD (1980). Macrophage damage in relation to the pathogenesis of lung diseases. Environ Health Persp 35, 21–28.

Brain JD (1992). Mechanisms, measurement and significance of lung macrophage function. Environ Health Persp 97, 5–10.

Castello PR, Drechsel DA, Patel M (2007). Mitochondria are a major source of paraquat-induced reactive oxygen species production in the brain. J Biol Chem 282, 14186–14193.

Clark DG, McElligott TF, Hurst EW (1966). The toxicity of paraquat. Br J Ind Med 23, 126–132.

Dormans JAMA, Van Bree L (1995). Function and response of type II cells to inhaled toxicants. Inhal Toxicol 7, 319–342.

Driscoll KE, Hassenbein DG, Carter J, et al. (1993). Macrophage inflammatory proteins 1 and 2: Expression by rat alveolar macrophages, fibroblasts, and epithelial cells and in rat lung after minimal dust exposure. Am J Respir Cell Mol Biol 8, 311–318.

Gordon T, Amdur MO (1994). Responses of the respiratory system to toxic agents. In: Amdur MO, Doull J, Klaassen CD, eds. Casarett and Doull's Toxicology: The Basic Science of Poisons, 4th edn. New York, NY: McGraw-Hill, 443–462.

Halliwell B, Cross CE (1994). Oxygen-derived species: Their relation to human disease and environmental stress. Environ Health Persp 102(Suppl 10), 5–12.

Hoffmann D, Hoffmann I (1997). The changing cigarette, 1950–1995. J Toxicol Environ Health 50, 307–364.

Hruban Z (1984). Pulmonary and generalized lysosomal storage induced by amphiphilic drugs. Environ Health Persp 55, 53–76.

Karol MH, Jin R (1991). Mechanism of immunotoxicity to isocyanates. Chem Res Toxicol 4, 503–509.

Kuhn DC, Stauffer JL, Gaydos LJ, et al. (1995). Inflammatory and fibrotic mediator release by alveoli macrophages from coal miners. J Toxicol Environ Health 45, 9–21.

Mast RW, McConnell EE, Anderson R, et al. (1995). Studies on the chronic toxicity (inhalation) of four types of refractory ceramic fiber in male Fischer 344 rats. Inhal Toxicol 7, 425–467.

National Academy of Sciences (NAS) (1975). Nickel. Washington, DC.: National Academy of Sciences.

Nikasinovic L, Momas I, Just J (2004). A review of experimental studies on diesel exhaust particles and nasal epithelium alterations. J Toxicol Environ Health B 7(2), 81–104.

Schultze AE, Roth RA (1998). Chronic pulmonary hypertension-The monocrotaline model and involvement of the hemostatic system. J Toxicol Environ Health B 1, 271–346.

Schuyler M, Gott K, Cherne A (1998). Effect of glucan on murine lungs. J Toxicol Environ Health A 53, 493–505.

Spitznagel JK, Moderzakowski MC, Pryzwansky KB, et al. (1980) Neutral proteases of human polymorphonuclear granulocytes: Putative mediators of pulmonary damage. Environ Health Persp 35, 29–38.

Timbrell JA (1991). Principles of Biochemical Toxicology. London, U.K.: Taylor & Francis.

Appendix 1   Site of Action and Pulmonary Disease Produced by Selected Occupationally Inhaled Toxicants

Toxicant	Common Name of the Disease	Acute Effect	Chronic Effect
Aluminum dust	Aluminosis	Cough, shortness of breath	Interstitial fibrosis
Aluminum abrasives	Shaver's disease, corundum smelter's lung, bauxite lung	Alveolar edema	Fibrotic thickening of alveolar walls, interstitial fibrosis, emphysema
Ammonia		Immediate upper and lower respiratory tract irritation, edema	Chronic bronchitis
Arsenic			Lung cancer, bronchitis, laryngitis
Asbestos	Asbestosis	Bronchitis	Pulmonary fibrosis, pleural calcification, lung cancer, pleural mesothelioma
Beryllium	Berylliosis	Edema, pneumonia	Pulmonary fibrosis, progressive dyspnea, interstitial granulomatosis, cor pulmonale
Cadmium oxide		Cough, pneumonia	Emphysema, cor pulmonale
Carbides of tungsten, titanium, tantalum	Hard metal disease	Hyperplasia and metaplasia of bronchial epithelium	Fibrosis, peribronchial and perivascular fibrosis
Chlorine		Cough, hemoptysis, dyspnea, tracheobronchitis, bronchopneumonia	
Chromium (VI)		Nasal irritation, bronchitis	Lung tumors and cancers
Coal dust	Pneumoconiosis (coal workers pneumoconiosis, anthracosis)		Pulmonary fibrosis
Coke oven emissions			Tracheobronchial cancers
Cotton dust	Byssinosis	Tightness in chest, wheezing, dyspnea	Reduced pulmonary function, chronic bronchitis

(continued)

Appendix 1 Site of Action and Pulmonary Disease Produced by Selected Occupationally Inhaled Toxicants (*continued*)

Toxicant	Common Name of the Disease	Acute Effect	Chronic Effect
Hydrogen fluoride		Respiratory irritation, hemorrhagic pulmonary edema	
Iron oxides	Siderotic lung disease Silver finisher's lung	Cough	Subpleural and perivascular aggregations of macrophages
	Hematite miner's lung Arc welder's lung		Diffuse fibrosis-like pneumoconiosis Bronchitis
Isocyanates		Cough, dyspnea	Asthma, reduced pulmonary function
Kaolin	Kaolinosis		Pulmonary fibrosis
Nickel		Pulmonary edema, delayed by 2 days (NiCO)	Squamous-cell carcinoma of nasal cavity and lungs
Oxides of nitrogen		Pulmonary congestion and edema	Emphysema
Ozone		Pulmonary edema	Emphysema
Phosgene		Edema	Bronchitis
Perchloroethylene		Pulmonary edema	
Silica	Silicosis, pneumoconiosis		Pulmonary fibrosis
Sulfur dioxide		Bronchoconstriction, cough, tightness in chest	
Talc	Talcosis		Pulmonary fibrosis
Tin	Stenosis		Widespread mottling of X-ray without clinical signs
Vanadium		Upper airway irritation and mucus production	Chronic bronchitis

Appendix 2   Mechanisms Underlying The Oxidative Stress Induced By Cigarette Smoke

1. Smoke contains many free radicals, especially peroxyl radicals that might attack biological molecules and deplete antioxidants, such as vitamin C and α-tocopherol.
2. Smoke contains oxides of nitrogen, including the unpleasant nitrogen dioxide (NO_2-).
3. The tar phase of smoke contains hydroquinones. These are lipid soluble and can redox cycle to form O_2- and H_2O_2. They can enter cells and may even reach the nucleus to cause oxidative DNA damage. Some hydroquinones may release iron from the iron-storage protein ferritin in lung cells and respiratory tract lining fluids.
4. Smoking may irritate lung macrophages, activating them to make O_2-.[a]
5. Smokers' lungs contain more neutrophils than the lungs of nonsmokers, and smoke might activate these cells to make O_2-.[a]
6. Smokers often eat poorly and drink more alcohol than nonsmokers and have a low intake of nutrient antioxidants.
7. Cigarette smoke contains large amounts of fine nanoparticles <50 nm, which generate reactive oxygen species.

[a]Superoxide anion.

13

Toxicology of the liver

GENERAL CONSIDERATIONS

The liver is the largest and metabolically the most complex organ in the body. It is involved in the metabolism of nutrients as well as most drugs and toxicants. The latter type of substances can usually be detoxified, but many of them can be bio-activated and become more toxic.

Hepatocytes (hepatic parenchymal cells) comprise the bulk of the organ. They are responsible for the liver's central role in metabolism. These cells lie between the blood-filled sinusoids and the biliary passages. Kupffer cells line the hepatic sinusoids and constitute an important part of the reticuloendothelial system of the body. The blood is supplied through the portal vein and hepatic artery, and it is drained through the central veins and then the hepatic vein into the vena cava. The biliary passages begin as tiny bile canaliculi formed by adjacent parenchymal cells. The canaliculi coalesce into ductules, interlobular bile ducts, and larger hepatic ducts (Fig. 13.1). The main hepatic duct joins the cystic duct from the gall-bladder to form the common bile duct, which drains into the duodenum.

The toxicology of liver is complicated by the variety of liver injuries and by the different mechanisms through which the injuries are induced. The types of injury, the underlying mechanisms, and the morphologic and biochemical changes are described and discussed.

The liver is often the target organ for a number of reasons. Most toxicants enter the body via the gastrointestinal tract, and after absorption they are carried by the hepatic portal vein to the liver. The liver has a high concentration of binding sites. It also has a high concentration of xenobiotic-metabolizing enzymes (mainly cytochrome P-450), which render most toxicants less toxic and more water solu-ble, and thus more readily excretable. But in some cases the toxicants are activated to be capable of inducing lesions (see also chap. 3). The fact that hepatic lesions are often centrilobular has been attributed to the higher concentration of cyto-chrome P-450 there. In addition, the relatively lower concentration of glutathione there, compared with that in other parts of the liver, may also play a role (Smith et al., 1979).

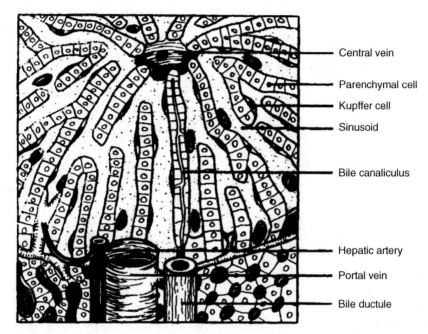

Central vein
Parenchymal cell
Kupffer cell
Sinusoid
Bile canaliculus
Hepatic artery
Portal vein
Bile ductule

Figure 13.1   Schematic structure of the liver indicating the relationship between paren-chymal cells and vascular and ductal systems. *Source*: Klaassen and Watkins (1984).

TYPES OF LIVER INJURY

Toxicants can induce a variety of toxic effects on different organelles in the cells in liver (as shown in Table 13.1), exhibiting different types of liver injury as described subsequently. These liver injuries are mediated through a number of biochemical reactions, such as lipid peroxidation, covalent binding, inhibition of protein syn-thesis, disturbance of biliary production and/or flow, immunologic reaction, and perturbation of calcium homeostasis.

Fatty Liver (Steatosis)

A fatty liver also known as fatty liver disease (FLD) is one that contains more than 5% lipid by weight. The presence of an excess stainable fat in such liver is demon-strable histochemically. The lesion can be acute, such as that induced by ethionine, phosphorus, or tetracycline. Ethanol and methotrexate may produce either acute or chronic lesions. Some toxicants, such as tetracycline, produce many small fat droplets in a cell, whereas others, such as ethanol, induce large fat droplets, which displace the nucleus. Metabolic syndrome (e.g., diabetes, hypertension, obesity, etc.) can also cause FLD. FLD is classified into alcoholic fatty liver disease

Table 13.1   Effects of Toxicants on Subcellular Organelles in Liver Cells

Organelle	Effect	Examples of Toxicants
Plasma membrane	Enzyme leakage	Acetaminophen, carbon tetrachloride, phalloidin
Nucleus	Neoplasia	Aflatoxin, beryllium, cycasin, dimethyl-nitrosamine, tannic acid
Mitochondria	Swelling	Carbon tetrachloride, cycasin, dimethyl-nitrosamine, diquat, ethionine, phosphorus
Lysosomes	Accumulation	Beryllium, carbon tetrachloride, ethionine, phosphorus
Peroxisomes	Proliferation	Clofibrate, trichloroethylene, high-fat diet
Endoplasmic reticulum	Degranulation; proliferation	Carbon tetrachloride, dimethyl-nitrosamine, ethionine, phosphorus
Cytoskeleton	Derangement	Cytochalasin B, phalloidin
Bile canaliculi	Dilatation	Lithocholate, taurocholate

Source: From Ref. de la Iglesia et al. (1982), Stott (1988), and Plaa (1993).

(AFLD) and non-alcoholic fatty liver disease (NAFLD). NAFLD is considered the most common of all liver disorders and the most frequent cause of chronic liver disease (Youssef and McCullough, 2002).

Although lipid accumulation in the liver is the common endpoint of these toxicants, the underlying mechanisms are varied. One of the mechanisms is an increased synthesis of triglyceride and the other lipid moieties. However, the most common mechanism is the impairment of the release of hepatic triglyceride to the plasma. Since hepatic triglyceride is secreted only when it is combined with lipoprotein (forming very low density lipoprotein), accumulation of hepatic lipid can occur as a result of a number of mechanisms:

1. inhibition of the synthesis of the protein moiety of lipoprotein;
2. reduced conjugation of triglycerides with lipoproteins;
3. loss of potassium from hepatocytes, resulting in an interference of transfer of the very low density lipoprotein across the cell membrane (Plaa, 1993).

Liver Necrosis

Liver necrosis involves the death of hepatocytes. The necrosis can be focal (central, mid-zonal, and peripheral) or massive. It is usually an acute injury. A number of chemicals have been demonstrated or reported to produce liver necrosis. It is a serious toxic manifestation but is not necessarily critical because of the remarkable regenerating capacity of the liver.

Cell death occurs along with rupture of the plasma membrane. No ultrastructural changes of the membrane per se have been detected prior to its rupture. There are, however, a number of changes that precede cell death. Early morphologic changes include cytoplasmic edema, dilatation of endoplasmic reticulum, and dis-aggregation of polysomes. There is an accumulation of triglycerides as fat droplets in the cells. Late changes are progressive swelling of mitochondria with cristae disruption, cytoplasmic swelling, dissolution of organelles and nucleus, and rupture of plasma membrane (Bridges et al., 1983). Cyanobacterial blooms are known to produce a variety of toxins including microcystins, which subsequently attack the liver. Microcystins were reported to produce severe deformations such as plasma membrane bleb formation and loss of microvilli. In addition, micro-cystins produce severe hypoglycemia attributed to the failure of hepatic gluconeo-genesis (Zurawell et al., 2005).

The biochemical changes are complex, and various hepatotoxicants appar-ently act through different mechanisms. Carbon tetrachloride (CCl_4) has been shown to act primarily through its reactive metabolite, the trichloromethyl radical CCl_3 (Recknagel and Glende, 1973), which covalently binds to proteins and unsaturated lipids and induces lipid peroxidation. Subcellular membranes are rich in such lipids and are, therefore, susceptible (Table 13.1). Recknagel et al. (1982), however, suggested that microsomal lipid peroxidation might lead to a depression of microsomal Ca^{2+} pump resulting in an early disturbance of liver cell Ca^{2+} homeostasis, which might then induce cell death. In addition, Shah et al. (1979) suggested that the toxicity of CCl_4 might be mediated through another metabolite, namely, phosgene. It is noteworthy that other drugs may act in a synergistic fashion. Chan et al. (2005) demonstrated that ketamine, an anesthetic, when administered to animals being given CCl_4 as a model drug to study liver functions shows that hepatotoxicity was more severe and occurred earlier (a synergistic response).

A number of chemically related compounds, such as chloroform, tetrachlo-roethane, and carbon tetrabromide, as well as phosphorus, appear to act in similar ways. Acetaminophen also induces liver necrosis but apparently not through lipid peroxidation (Kamiyama et al., 1993). At low doses, its reactive metabolite con-jugates with sulfate and glutathione. With increasing doses, the level of glutathi-one reduces, and the covalent binding of the chemical to the proteins rises, as shown in Figure 3.2 of chapter 3. Bromobenzene is also bioactivated in the liver. Its 3,4-epoxide covalently binds to proteins and lipids and produces necrosis (see also chap. 3). Other examples include isoniazid and iproniazid, both of which undergo bioactivation and form metabolites that bind to macromolecules and pro-duce necrosis (Mitchell et al., 1976).

Disturbance of Ca^{2+} homeostasis may also play an important role through an activation of molecular oxygen resulting in an oxidative stress, as discussed in chapter 4 (Thomas and Reed, 1989).

Other biochemical changes include depletion of adenosine triphosphate (ATP), shifts of the Na^+ and K^+ balance between hepatocytes and blood, depletion of glutathione, damage to cytochrome P-450, and loss of nicotinamide adenine dinucleotide (NAD) and nicotinamide adenine dinucleotide phosphate (NADP) (Kulkarni and Hodgson, 1980).

Cholestasis

Cholestasis is a hepatic disorder that the normal flow of bile and/or the secretion of bile in the liver cells is reduced or impaired, which results in intrahepatic accumulation of bile acids. This type of liver damage, usually acute, is less common than fatty liver and necrosis, and it is more difficult to induce in animals with the possible exception of the steroids. The cholestatic agents appear to act through several mechanisms. For example, α-naphthylisocyanate (ANIT) can induce cholestasis, hyperbilirubinemia, and inhibition of microsomal mixed-function oxygenases. Reduction of biliary excretory activity of the canalicular membrane appears to be the predominant mechanism for cholestasis. Furthermore, ANIT seems to alter ductular cell permeability. Bailie et al. (1994) showed that platelets seem to contribute to ANIT-induced liver injury. In addition, cholestasis is associated with complex transcriptional and post-transcriptional alterations of hepatobiliary transporters [e.g., ATP-binding cassette transporters] and enzymes participating in bile formation (Wagner et al., 2009).

A number of anabolic and contraceptive steroids as well as taurocholate, chlorpromazine, and erythromycin lactobionate have been found to cause cholestasis and hyperbilirubinemia associated with canalicular bile plugs. Ethinyl estradiol and chlorpromazine seem to impair the permeability of the biliary tract, thus reducing bile salt–independent bile flow Plaa (1976, 1993). Ampicillin, rifampin, imipramin, and tetracycline produce cholestasis, but this kind of drug-induced cholestasis can be recovered shortly when medications are discontinued. Other types of cholestasis include hereditary cholestasis, extrahepatic cholestasis, intrahepatic cholestasis of pregnancy, and inflammatory cholestasis (Zollner and Trauner, 2008).

Cirrhosis

Cirrhosis is characterized by the presence of septae of collagen distributed throughout most of the liver. Separated by these fibrous sheaths, clusters of hepatocytes appear as nodules.

The pathogenesis is not fully understood, but in a majority of cases, cirrhosis seems to originate from single-cell necrosis associated with a deficiency in the repair mechanism. This condition then leads to fibroblastic activity and scar formation. Inadequate blood flow in the liver may be a contributing factor.

Several chemical carcinogens and long-term administration of CCl_4 can induce cirrhosis in animals. The most important cause of human cirrhosis is chronic ingestion of alcoholic beverages. The mechanism is not fully understood, but ethanol may damage mitochondria and increase local production of reactive oxygen species. These may lead to steatosis, necrosis, and cirrhosis. This pathologic condition can be induced in animals only with ethanol in combination with diets deficient in choline, proteins, methionine, vitamin B_{12}, and folic acid. Because this type of nutritional deficiency is common in alcoholism, Hartroft

(1975) suggested the nutritional deficiency as the primary cause. Lieber and DiCarli (1976) were able to induce cirrhosis in baboons with ethanol alone and claimed, therefore, that alcohol has direct hepatotoxicity. For the etiology of cirrhosis, alcohol contributes about 60–70%, viral hepatitis 10%, and biliary disease 5–10%. In addition, vitamin D deficiency may be associated with more frequent and severe degree of liver dysfunction in patients with alcoholic liver cirrhosis than in patients with primary biliary cirrhosis, rather than the etiology of cirrhosis (Malham et al., 2011).

Viral-Like Hepatitis

A clinical syndrome indistinguishable from viral hepatitis has been known to be associated with various drugs. In general, they have the following characteristics (Plaa, 1993):

1. Such liver injuries are not demonstrable in animals.
2. Effects in humans do not seem to be related to the dose.
3. Latent period varies greatly.
4. Toxicity is manifest in only a few susceptible individuals.
5. Histologic picture is more variable.
6. Patients usually show other signs of hypersensitivity and sometimes respond to a challenge dose.
7. Fever, rash, and eosinophilia are present in many cases.

The clinical picture may vary from patient to patient. For example, among those with halothane-induced hepatotoxicity, 50% of the patients had signs of typical immunologic reaction: fever, eosinophilia, and prior exposure to this anesthetic. Others did not exhibit these signs, and the livers of fatal cases showed lesions similar to those induced by CCl_4 (Lewis and Zimmerman, 1989).

Halothane may induce a mild hepatotoxicity, which is reproducible in animals. In addition, it may act through an immune-mediated mechanism to produce the viral-like liver toxicity, which is more severe and delayed in onset (Hubbard et al., 1988).

Carcinogenesis

Hepatocellular carcinoma and cholangiocarcinoma are the most common types of primary malignant neoplasms of the liver. Others include angiosarcoma, glandular carcinoma, trabecular carcinoma, and undifferentiated liver cell carcinoma. The significance of adenoma, focal basophilic hyperplasia, and hyperplastic nodule is as yet uncertain, whereas bile duct hyperplasia is likely to be a physiologic response to toxic exposure (Newberne, 1982).

As discussed in chapter 7, a large number of toxicants are known to induce liver cancers in animals. However, the carcinogenicity of these chemicals in humans with respect to liver has not been well established (Wogan, 1976).

Dieldrin induces hepatocarcinogenesis via a nongenotoxic mechanism only in the mouse but not in the rat (Kamendulis et al., 2001). Although the precise mechanisms are not known, fumonisin B, in addition to producing hepatotoxicity, induces also hepatocellular adenoma and carcinoma (Li et al., 2000). On the other hand, the role of vinyl chloride in inducing angiosarcoma in humans is beyond doubt.

HEPATOTOXICANTS

Some of the liver injuries described, namely, steatosis, necrosis, cirrhosis, and neoplasia have a number of common features. (i) These injuries are relatively easily produced in experimental animals. (ii) Many toxicants can induce several types of such injuries. For example, steatosis, necrosis, and cirrhosis can result from exposure to CCl_4 (and related chemicals such as chloroform), aflatoxins, and phosphorus. Aflatoxins and dioxins induce necrosis, cirrhosis, and neoplasm. Steatosis and cirrhosis are seen after exposure to ethanol; bromobenzene is known to induce necrosis and cirrhosis. Recently, chloroform was shown to produce liver cell death by depletion of glutathione and an oxidative phase characterized by mitochondrial permeability transition and protein nitration (Burke et al., 2007). Comfrey, a herbal medicine containing pyrrolizidine alkaloids, produces hepatotoxicity in humans and livestock, and carcinogenicity by interacting with DNA in hepatocytes (Mei et al., 2010)

Cholestasis is induced mainly by certain bile salts, α-naphthylisocyanate, certain anabolic and contraceptive steroids, manganese, and a number of drugs. Some of these drugs and other substances are also known to induce viral-like hepatitis. For example, *p*-aminosalicylic acid, chlorpromazine, erythromycin, and phenytoin (diphenylhydantoin) appear to produce viral-like hepatitis through a type of hypersensitivity reaction. On the other hand, iproniazid, isoniazid, and hydrazine derivatives induce this effect perhaps through a metabolic abnormality.

Examples of the various types of hepatotoxicants are listed in Appendix 1.

CLINICAL BIOCHEMICAL TESTS

A number of serum enzymes have been used as indicators of hepatic injuries. These enzymes are released to the blood from the cytosol and subcellular organelles. The serum level of alanine aminotransferase (ALT) or aspartate aminotransferase (AST) is increased in reliable correlation with the severity of hepatic necrosis. It is, therefore, the choice test in liver necrosis. In addition, ornithine carbamoyl transferase (OCT) and sorbitol dehydrogenase (SDH) are more sensitive, but less specific, than ALT. They are therefore often used in conjunction with ALT when testing new toxicants. The enzyme levels in blood are often used as biomarkers among humans exposed to hepatotoxicants.

In cholestatic lesions, both ALT and alkaline phosphatase (AP) are greatly elevated. On the other hand, serum cholinesterase may be reduced in certain cases of liver diseases. For additional details, see Plaa and Charbonneau (1994).

Glutamate dehydrogenase, paraoxonase, malate dehydrogenase, and purine nucleoside phosphorylase can be used for biomarkers of hepatotoxicity by photometric methods (Ozer et al., 2008). In addition, other biomarkers such as serum F protein, arginase I, and glutathione-S-transferase alfa (GST-α) may be applictable, but have limitations due to antibody availability and high cost.

Other Tests

The liver is involved in the metabolism of carbohydrate, fat, and protein as well as in the formation of prothrombin and the excretion of bilirubin and certain foreign chemicals. It is also the major site of biotransformation of toxicants. Tests have thus been devised to determine these hepatic functions.

For example, bilirubin is excreted by the liver, hence its level in the blood is an index of liver function, but it is relatively insensitive. The rate of excretion of bromosulfophthalein is a more sensitive indicator of liver damage. Clinically, the prolongation of prothrombin time, after excluding vitamin K deficiency, has been used in detecting acute hepatic lesions. A chemical may either potentiate or inhibit the pharmacologic and toxicologic actions of another by stimulating the hepatic microsomal enzymes (see chap. 5). Measurements of barbiturate-induced sleeping time and the duration of zoxazolamine-induced paralysis have been used as indications of hepatic effects.

In addition, a number of biochemical tests can be performed on the liver tissue:

1. level of triglycerides;
2. activity of glucose 6-phosphatase;
3. level of microsomal conjugated dienes, resulting from the peroxidation of microsomal lipids;
4. covalent binding of reactive metabolites to tissue macromolecules;
5. arylation or alkylation of purine and pyrimidine components of DNA and RNA (carcinogenicity);
6. arylation or alkylation of other macromolecules (necrosis).

Because of the importance of lipid peroxidation in liver lesions, the extent of this reaction is often determined by using thiobarbituric acid. It combines with malonaldehyde, a degradation product of the lipid, to form a colored complex, which can be measured quantitatively.

REFERENCES

Bailie MB, Pearson JM, Lappin PB, et al. (1994). Platelets and α-naphthylisothiocyanate-induced liver injury. Toxicol Appl Pharmacol 129, 207–213.

Bass NM (1996). Toxic and drug induced liver disease. In: Bennett JC, Plumm F, eds. Cecil's Textbook of Medicine. Philadelphia, PA: W.B. Saunders, 772–776.

Bridges JW, Benford DJ, Hubbard SA (1983). Mechanisms of toxic injury. Ann N Y Acad Sci 407, 42–63.

Burke AS, Redeker K, Kurten RC, et al. (2007). Mechanisms of chloroform-induced hepatotoxicity: Oxidative stress and mitochondrial permeability transition in freshly isolated mouse hepatocytes. J Toxicol Environ Health A 70, 1936–1945.

Chan W-H, Sun W-Z, Ueng T-H (2005). Induction of rat hepatic cytochrome P450 by ketamine and its toxicological implications. J Toxicol Environ Health A 68, 1581–1597.

de la Iglesia F, Sturgess JM, Feuer G (1982). New approaches for assessment of hepatotoxicity by means of quantitative functional–morphological interrelationship. In: Plaa GL, Hewitt WR, eds. Toxicology of the Liver. New York, NY: Raven Press.

Deng DJ, Yang SM, Li T, et al. (1999). Confirmation of N-(nitrosomethyl)urea as a nitrosourea derived by nitrosation of fish sauce. Biomed Environ Sci 12, 54–61.

Hartroft WS (1975). On the etiology of alcoholic liver cirrhosis. In: Khanna JM, Israel Y, Kalant H, eds. Alcoholic Liver Pathology. Toronto, Canada: Addiction Research Foundation.

Hubbard AK, Gandolfi AJ, Brown RR (1988). Immunological basis of anesthetic-induced hepatotoxicity. Anesthesiol 69, 814–817.

Kamendulis LM, Kolaja KL, Stevenson DE, et al. (2001). Comparative effects of dieldrin on hepatic ploidy, cell proliferation, and apoptosis. J Toxicol Environ Health A 62, 127–141.

Kamiyama T, Sato C, Liu J, et al. (1993). Role of peroxidation in acetaminophen-induced hepatotoxicity: Comparison with carbon tetrachloride. Toxicol Lett 66, 7–12.

Klaassen CD, Watkins JB (1984). Mechanisms of bile formation, hepatic uptake and biliary excretion. Pharmacol Rev 36, 1–67.

Kulkarni AP, Hodgson E (1980). Hepatoxicity. In: Hodgson E, Guthrie FE, eds. Introduction to Biochemical Toxicology. New York, NY: Elsevier.

Levi PE (1987). Types of liver injury. In: Hodgson E, Levi PE, eds. A Textbook of Modern Toxicology. New York, NY: Elsevier.

Lewis JH, Zimmerman HJ (1989). Drug-induced liver disease. Med Clin North Am 73, 775–792.

Li W, Riley RT, Voss KA, et al. (2000). Role of proliferation in the toxicity of fumonisin B: Enhanced hepatoxic response in the partially hepatectomized rat. J Toxicol Environ Health A 60, 441–457.

Lieber CS, DiCarli LM (1976). Animal models of ethanol dependence of liver injury in rats and baboons. Fed Proc 35, 1232–1236.

Malham M, Jørgensen SP, Ott P et al. (2011). Vitamin D deficiency in cirrhosis relates to liver dysfunction rather than aetiology. World J Gastroenterol 17, 922–925.

Mei N, Guo P, Fu PP, et al. (2010). Metabolism, genotoxicity and carcinogenicity of comfrey. J. Toxicol. Environ, Health B 13, 509–526.

Mitchell JR, Snodgrass WR, Gillette JR(1976). The role of biotransformation in chemical-induced liver injury. Environ Health Persp 15, 27–38.

Newberne PM (1982). Assessment of the hepatocarcinogenic potential of chemicals: Response of the liver. In: Plaa GL, Hewitt WR, eds., Toxicology of the Liver. New York, NY: Raven Press.

Ozer J, Ratner M, Shaw M, et al. (2008). The current state of serum biomarkers of hepatotoxicity. Toxicology 245, 194–205.

Plaa GL (1976). Quantitative aspects in the assessment of liver injury. Environ Health Persp 15, 39–46.

Plaa GL (1993). Toxic responses of the liver. In: Amdur MO, Doull J, Klaassen CD, eds. Casarett and Doull's Toxicology, 4th edn. New York, NY: McGraw-Hill, 334–353.

Plaa GL, Charbonneau M (1994). Detection and evaluation of chemically induced liver injury. In: Hayes AW, ed. Principles and Methods of Toxicology. New York, NY: Raven Press, 839–870.

Recknagel RO, Glende EA Jr (1973). Carbon tetrachloride hepatotoxicity: An example of lethal cleavage. CRC Crit Rev Toxicol 2, 263–297.

Recknagel RO, Glende EA, Waller RL, et al. (1982). Lipid peroxidation: Biochemistry, measurement, and significance in liver cell injury. In: Plaa GL, Hewitt WR, eds. Toxicology of the Liver. New York, NY: Raven Press.

Shah H, Martman SP, Weinhouse S (1979). Formation of carbonyl chloride in carbon tetrachloride metabolism by rat liver in vitro. Cancer Res 39, 3942–3947.

Smith ML, Loveridge N, Wills ED, et al. (1979). The distribution of glutathione in rat liver lobule. Biochem J. 182, 103–108.

Stott WT (1988). Chemically induced proliferation of peroxisomes: Implications for risk assessment. Reg Toxicol Pharmacol 8, 125–159.

Thomas CE, Reed DJ (1989). Current status of calcium in hepatocellular injury. Hepatology 10, 375–384.

Wagner M., Zollner G, Trauner, M (2009). New molecular insights into the mechanisms of cholestasis. J Hepatol 51, 565–580.

Wogan CN (1976). The induction of liver cell cancer by chemicals. In: Cameron HM, Linsell DA, Warwick GP, eds. Liver Cell Cancer. Amsterdam, The Netherlands: Elsevier.

Youssef WI, McCullough AJ (2002). Steatohepatitis in obese individuals. Best Pract and Res in Clinical Gastroenterol 16, 733–747.

Zollner G, Trauner M (2008). Mechanisms of cholestasis. Clin Liver Dis. 12, 1–26.

Zurawell RW, Chen H, Burke JM, et al. (2005). Hepatotoxic cyanobacteria: A review of the biological importance of microcystins in freshwater environments. J Toxicol Environ Health B 8, 1–37.

Appendix 1   Examples of Hepatotoxic Agents and Associated Liver Injury

Necrosis and fatty liver

Acetaminophen[a]	Ethanol[b]
Aflatoxin	Ethionine[b]
Allyl alcohol[a]	Fumonisin B
	Furosemide[a]
Azaserine	Galactosamine
Beryllium[a]	Phosphorus
Bromobenzene[a]	Puromycin[b]
Carbon disulfide	Pyrrolizidine alkaloids
Carbon tetrachloride	Tannic acid[a]
Chloroform	Tetrachloroethane
Corticosteroid	Tetracycline[b]
Cycloheximide[b]	Thioacetamide[a]
Dichlorobenzene	Trichloroethylene
Dimethylnitrosamine	Valproic acid[b]
Diquat	

Cholestasis (drug-induced)

p-Aminosalicylic acid[c]	Mestranol
Amitriptyline	Methandrolone
Carbamazepine[c]	Methimazole
Carbarsone	Oxyphenisatin[c]
Chlorpromazine[c]	Perphenazine
Chlorthiazide	Phenindione[c]
Diazepam	Promazine
Erythromycin estolate[c]	Steroids, androgenic, and anabolic
Estradiol	Sulfanilamide
Ethacrynic acid[c]	Thiabendazole
Imipramine[c]	Thioridazine
Mepazine	

Viral-like hepatitis (drug induced)

Colchicine	Methoxyflurane
Halothane	α-Methyldopa
Imipramine	Papaverine
Indomethacin	Phenylbutazone
Iproniazid	Phenytoin
Isoniazid	Sulfonamides
6-Mercaptopurine	Zoxazolamine

Carcinogenesis (in experimental animals)

Acetylaminofluorene	Polychlorinated biphenyls
Aflatoxin B1[d]	Pyrrolizidine alkaloids
Cycasin	Safrole
Dialkyl nitrosamines	Urethane
N(nitrosomethyl)urea[d]	Vinyl chloride[d]

[a]Primary effect is necrosis.
[b]Primary effect is fatty liver.
[c]Also induces viral-like hepatitis.

14

Toxicology of the kidney

INTRODUCTION

As noted in chapter 2, urine is the principal route by which most toxicants are excreted. As a result, the kidney has a high volume of blood flow, concentrates the toxicants in the filtrate, transports them across the tubular cells, and bioactivates or detoxifies certain toxicants. It is therefore a major target organ for adverse effects. To facilitate discussions on these effects, the renal structure and functions are briefly reviewed.

The Structure

The predominant structures in the kidney are the nephrons, numbering approximately 1.3×10^6. Each nephron consists of a glomerulus and a series of tubules (Fig. 14.1). The glomerulus is supplied with a high-pressure capillary system that produces an ultrafiltrate from the plasma. The filtrate collected in the Bowman's capsule flows through the proximal convoluted tubule, the loop of Henle, and the distal convoluted tubule, and then drains through a collecting tubule into the renal pelvis for excretion as urine.

The proximal tubule is divided into three sections (S_1, S_2, and S_3). S_1 and S_3 consist of major portions of the convoluted tubule and the straight portion, respectively. S_2 consists of the end of the convoluted portion and the beginning of the straight portion.

The major function of the kidney is to eliminate wastes resulting from normal metabolism and to excrete xenobiotics and their metabolites. These functions occur through the production of urine, a process that also contributes to the maintenance of the homeostatic status of the body. In addition, it has several non-excretory functions.

The Production of Urine

The production of urine is a complex process. It begins with filtration in the glomeruli. In humans, approximately 180 L of filtrate is formed per day. As only 500–2500 ml of urine is excreted, some 99% of the filtered water is reabsorbed.

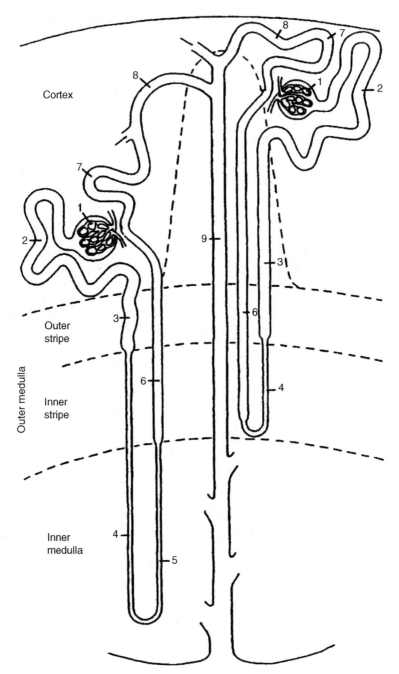

Figure 14.1 Schematic presentation of a cortical (short-looped) and a juxtamedallary (long-looped) nephron together with the collecting system. 1, glomerulus with Bowman's capsule; 2, proximal tubule (*convoluted portion*); 3, proximal tubule (*straight portion*); 4, descending thin limb (loop of Henle); 5, ascending limb (loop of Henle); 6, thick ascending limb; 7, distal convoluted tubule; 8, connecting tubule; 9, collecting tubule. *Source*: From Kriz and Bankir (1988).

The reabsorption of water, through diffusion, takes place first at the proximal tubules, where Na^+ is actively reabsorbed. Further diffusion of water takes place at the descending limb of the loop of Henle to the hyperosmolar interstitium. The hyperosmolarity is produced by the active reabsorption of Cl^- (along with Na^+) at the ascending limb of the loop. The spatial arrangement of the loops and the vasa recta provides an effective countercurrent multiplier mechanism.

Additional water is removed from the filtrate in the distal and the collecting tubules, as Na^+ is actively reabsorbed. The extent of the removal of water from these tubules depends on the activity of antidiuretic hormone (ADH). ADH reduces the urine volume by increasing the permeability of these structures to water.

Tubular Resorption and Secretion

As the glomerular capillaries have large pores (70 nm), substances with molecular weights under 60,000 Da are filtered into Bowman's capsules. Some of the filtered substances such as glucose and amino acids, which are vital to the body, are reabsorbed by the tubules. On the other hand, ammonia (NH_3), a metabolic waste of amino acids, diffuses through the cells to the filtrate, where it reacts with H^+ to form NH_4^+, which is nondiffusible, hence excreted.

To facilitate the passive reabsorption of water and to maintain homeostasis, various electrolytes in the glomerular filtrate are reabsorbed nearly completely or to a great extent. The reabsorption of Na^+ at the distal and collecting tubules is regulated by mineralocorticoids, that of phosphorus by parathyroid hormone, and that of bicarbonate (HCO_3^-) by the acid–base balance. In addition, K^+ and H^+ are secreted by the tubules.

Non-excretory Functions

The kidney possesses other functions such as the regulation of blood pressure and volume. This is mediated through the renin–angiotensin–aldosterone system. Renin, a proteolytic enzyme, is formed in the cells of the juxtaglomerular apparatus and catalyzes the conversion of a plasma angiotensin prohormone to angiotensin I. The latter, a decapeptide, is converted in the lungs to angiotensin II by an enzyme that removes a dipeptide from the C-terminal end.

A renal erythropoietic factor also acts on a plasma protein to form erythropoietin, which increases the production of normoblasts and the synthesis of hemoglobin. Renal prostaglandins are produced in the interstitial cells in the medulla and appear to have the capability of regulating renal blood flow and the excretion of Na^+ and urine. The kidney is also involved in the conversion of the relatively inactive 25-hydroxy-vitamin D_3 to the active 1,25-dihydroxyvitamin D_3.

NEPHROTOXICANTS: MECHANISM AND SITE OF ACTION

The major groups of nephrotoxicants are heavy metals, antibiotics, analgesics, and certain halogenated hydrocarbons (Table 14.1). All parts of the nephron are

Table 14.1   Nephrotoxicants

Toxicants	Site of Action
Heavy Metals	
Cadmium	Proximal tubules
Chromium	Proximal tubules
Gold	Glomeruli
Lead	Proximal tubules and blood vessels
Mercury, inorganic	Proximal tubules and glomeruli
Antibiotics	
Aminoglycosides	Glomeruli and proximal tubules
Amphotericin-B	Glomerular blood vessels and distal tubules
Cephaloridine	Proximal tubules
Gentamicin	Glomeruli and proximal tubules
Puromycin	Glomeruli
Tetracycline	Interstitial tissues in medulla
Halogenated Hydrocarbons	
Bromobenzene	Proximal tubules
Carbon tetrachloride	Proximal tubules
Chloroform	Proximal tubules
Decalin	Proximal tubules
Hexachlorobutadiene	Pars recta
Hydroquinone	Proximal tubules
Analgesics/anesthetics	
Acetaminophen	Various parts of a nephron and blood vessel
Ibuprofen	Glomeruli and proximal tubules
Methoxyflurane	Various parts of a nephron
Antineoplastics	
Adriamycin	Glomeruli
Cisplatin	Pars recta and other parts of a nephron proximal tubules
Immunosuppressants	
Cyclosporin	Blood vessels and interstitial tissue
	Proximal tubules and distal tubules
Miscellaneous	
Glycol	Tubular blockade
Sulfapyridine	Tubular blockade

potentially subject to the detrimental effects of toxicants. However, most toxicants preferentially affect specific parts of the kidney. The mechanisms of action of nephrotoxicants include interaction with receptors, inhibition of oxidative phosphorylation, disturbance of Ca^{2+} homeostasis, and adverse effects in plasma and subcellular membranes. Certain chemicals may affect one area predominantly, but the entire nephron is subject to damage. Analgesics induce a nephropathy with decease in renal volume, but histologically there is thickening of the basement membrane of the loop of Henle, isolated necrosis of interstitial and papillary tubular cells followed by fibrosis and cortical interstitial nephritis (Schnellmann, 1998). High-molecular-weight organic compounds such as humic or fulvic acid, which occur naturally in lignite beds, induce a nephropathy that resembles Balkan endemic nephropathy (BEN). Ochratoxin A, a naturally occurring mycotoxin also produced BEN as well as renal tumors (Clark and Snedeker, 2006). This is an irreversible disease and results in end-stage renal failure (Bunnell et al., 2007). The *n*-arylsuccinimides produce a chronic interstitial nephritis characterized by polyuric renal failure (Rankin, 2004). Details of these are provided in a review article (Commandeur and Vermeulen, 1990). In general, men are more susceptible to chemical-induced nephrotoxicity. This is especially true among geriatric patients (Kacew et al., 1995).

Glomeruli

The antibiotic puromycin can increase the permeability of the glomerulus to proteins such as albumin. This has been attributed to an alteration in the electrical charge of glomerular basement membrane (Brenner et al., 1977). On the other hand, the aminoglycoside antibiotics, such as gentamicin and kanamycin, decrease the glomerular filtration, in addition to their effects on renal tubules (Humes and O'Connor, 1988). Certain toxicants, for example, gold, mercury, and penicillamine, may induce membranous glomerulonephritis by the deposition of antigen–antibody conjugates in the glomerular basement membrane. Deoxynivalenol, a mycotoxin commonly found in cereal-based foods, produces deposition of immunoglobin A in the kidney, which resembles human glomerulonephritis nephropathy (Pestka and Smolinski, 2005). Ibuprofen decreases the renal blood flow and glomerular filtration rate (GFR) (Kent et al., 2007).

Proximal Tubules

Because of their active absorptive and secretory activities, the proximal tubules often have higher concentrations of toxicants. Furthermore, proximal tubules have higher levels of cytochrome P-450 to detoxify or activate toxicants and are thus often the site of adverse effects. Heavy metals, such as mercury, chromium, cadmium, and lead, can alter the functions of the tubules, characterized by glycosuria, aminoaciduria, and polyuria. However, one needs to be cautious with respect to concentration or dose in terms of exposure. Diamond et al. (2003) clearly showed that exposure to cadmium produced renal toxicity as evidenced by proteinuria, but the source of cadmium inducing this effect was not derived from the diet. After higher doses, they cause tubular cell death, elevated blood urea nitrogen (BUN), and anuria. The straight portion (pars recta) of the proximal tubules appears more susceptible than the convoluted portion to the toxicity of mercury (Phillips et al., 1977). The nephrotoxicity may result from a combination of direct cellular toxicity and ischemia secondary to vasoconstriction. Additional information on renal toxicity of metals is given in chapter 23.

As noted above, certain antibiotics affect the glomerular filtration. In addition, many antibiotics are also secreted by the proximal tubules and can induce alterations in the tubular functions. Various aminoglycoside antibiotics (streptomycin, neomycin, kanamycin, gentamicin, and amphotericin-B) have been reported to affect the proximal tubules. These drugs alter membrane phospholipid compositions, permeability, Na^+–K^+–ATPase activity, adenylate cyclase activity, and transport of K^+, Ca^{2+}, and Mg^{2+} (Kaloyanides, 1984; Mingeot-Leclercq et al., 1995). Cephaloridine, unlike the antibiotics named above, is not secreted from the proximal tubules but is accumulated in these cells, thereby producing damage.

Halogenated hydrocarbons such as carbon tetrachloride and chloroform are mainly hepatotoxic, but in certain animal species they may also exert toxic effects on the kidney, especially on the proximal tubules, as reflected in functional changes. At higher doses, however, morphological changes may be produced in other parts of the nephron. Hexachlorobutadiene damages mainly the pars recta of the proximal tubules, resulting in a decreased urinary concentrating ability. Bromobenzene as hexachlorobutadiene is also nephrotoxic, acting on the proximal tubules; while the former is bioactivated in the liver, the latter is bioactivated in the kidney, via a renal enzyme (C-S lyase) after biotransformation in the liver (Hook et al., 1982).

Other Sites

Tetracycline, especially outdated products, may affect the renal medulla and induce interstitial nephritis. Amphotericin-B induces renal toxicity in a majority of the patients, affecting various renal structures.

Methoxyflurane, an anesthetic, is known to be nephrotoxic in humans and certain animals, producing *high-output* renal failure. This chemical was shown to be biotransformed to inorganic fluoride and oxalate. Experimental data suggest that the F^- acts on several parts of the nephron to reduce the reabsorption of water. First, it interferes with the capability of the proximal tubules to reabsorb water. Second, methoxyflurane inhibits the enzymes involved in the transport of ions at the ascending limb of the loop of Henle, thus reducing the interstitial osmolarity, thereby decreasing water reabsorption. This chemical also damages the collecting tubules, rendering them insensitive to ADH (Mazze, 1976).

Analgesic mixtures containing aspirin and phenacetin, a derivative of acetaminophen, produce chronic renal failure, with adverse effects located predominantly in the medulla, that is, loop of Henle, vasa recta, interstitial cells, and collecting tubules (Schnellmann, 1998). The effects might be a result of vasoconstriction of the vasa recta (the blood vessels surrounding the loop of Henle) due to an inhibition of the synthesis of vasodilator prostaglandin (Nanra, 1974). Cisplatin affects many parts of the tubules in patients taking this chemotherapeutic agent (Tanaka et al., 1986). Cyclosporin produces acute thrombotic microangiopathy and chronic nephropathy with interstitial fibrosis (Racusen and Solez, 1988).

Other types of toxicity include renal carcinogenicity of DMN (dimethyl nitrosamine), and tubular blockade induced by the metabolites of sulfapyridine (acetylsulfapyridine) and glycols (oxalic acid). Penicillins and sulfonamides were reported to produce inflammatory interstitial nephritis in humans. An immunological mechanism was suggested as responsible for this toxicity (Appel and Neu, 1977). High concentrations of calcium may lead to calcification in the kidney and subsequent renal failure (Hwang et al., 2003).

TESTING PROCEDURE

Functional and morphological examinations of the kidney are routinely carried out as an integral part of short-term and long-term toxicity studies. The types of examinations involved are described in chapter 6 and are further elaborated here.

In studies designed specifically for nephrotoxicity, dogs, rabbits, and rats are the commonly used animals. Examinations of kidney functions may be done in a number of ways.

Urinalysis

Proteinuria

Because of the size of their molecules, only a very small amount of proteins of low molecular weight pass through the glomerular filter. The low-molecular-weight proteins are readily reabsorbed by the proximal tubules. The occurrence of large amounts of such proteins in the urine is thus an indication of a loss of tubular reabsorptive function, as in cadmium poisoning (Diamond et al., 2003). On the other hand, excretion of high-molecular-weight protein indicates a loss of integrity of glomeruli. It is to be noted that normal rat urine may contain some protein. A critical comparison of the treated animals with the controls is therefore important.

Glycosuria

Glucose in the glomerular filtrate is completely reabsorbed in the tubules, provided the amount of glucose to be reabsorbed does not exceed the *transport maximum* (Tm). Glycosuria in the absence of hyperglycemia thus indicates tubular dysfunction.

Urine Volume and Osmolarity

These two values are usually inversely related and are useful indicators of renal function in a *concentration test*, wherein water is withheld from the animal, and also in a *dilution test*, wherein a large amount of water is given to the animal. The osmolarity can be estimated from the specific gravity, but the freezing point of urine provides a more accurate measurement. A toxicant may produce high-output renal failure as noted above. On the other hand, it may cause oliguria or even anuria, resulting from tubular injury, with concomitant interstitial edema and intraluminal sediment or debris, which blocks urine flow.

Acidifying Capacity

This can be assessed from urine pH, titratable acids, and NH_4^+. This capacity is reduced when there is distal tubular dysfunction.

Enzymes

Enzymes such as maltase and acid phosphatase in urine may indicate destruction of proximal tubules. Urine alkaline phosphatase, on the other hand, may be renal or hepatic in origin. Plummer (1981) suggested that the urinary enzymes not only are useful indicators of renal damage but also indicate the subcellular site of origin. For example, alkaline phosphatase is located in the endoplasmic reticulum, glutamate dehydrogenase in mitochondria, and lactate dehydrogenase in cytoplasm. In general, urinary enzymes are more useful measures in acute nephrotoxic conditions.

New Biomarkers

Next generation of biomarkers for detecting nephrotoxicity has been investigated (Bonventre et al., 2010; Waring and Moonie, 2011). Potential renal biomarkers include urinary kidney injury molecule-1, neutrophil gelatinase-associated lipocalin, interleukin-18, cystatin C, clusterin, and fatty acid binding protein–liver type. However, these new biomarkers require validation for successful application.

Blood Analysis

Blood Urea Nitrogen

BUN is derived from normal metabolism of protein and is excreted in the urine. Elevated BUN usually indicates glomerular damage and decreased kidney function. However, its level can also be affected by poor nutrition and hepatotoxicity, which are common effects of many toxicants.

Creatinine

Creatinine is a metabolite of creatine and is excreted completely in the urine via glomerular filtration. An elevation of its level in the blood is thus an indication of impaired kidney function. Furthermore, data on its level in blood and its amounts in urine can be used to estimate the glomerular filtration rate. One drawback with this procedure is the fact that the tubules secrete some creatinine.

Special Tests

Glomerular Filtration Rate

GFR can be more accurately determined by the clearance of inulin, a polysaccharide. It is diffused into the glomerular filtrate and is neither reabsorbed nor secreted by the tubules. Reduced GFR indicates impairment of glomerular filtration.

Renal Clearance

This is the volume of plasma that is completely cleared of a substance in a unit of time. The renal clearance of p-aminohippuric acid (PAH) exceeds that of inulin because it is not only filtered through the glomeruli but also secreted by the tubules. A reduction of PAH elimination without a concomitant decrease of GFR indicates tubular dysfunction. PAH is nearly completely (up to 90%) removed from the blood in one passage. The rate of its clearance is therefore useful in determining the effective renal plasma flow. The renal blood flow can also be determined by the use of radiolabeled microspheres or an electromagnetic flow meter.

Phenol Sulfonphthalein Excretion Test

The rate of excretion of phenol sulfonphthalein is related to renal blood flow. It is, therefore, often used in the assessment of renal function. However, a reduced secretion rate can also result from cardiovascular diseases.

NATURE OF TOXICITY

The kidney has a remarkable compensatory capability. Even after appreciable changes in renal functions and morphology, the kidney may compensate and regain normal functions. Therefore, it is important to perform tests at repeated and appropriate time intervals.

Nephrotoxicants can exert adverse effects on various parts of the kidney, resulting in alterations of different functions. A variety of tests should therefore be performed. The most sensitive and reliable tests appear to vary depending on the nature of the nephrotoxicants as well as the experimental conditions (e.g., animal species, duration of exposure). Kluwe (1981) concluded from his studies that in-vitro accumulation of organic ions (e.g., PAH, TEA etc.), urinary concentrating ability, and kidney weight were the most sensitive and consistent indicators of nephrotoxicity. Standard urinalysis, serum analyses, qualitative enzymuria, and histopathological changes were less sensitive and less consistent. It was observed that urine osmolarity was the most sensitive indicator of the nephrotoxicity of a platinum complex, whereas GFR and effective renal plasma flow were affected only later and at higher doses.

In assessing the renal effects of a toxicant, extrarenal factors that might affect the blood volume or blood pressure should be taken into account, since they may indirectly impair renal functions. Furthermore, kidney diseases, such as those associated with aging, may be prevalent and should also be considered.

REFERENCES

Appel GB, Neu HC (1977). The nephrotoxicity of antimicrobial agents (parts 1 and 2). N Engl J Med 296, 663–670, 722–728.

Bonventre JV, Vaidya VS, Schmouder R, et al. (2010). Next-generation biomarkers for detecting kidney toxicity. Nat Biotechnol 28, 436–440.

Brenner BM, Bohrer MP, Baglis C, et al. (1977). Determinants of glomerular permselectivity: Insights derived from observations in vivo. Kidney Int 12, 229–257.

Bunnell JE, Tatu CA, Lerch HE, et al. (2007). Evaluating nephrotoxicity of high-molecular weight organic compounds in drinking water from lignite aquifiers. J Toxicol Environ Health A 70, 2089–2091.

Clark, H.A.. Snedeker, S.M. (2006). Ochratoxin A: Its cancer risk and potentiation for exposure. J Toxicol. Environ Health B 9, 265–296.

Commandeur JNM, Vermeulen NPE (1990). Molecular and biochemical mechanisms of chemically induced nephrotoxicity: A review. Chem Res Toxicol 3, 171–194.

Diamond GL, Thayer WC, Choudhury H (2003). Pharmacokinetics/pharmacodynamics (PK/PD) modeling of risks of kidney toxicity from exposure to cadmium: Estimates of dietary risks in the US population. J Toxicol Environ Health A 66, 2141–2164.

Hook JB, Rose MS, Lock EA (1982). The nephrotoxicity of hexachloro-1:3-butadiene in the rat: Studies of organic anion and cation transport in renal slices and the effects of monoxygenase inducers. Toxicol Appl Pharmacol 65, 373–382.

Humes HD, O'Connor RP (1988). Aminoglycoside nephrotoxicity. In: Shrier RW, Gottschalk CW, eds. Diseases of the Kidney, 4th edn., vol. 2. Boston, MA: Little, Brown.

Hwang S-J, Lai Y-H, Chiu H-F, et al. (2003). Association of death from renal failure with calcium levels in drinking water. J Toxicol Environ Health A 66, 2327–2335.

Kacew S, Ruben Z, McConnell RF (1995). Strain as a determinant factor in the differential responsiveness of rats to chemicals. Toxicol Pathol 23, 701–714.

Kaloyanides GJ (1984). Aminoglycoside-induced functional and biochemical defects in the renal cortex. Fundam Appl Toxicol 4, 930–943.

Kent AL, Maxwell LE, Koina ME, et al. (2007). Renal glomeruli and tubular injury following indomethacin, ibuprofen, and gentamicin exposure in a neonatal rat model. Pediatr Res 62, 307–312.

Kluwe WM (1981). Renal function tests as indicators of kidney injury in subacute toxicity studies. Toxicol Appl Pharmacol 57, 414–424.

Kriz W, Bankir L (1988). A standard nomenclature for structures of the kidney. Am J Physiol 254, F1–F8.

Mazze RI (1976). Methoxyflurane nephropathy. Environ Health Perspect 15, 111–120.

Mingeot-Leclercq MP, Brasseur R, Schank A (1995). Molecular parameters involved in aminoglycoside nephrotoxicity. J Toxicol Environ Health 44, 263–300.

Nanra RS (1974). Pathology, etiology and pathogenesis of analgesic nephropathy. Aust NZJ Med 4, 602–603.

Pestka JJ, Smolinski AT (2005). Deoxynivalenol: Toxicology and potential effects on humans. J Toxicol Environ Health B 8, 39–69.

Phillips R, Yamaguchi M, Cote MG, et al. (1977). Assessment of mercuric chloride-induced nephrotoxicity by p-aminohippuric acid uptake and the activity of four gluconeogenic enzymes in rat renal cortex. Toxicol Appl Pharmacol 41, 407–422.

Plummer DT (1981). Urinary enzyme in drug toxicity. In: Gorrod JW, ed. Testing for Toxicity. London, U.K.: Taylor & Francis.

Racusen LC, Solez K (1988). Cyclosporine nephrotoxicity. Int Rev Expo Pathol 30, 107–157.

Rankin GO (2004). Nephrotoxicity induced by C- and N-arylsuccinimides. J Toxicol Environ Health B 7, 399–416.

Schnellmann RG (1998). Analgesic nephropathy in rodents. J Toxicol Environ Health B 1, 81–90.

Tanaka H, Ishikawa E, Teshima S, et al. (1986). Histopathological study of human cisplatin nephrotoxicity. Toxicol Pathol 14, 247–257.

Waring WS, Moonie A (2011). Earlier recognition of nephrotoxicity using novel biomarkers of acute kidney injury. Clin Toxicol 49, 720–728.

FURTHER READING

WHO (1991). Principles and methods for the assessment of nephrotoxicity associated with exposure to chemicals. Environ Health Criteria 119.

15

Toxicology of the skin

GENERAL CONSIDERATIONS

The body of humans, as well as that of other animals, is almost entirely covered by skin. As a result, it is exposed to a variety of chemicals such as cosmetics, household products, topical medication, heavy metals, and industrial pollutants, especially in certain workplaces. Dermal exposure to chemicals can result in various types of lesions. Furthermore, skin lesions may occur following systemic exposure to chemicals.

The skin consists of the epidermis and the dermis, which rests over the subcutaneous tissue (Fig. 15.1). The epidermis is relatively thin, averaging 0.1–0.2 mm in thickness, whereas the dermis is about 2 mm thick. These two layers are separated by a basement membrane.

The living layer of epidermis in turn consists of a basal cell layer (stratum germinativum), which provides the other layers with new cells. These new cells become prickle cells (stratum spinosum) and, later, the granular cells (stratum granulosum). The nuclei in these cells disintegrate and dissolve. In addition, these cells produce keratohydrin, which later becomes keratin in the outermost stratum corneum, the horny layer. This layer is gradually shed. This development process takes about four weeks. The epidermis also contains melanocytes, which produce pigments; the Langerhans cells, which act as macrophages; and lymphocytes. The latter two types of cells are involved in immune responses. The epidermis thus forms an important protective cover of the body.

The dermis is mainly composed of collagen and elastin, which are important structures for the support of the skin. This layer consists of several types of cells, the most abundant being the fibroblasts, which are involved in the biosynthesis of the fibrous proteins and ground substances such as hyaluronic acid, chondroitin sulfates, and mucopolysaccharides. The other types of cells include fat cells, macrophages, histiocytes, and mast cells. Underneath the dermis is the subcutaneous tissue.

There are, in addition, a number of other structures, such as hair follicles, sweat glands (the exocrine glands), sebaceous glands, small blood vessels, and neural elements.

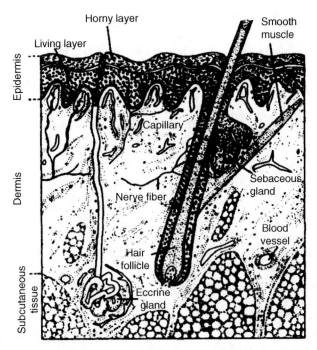

Figure 15.1 Cross section of the skin showing the two major layers of epidermis and dermis, and the various structures in the dermis. *Source*: From Montagna (1965).

The possibility of systemic toxicity following dermal exposure to toxicants is discussed in chapter 2. In addition, dermal reactions may appear following a systemic administration of toxicants. Various types of toxicity of pesticides, industrial chemicals, heavy metals, and industrial chemicals from dermal exposure are discussed in chapters 21, 23, and 26.

TYPES OF TOXIC EFFECTS AND DERMATOTOXICANTS

A variety of effects can result from dermal exposures to toxicants. Most of the effects involve the skin itself, but some of them affect its appendages—hair, sebaceous glands, and sweat glands.

Primary Irritation

Irritation is a reaction of the skin to chemicals such as strong alkalis, acids, solvents, and detergents. Irritation ranges in severity from hyperemia, edema, and vesiculation to ulceration (corrosion). Primary irritations occur at the site of contact and, in general, on the first contact. Irritation is thus different from sensitization.

Table 15.1   Selected Dermal Sensitizers

Antibiotics	Neomycin
Hair dye ingredient	*p*-Phenylenediamine
Local anesthetics	Benzocaine
Metals	Nickel and nickel salts, beryllium, chromium salts, organomercurials (thimerosal)
Pesticides	Captan, ethylenediamine
Poisonous plants	Poison ivy, poison oak

Sensitization Reaction

The skin may show little or no reaction on the first contact with a chemical. However, a reaction or a more severe reaction occurs after a subsequent exposure to the chemical. The induction period ranges from a few days to years. A subsequent exposure to the specific toxicant will elicit a reaction after a delay of 12–48 hours. It is therefore known as "delayed hypersensitivity." A complex immune mechanism is involved in this reaction. Briefly, the toxicant, upon entering the skin, becomes bonded to the surface of certain cells (the antigen presenting cells), which will process it for reaction with T lymphocytes. After such reaction, the sensitized T lymphocytes may release a variety of substances upon re-exposure to the same toxicant and result in hyperemia and edema (see also chaps. 4 and 11).

A variety of chemicals, including topical medicaments, can induce sensitization reactions. Table 15.1 lists a number of them. The chemicals produce a positive response in human patch test with a frequency of 5–11% (Nethercott et al., 1994).

Toluene diisocyanate (TDI), as noted in chapter 12, is an allergenic agent, producing asthma and other effects in the respiratory tract. In addition, it may induce skin sensitization after inhalation (Ebino et al., 2001).TDI is used in the pharmaceutical industry for development of anti-asthmatic medications.

Phototoxicity and Photoallergy

These two types of skin reaction are similar in that both are light induced and may follow either systemic administration or topical application of the offending chemical. However, photoallergy involves immune reactions, whereas phototoxicity does not. This and other differences have been summarized by Harber and Baer (1972) (Table 15.2).

Phototoxicity is more common than photoallergy. The commonly reported phototoxic chemicals in humans, according to Harber et al. (1987), are aminobenzoic acid derivatives, anthraquinone dyes, chlorpromazine, chlorothiazides, phenothiazines, sulfanilamide, and coal tar derivatives (e.g., anthracene, pyridine, acridine, and phenanthrene). The skin reaction consists of a delayed erythema, followed by hyperpigmentation and desquamation.

Table 15.2   Comparison of Phototoxic and Photoallergic Reactions

Reaction	Phototoxic	Photoallergic
Reaction possible on first exposure	Yes	No
Incubation period necessary after first exposure	No	Yes
Chemical alteration of photosensitizer	No	Yes
Covalent binding with carrier	No	Yes
Clinical changes	Usually like sunburn	Varied morphology
Flares at distant previously involved sites possible	No	Yes
Persistent light reactions can develop	No	Yes
Cross-reactions to structurally related agents	Infrequent	Frequent
Concentration of drug necessary for reaction	High	Low
Incidence	Usually relatively high	Usually very low
Passive transfer	No	Possible
Lymphocyte stimulation test	No	Possible
Macrophage migration inhibition test	No	Possible

Source: From Harber and Baer (1972).

The commonly reported photoallergic chemicals include aminobenzoic acids, chlorpromazine, chlorpropamide, 2,2-thiobis(4-chlorophenol) (Fentichlor), halogenated salicylanilides, promethazine, sulfanilamide, and thiazides (Harber et al., 1987) (Table 15.3). Many compounds are, therefore, both phototoxic and photoallergic. Clinically, photoallergy usually manifests as delayed papules and eczema, but it may also appear as immediate urticarial reaction. Histologically, it is characterized by a dense perivascular round cell infiltrate in the dermis. The delayed reactions are Type IV T-cell–mediated immune response, whereas the immediate reaction is probably antibody mediated (chap. 11).

The most biologically active rays that produce erythema and pigmentation are in the shorter ultraviolet range, that is, wavelengths below 320 nm. The sunlight ranges from 290 nm upward, but the UV rays emitted by artificial light sources may be shorter. However, the longer UV rays (320–400 nm) per se are less erythrogenic, but are responsible for both phototoxic and photoallergic reactions to chemicals (see the section "Testing Procedures").

Contact Urticaria/Urticarial Reactions

These skin reactions, in the form of urticaria or eczema, appear within minutes to an hour after contact with the offending substance. Hence they are different from the sensitization reaction described above. The mechanism may be non-immunological, such as the case with aspirin and methyl nicotinate. In other cases, for example, latex rubber and penicillin, an immunologic mechanism is involved. However, unlike the sensitization reaction described earlier, an antibody (IgE),

Table 15.3   Examples of Phototoxic Photoallergic Chemicals

Chemicals	Phototoxicity	Photoallergy
Aminobenzoic acid derivatives	+	+
Chlorpromazine	+	+
Chlorothiazide	+	+
Methoxy psoralens	+	−
Psoralens	+	−
Sulfonamides	+	+
Tetracyclines	+	−
Coal tar derivatives	+	−
Nonsteroidal anti inflammatory drugs	+	−

rather than T cell, is involved. In both immunological and non-immunological cases, the dermal reactions are elicited by vasoactive substances, for example, histamine along with prostaglandins, leukotrienes, and kinins. A great variety of substances have been reported to induce these reactions, including metals (copper and platinum), medicaments (antibiotics and local anesthetics), and biogenic polymers released from arthropods (jellyfish). Amin et al. (1995) provided extensive lists of agents that induce immunological and non-immunological immediate contact reactions. Urticarial actions may also follow ingested or parenterally administered agents.

Cutaneous Cancer

It has been known for over two centuries that soots produce skin cancer (chap. 7). More recent studies confirm that soots and related substances, such as coal tars, creosote oils, shale oils, and cutting oil, induce cancers of the skin and other sites in animals and humans. In addition, arsenic and certain arsenic compounds have been reported to be associated with skin cancer in humans (chap. 21).

A number of polycyclic aromatic hydrocarbons (e.g., benzo[*a*]pyrene) and heterocyclic compounds (e.g., benz[*c*]acridine) are known to induce skin cancer after topical applications on animals (IARC, 1973). UV radiation is an important cause of skin cancer in humans, and a number of chemicals influence the effect of UV light and vice versa (Forbes, 1995; Brozyna and Chwirot, 2006). Other risk factors for skin cancer include chronic wounds, inflammation, irritation, acute trauma, and a history of sunburns early in life (Kasper et al., 2011),

Effects on Epidermal Adnexa

Hair

Loss of hair may result from various antimitotic agents used in cancer chemotherapy. These agents affect the anagen phase of hair growth. The affected hair starts to shed after about two weeks of therapy, but hair growth resumes about two months after the suspension of therapy.

A number of other medications are known to cause hair loss by converting hair follicles in the anagen phase to telogen phase. In such cases, hair shedding generally starts 24 months after therapy. The medications involved in this type of hair loss include oral contraceptives, anticoagulants, propranolol, and triparanol.

Sebaceous Glands

These glands secrete lipid through expulsion of their lipid-laden cells and are therefore known as *holocrine*. Their activity is hormone dependent. For example, androgens stimulate and estrogens inhibit the excretion. Adrenocortical steroids and thyroid hormones also have some stimulatory activity. Acne may be formed as a result of proliferation of the follicular epithelium of the sebaceous gland. Topically applied substances such as greases and oils, and systemically administered substances such as iodides and bromides, may increase the formation of acnes.

A number of chlorinated aromatic hydrocarbons produce various skin lesions, including *chloracne*, which is characterized by small straw-colored cysts and comedones in which the sebaceous gland is replaced by a keratinous cyst. The severity of chloracne varies, but it has been noted among occupational workers. However, it was more notable in the outbreaks in Japan among individuals after their consumption of a batch of rice oil contaminated with polychlorinated biphenyls (WHO, 1976), and in Seveso, Italy, among residents near a factory that accidentally released a large amount of 2,3,7,8-tetrachlorodibenzo-*p*-dioxin (Pocchiari, 1980).

Sweat Glands

Sweating serves useful physiological functions such as regulation of body temperature. Blockage of the sweat ducts, a disorder known as miliaria, may occur after topical application of 95% phenol and chloroform (Shelley and Horvath, 1950).

TESTING PROCEDURES

Primary Irritation

This effect is in general measured by a patch test on the skin of rabbits (Draize, 1959). A small amount (0.5 g or 0.5 mL) of the chemical to be tested is introduced under a 1-sq.inch gauze pad that is placed over a shaved part of the skin. The pad is suitably fastened over the animal for 24 hours. At the end of this period, the pad is removed and the skin reaction is graded according to the extent of (i) erythema and eschar formation and (ii) edema formation. The skin reaction is read again at the end of 72 hours. The same test is done on other rabbits, except that the skin has been abraded. The 24- and 72-hour readings from both groups are added to obtain the *primary irritation index* (PII). The test procedure, grading of skin reaction, and interpretation of the grading are given in Appendix 1.

There are a number of modified skin irritation tests based on the Draize procedure. The modifications involve the animal species and the number of animals used; quantity of the test material applied; repetitive applications; and types of examinations.

Sensitization Reaction

The procedure described by Draize (1959) calls for the use of guinea pigs that are given the chemical by 10 repeated intradermal injections on one flank and a challenging dose on the other flank after a 10- to 14-day resting period. A greater reaction after the challenging dose, in comparison with that after the sensitizing doses, indicates sensitization.

The *Draize test* is generally considered insufficiently sensitive to identify allergic potential. Magnusson and Kligman (1969), therefore, recommended the use of the *maximization test* in which the guinea pigs are given intradermally on day 0 the test substance with and without Freund's complete adjuvant. On day 7, the substance is applied at the same site occlusively. Two weeks later, the test substance is applied topically over the pretreated areas in these animals. Different concentrations of the agent are used in the challenge. Recently, OECD (1992) has adopted this and the Buehler test which requires the application of the chemical under closed patches.

Human experience is obtained either in patch tests or in a controlled population. In the latter case, the substance is widely distributed to the target population for use as directed. Their skin reactions are examined and evaluated. A patch test usually involves 100 men and 100 women, covering a wide age range. The test material (0.5 mL or 0.5 g) is applied by patch to an area on the arm or back. The skin reaction is examined on the following day after the removal of the patch.

Phototoxicity and Photoallergy

Phototoxicity appears to be more readily demonstrable in the hairless mouse, the rabbit, and the guinea pig. The substance to be tested may be administered topically or by a systemic route. The reaction of the skin to non-erythrogenic light (wavelength greater than 320 nm) is then determined. Significant erythema, compared with controls, indicates phototoxicity.

For the detection of photoallergy, albino guinea pigs are especially useful. The procedure involves, in principle, an induction of photosensitization by repeatedly applying a small amount of the chemical on a shaved and depilated area of the skin and exposing that area to appropriate UV rays. After a three-week interval, the guinea pigs are exposed to the chemical and the UV rays to elicit photoallergy.

Contact Urticaria

A number of animal models have been proposed based on the procedure devised by Jacobs (1940). These generally involve a patch test on the flank and nipples of guinea pigs. Recently, a test using guinea pig ears has been found satisfactory in screening human contact with urticarigenic substances (Lahti and Maibach, 1984).

The open patch test can be applied to human volunteers or to patients suspected of being susceptible to the chemical. In the latter case, all necessary resuscitation equipment and qualified personnel should be available to respond to anaphylactoid reaction.

Any immunological involvement can be demonstrated by the passive transfer test in which 0.1 mL fresh serum from the patient is injected intradermally into the forearm of a volunteer and challenged 24 hours later by applying the suspect chemical to the injection site.

Cutaneous Cancer

The procedure involves topical application of the substance on a shaved area of the skin. The substance per se, if a liquid, is applied directly. Otherwise, it is dissolved or suspended in a suitable vehicle. The skin painting is usually done once a week or more frequently. The commonly used animal is the mouse. It is advisable to include a vehicle control group as well as a positive control group, which is treated with a known skin carcinogen such as benzo[a]pyrene.

REFERENCES

Amin S, Lahti A, Maibach HI (1995). Immediate contact reactions: Contact urticaria and the contact urticaria syndrome. In: Marzulli FN, Maibach HI, eds. Dermatotoxicology, 5th ed. Washington, DC.: Taylor & Francis.

Brozyna A, Chwirot BW (2006). Porcine skin as a model system for studies of ultraviolet effects in human skin. J Toxicol Environ Health A 69, 1155–1165.

Draize JH (1959). Dermal toxicity. In: Editorial Committee of the Association of Food and Drug Officials of the United States, eds. Appraisal of the Safety of Chemicals in Foods, Drugs and Cosmetics. Association of Food & Drug Officials of the United States

Ebino K, Ueda H, Kawakatsu H, et al. (2001). Isolated airway exposure to toluene diisocyate results skin sensitization. Toxicol Lett 121, 79–85.

Forbes PD (1995). Carcinogenesis and photocarcinogenesis test methods. In: Marzull FN, Maibach HI, eds. Dermatotoxicology. Washington, DC.: Taylor & Francis.

Harber LC, Baer RL (1972). Pathogenic mechanisms of drug-induced photosensitivity. J Invest Dermatol 58, 327–342.

Harber LS, Shalita AR, Armstrong RB (1987). Immunologically mediated contact photosensitivity in guinea pigs. In: Marzulli FN, Maibach HI, eds. Dermatotoxicology. Washington, DC.: Hemisphere, 413–430.

IARC (1973). Certain polycyclic aromatic hydrocarbons and heterocyclic compounds. IARC Monographs on the Evaluation of Carcinogenic Risk of the Chemical to Man, vol. 3. Lyon, France: International Agency for Research on Cancer.

Jacobs JL (1940). Immediate generalized skin reactions in hypersensitive guinea pigs. ProcSoc Exp Biol Med 43, 641–643.

Kasper M, Jaks V, Are A, et al. (2011). Wounding enhances epidermal tumorigenesis by recruiting hair follicle keratinocytes. Proc Natl Acad Sci 108, 4099–4104.

Lahti A, Maibach HI (1984). An animal model for nonimmunologic contact urticaria. Toxicol Appl Pharmacol 76, 219–224.

Magnusson B, Kligman AM (1969). The identification of contact allergens by animal assay. The guinea pig maximization test. J Invest Dermatol 52, 268–276.

Montagna W (1965). The skin. Sci Am 212: 56–65.

Nethercott JR, Holness DL, Adams RM, et al. (1994). Multivariate analysis of the effect of selected factors on the elicitation of patch test response to 28 common environmental contactants in North America. Am J Contact Dermatitis 5, 13–18.

OECD (1992). OECD Guidelines for Testing Chemicals. Paris: Organization for Economic Cooperation and Development.

Pocchiari F (1980). Accidental release of 2,3,7,8-tetrachlorodibenzo-*p*-dioxin (TCDD) at Seveso, Italy. Ecotoxicol Environ Saf 4, 282.

Shelley WB, Horvath PN (1950). Experimental miliaria in man. II. Production of sweat retention anhidrosis and miliaria crystallina by various kinds of injury. J Invest Dermatol 1, 9–20.

WHO (1976). Polychlorinated biphenyls and terphenyls. Environ Health Criteria, 2nd edn. Geneva, Switzerland: World Health Organization.

APPENDIX 1   PRIMARY IRRITATION

Primary irritation of the skin is measured by a patch-test technique on the abraded and intact skin of the albino rabbit clipped free of hair. A minimum of six subjects is used per preparation tested. The method consists of introducing under a 1-inch patch 0.5 mL (in case of liquids) or 0.5 g (in cases of solids and semisolids) of the test substance to an area of skin approximately 1 inch × 1 inch (2.54 cm × 2.54 cm) square and to each site (two sites per rabbit). It is also desirable in the case of solids to attempt solubilizing in an appropriate solvent and to apply the solution as for liquids. The animals are immobilized in an animal holder with patches secured in place by adhesive tape. The entire trunk of the animal is then wrapped with a rubberized cloth for the entire 24-hour period of exposure. This latter procedure aids in maintaining the test patches in position, and, in addition, retards the evaporation of volatile substances. After the 24 hours of exposure, the patches are removed and the resulting reactions are evaluated on the basis of scores in Table A1. Readings are also made after 72 hours, and the final score represents an average of 24- and 72-hour readings. An equal number of exposures are made on areas of skin, which have been previously abraded. The abrasions are minor incisions through the stratum corneum, but not sufficiently deep to disturb the derma (i.e., not sufficiently deep to produce bleeding).

The total erythema and edema scores are added in both the 24- and 72-hour readings, and the averages of the scores for intact and abraded skin are combined. This combined average is referred to as the PII. It is useful for placing compounds in general groups with reference to irritant properties.

Compounds producing combined averages (PIIs) of 2 or less are only mildly irritating; whereas those with indexes from 2 to 5 are moderate irritants, and those with scores above 6 are considered severe irritants.

Table A1   Evaluation of Skin Reactions

Erythema and Eschar Formation	Score
No erythema	0
Very slight erythema (barely perceptible)	1
Well-defined erythema	2
Moderate-to-severe erythema	3
Severe erythema (beet redness) to slight eschar formation (injuries in depth)	4
Total possible erythema score	4
Edema formation	
No edema	0
Very slight edema (barely perceptible)	1
Slight edema (edges of area well defined by definite raising)	2
Moderate edema (raised approximately 1 mm)	3
Severe edema (raised more than 1 mm and extending beyond the area of exposure)	4
Total possible edema score	4

Source: From Draize (1959).

16

Toxicology of the eye

GENERAL CONSIDERATIONS

Although the eyes are relatively small, they are important to one's well-being and they are complex in structure.

The eye is a spherical body that is covered mainly by three coats of tissues: the sclera, choroids, and retina. These coats mainly consist of, respectively, fibrous tissues; pigments and blood vessels; and nerve fibers, cells, and special receptors. They are nontransparent. However, light is admitted through the front of the eye, where the three coats are replaced by a number of tissues, notably the cornea and the lens (Fig. 16.1(A)).

The cornea is a continuum of the sclera. It consists of a relatively thick stroma and is covered, in front, by an epithelium, consisting of several layers of cells and Bowman's membranes, and, behind, by Descemet's membrane and an endothelium. The cornea and the front portion of the sclera as well as the inside of the eyelids are covered by a thin layer of conjunctiva.

The lens consists of transparent fibers enclosed in the lens capsule. It is suspended by the ciliary zonule to the ciliary body and its curvature is adjustable by the contraction and relaxation of the ciliary muscle.

The space between the lens and the cornea is filled with the aqueous humor. Also in this space and immediately in front of the lens is the iris. It is rich in blood vessels and heavily pigmented. The iris has a central opening, the pupil. Filling the space between the lens and retina is the vitreous humor.

The retina is the ocular structure that responds to light stimuli. It consists of several layers (Fig. 16.1(B)). The outermost is a pigmented epithelium. Next to it are the retinal rods and cones, which are the light-responsive neural structures. They are connected via the bipolar cells to the ganglion cells. The axons from the latter cells converge and exit from the eye at the optic papilla as the optic nerve.

Because of their diverse physiological nature and spatial relations, these various ocular structures may exhibit a variety of effects as a result of exposure to toxicants.

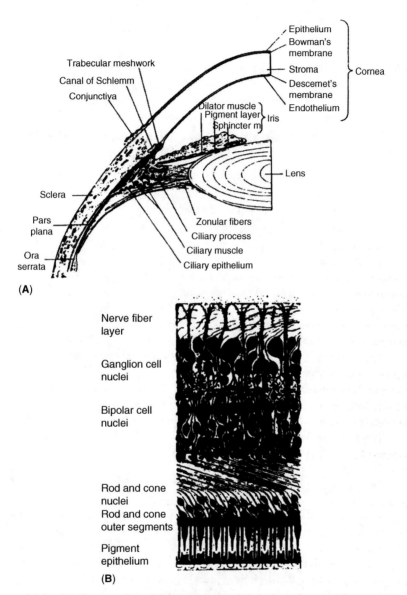

Figure 16.1 (**A**) Cross section of the anterior chamber angle and surrounding structures. (**B**) Cross section of the retina. *Source*: From Vaughan and Asbury (1983) and Polyak (1940) respectively.

TOXICANTS AND THE SITES THEY CAN AFFECT

Cornea

The cornea is a delicate structure and is subject to toxic effects of chemicals, mainly from external exposure. Chemicals that affect the cornea include acids, alkalies, detergents, organic solvents, and smog. Acids and alkalies can readily damage the cornea. The extent of damage ranges from minor, superficial destruction of the tissue, which heals completely, to opacity of the cornea or even perforation. Acid burns are related to the low pH as well as the affinity of the anion for the corneal tissue. The effects of alkalies usually have slower onset than those caused by acids and are essentially pH-dependent. However, ammonium ion, which is present in many household products, penetrates the cornea more readily and can thereby affect the iris (Potts, 1996).

Detergents are useful household and industrial products. In general, the nonionic detergents are less damaging than the ionic agents, and the cationics are more damaging than the anionics (Draize and Kelley, 1952). Organic solvents, such as acetone, hexane, and toluene, may enter the eye as a result of industrial or laboratory accidents. These substances can dissolve fat and damage the corneal epithelial cells.

Smog is a mixture of industrial smoke and fog. However, it now refers more often to the photochemical reaction products of automobile exhaust (see chap. 23). These products accumulate under certain meteorological conditions. They affect mainly the respiratory tract, but even at low concentrations they irritate the corneal sensory nerve endings and cause reflex lacrimation.

Other chemicals can affect the cornea following *systemic administration*. These include quinacrine, chloroquine, and chlorpromazine. Potts (1996) reviewed the corneal effects of these drugs and other chemicals. They affect the cornea via tears and/or after passing through the blood–aqueous barrier. However, they affect humans only rarely and only after large doses.

Iris, Aqueous Humor, and Ciliary Body

Because of its proximity to the cornea, the iris is susceptible to physical trauma and chemical irritation. The effects of such irritation consist of leakage of serum proteins and fibrin as well as leukocytes from the blood vessels. These may be followed by fibroblast metaplasia. Severe damages to the iris cause liberation of melanin granules from the posterior epithelium of the iris.

The iris is innervated by sympathetic nerves (for the dilator muscles) and parasympathetic nerves (for the constrictor muscles). Therefore, the pupil can be dilated by chemicals that are sympathomimetic or parasympatholytic and it can be constricted by parasympathomimetic and sympatholytic chemicals. Furthermore, the size of the pupil can be altered via the central nervous system by chemicals such as morphine and general anesthetics.

The aqueous humor is secreted by the epithelium of the ciliary body into the posterior chamber. It flows through the pupil into the anterior chamber and drains through the canal of Schlemm at the angle of the anterior chamber. Inflammatory changes of the iris can block the drainage of the fluid through the canal of Schlemm and raise the intraocular pressure, thereby inducing glaucoma. Atropine and other mydriatics may also precipitate glaucoma by dilating the pupil, thus blocking the drainage. Corticosteroids, applied topically or systemically, can also increase the intraocular pressure and cause glaucoma.

The ciliary muscle lies in the ciliary body. The contraction of the ciliary muscle allows relaxation of the ciliary zonule, which in turn allows the lens capsule to assume a more spherical form. This muscle is parasympathetically innervated; therefore, acetylcholinesterase inhibitors and parasympatholytic agents such as atropine can cause the lens to be fixed in different states of visual accommodation.

Lens

A number of chemicals are known to alter the lenticular transparency, resulting in the formation of cataract. Examples are 2,4-dinitrophenol, corticosteroids, busulfan, triparanol, and thallium. Their cataractogenic property has been noted in humans as well as in animals, such as the rabbit, rat, and young fowl. The effects generally follow systemic exposure, but with certain chemicals (e.g., corticosteroids and anticholinesterases), they may occur after topical application (Woods et al., 1967; Axelsson, 1968).

Diabetic patients are more likely to have cataracts, which can also be produced in rats and rabbits rendered diabetic with alloxan or streptozotocin (Heywood, 1982).

In addition, rats fed large amounts of galactose develop cataract (Sippel, 1966). This condition may be comparable to the cataract observed in infants with galactosemia. Such galactosemia results from a metabolic inability, inherited as an autosomal recessive trait, to convert galactose to glucose, because of the absence of the enzyme galactose-1-phosphate uridylyl transferase (Kinosita, 1965).

On the other hand, deficiencies of certain nutrients may also induce cataract. These nutrients include tryptophan, proteins, vitamin E, riboflavin, and folic acid (Gehring, 1971).

The mechanism underlying the formation of cataract is not fully understood. It is likely that it varies with the nature of the toxicant. For example, corticosteroid cataract may be mediated through an inhibition of protein synthesis in the lens (Ono, 1972). Busulfan may act through an interference of mitosis of the lenticular epithelial cells (Grimes and von Sallmann, 1966). Triparanol may interfere with the Na^+ pump, resulting in an increase of Na^+ and water in the lens (Harris and Gruber, 1972). The effect of dinitrophenol is likely to be mediated through the uncoupling of oxidative phosphorylation (see also chap. 4).

An extensive review of cataractogenic chemicals has been prepared by Gehring (1971). The cataractogenic chemicals are listed in Appendix 1.

Apart from cataractogenic effects, which are permanent, transient lens opacity has been noted in young beagle dogs following administration of some tranquilizers, some diuretics, and diisophenol. In addition, the transparency and refraction of the lens may also be altered by dimethyl sulfoxide and *p*-chlorophenylalanine (Heywood, 1982).

Ultraviolet (UV)-A or UV-B radiation can induce cataract, and lead to impaired vision and transient or permanent blindness (Roberts, 2011). Increased risks for cataracts were observed among Japanese A-bomb survivors and Chernobyl clean-up workers even at low to moderate radiation doses (Shore et al., 2010). Other risk factors include aging, women, smoking, heavy drinking, myopia, and long-term exposure to heavy metals (e.g., lead, gold, and copper).

Retina

Certain polycyclic compounds, such as chloroquine, hydroxychloroquine, and thioridazine, can induce retinopathy in humans and animals. They affect the visual acuity, dark adaptation, and retinal pigment pattern. Hyperoxia and iodate may also induce retinal changes.

Different mechanisms are involved in these retinal effects. Inhibition of protein metabolism in the pigment epithelium has been suggested as the primary toxic effect of chloroquine and hydroxychloroquine, which have strong affinity for melanin (Meier-Ruge, 1972). Increased oxygen supply to the retina induces vasoconstriction, which is associated with a decrease in the supply of nutrients. The latter effect is probably responsible for the hyperoxia-induced retinal changes. Iodate apparently affects the pigment epithelium, the derangement of which results in the degeneration of the rod layer. Various reviewed modes of action have been provided by Heywood (1982). These include the early formation of membranous cytoplasmic bodies (myeloid bodies), degenerative changes in the cell body of the rods and cones, derangement of the intracytoplasmic rods, and the appearance of vacuoles around these rods in the tapetum.

Leong et al. (1987) reported that an important chemical intermediate, 4,4-methylenedianiline, a well-known hepatotoxicant, induces degeneration of the inner and outer segments of the photoreceptor cells in albino and pigmented guinea pigs. Other retinal effects include hemorrhage from the rupture of blood vessels or disturbance of blood clotting mechanism and exudates, which may cause partial detachment of retina.

Hayasaka et al. (2011) reported that supplementation of long-term (exceeding a few years) ornithine and high blood concentrations (exceeding 600 μmol/L) of ornithine can induce retinal toxicity in gyrate atrophy of the choroid and retina (GA). Therefore, patients with GA were recommended to avoid taking ornithine; amino acid supplementation should be administered carefully for patients with the hyperornithinemia–hyperammonemia–homocitrullinuria syndrome.

Optic Nerve

As noted above, the retina contains, among other structures, the ganglion cells, the axons of which form the optic nerve. Toxicants can affect either the ganglion cells or the optic nerve. Damage to one of them often results in the degeneration of the other.

Some toxicants affect mainly the central vision. The most notable example is methanol. Others include carbon disulfide, disulfiram, ethambutol, and thallium. On the other hand, quinine, chloroquine, pentavalent arsenic, and carbon monoxide cause constriction of visual fields by damaging the structures responsible for peripheral vision. Interestingly, nitrobenzol affects both the central and peripheral vision (Harrington, 1976). While methyl mercury also causes constriction of the visual field, its toxic effect is on the visual cortex instead of the optic nerve (chap. 21).

These toxicants can also be classified according to their effects on other peripheral nerves. For example, quinine, ethambutol, and methanol generally do not affect other peripheral nerves, while carbon disulfide, disulfiram, and thallium cause both optic and peripheral neuropathies. It is worthy to note that certain organic solvents can induce peripheral neuropathy but spare the visual system. These include tri-o-cresyl phosphate, acrylamide, n-hexane, and methyl n-butyl ketone (Grant, 1980).

Clioquinol (also known as Vioform and Entero-Vioform) was widely used for the prevention and treatment of "traveler's diarrhea." It has reportedly caused more than 10,000 cases of subacute myelo-opticoneuropathy, a disease affecting the optic nerves, spinal tracts, and peripheral nerves (Potts, 1996).

TESTING PROCEDURES

Effects on the eye can be examined after topical application of the toxicants. In addition, systemic administration can also result in ocular alterations. Several types of examinations are available.

Albino rabbits are commonly used to determine the ocular irritancy of ophthalmic medications and other chemicals that might come in contact with the eye. Dogs and nonhuman primates (rhesus monkeys) have also been used. For studying the effects of toxicants on the lens, retina, and optical nerve, many species of animals are used such as rat, rabbit, cat, dog, monkey, and pig.

Gross Examination

The test described by Draize and Kelley (1952) has been a standard procedure for testing ocular irritancy. It specifies the use of nine rabbits. Into one eye of each rabbit, 0.1 mL of the test material is instilled. In three of the nine rabbits, the test material is washed with 20 mL lukewarm water two seconds after the instillation, and in three others, the washing is done with a four-second delay. In the three remaining rabbits, the material is left in the eye. The ocular reactions are read with the unaided eye or with the aid of a slit-lamp at 24, 48, and 72 hours and at four and seven days after treatment. The reactions on the conjunctiva (redness, chemosis, and discharge), cornea (the degree and extent of opacity), and iris (congestion, swelling, and circumcorneal injection) are scored according to a specified scale.

A series of colored pictures, originally provided by the U.S. Food and Drug Administration in 1965 as a guide for grading eye irritation, are available from the U.S. Consumer Product Safety Commission, Washington, D.C. Samples were reproduced in Hackett and McDonald (1995).

Several modified versions of the Draize and Kelley test have been proposed. Griffith et al. (1980) reported on their results of assessing eye irritancy of a large number of substances. The irritancy ranged from nil to corrosive. The authors recommend that the following points should be taken into account in conducting eye irritation tests:

1. A 0.01 mL dose, or its weight equivalent for solids and powders, should be applied directly to the central corneal surface of at least six eyes without subsequent rinsing or manipulation of the eyelids.
2. Evaluation of the irritancy should be based on the median duration for the eyes to return to normal, instead of using a scoring system based on the type and extent of the effects.

The latest U.S. federal agency regulation (CPSC, 1988) requires the use of six albino rabbits for each test substance. For test liquids, 0.1 mL of the test material is used, and for solids and pastes, 100 mg of the test material is used. The test material is instilled into one eye of each rabbit without washing. Ocular examinations are done after 24, 48, and 72 hours. A rabbit is considered as having positive reaction if the eye shows, on any examination, ulceration or opacity of the cornea, inflammation of the iris, or swelling of the conjunctiva with partial eversion of the eyelids.

Another variation of the Draize procedure calls for the use of three rabbits whose eyes are examined at 1, 24, 48, and 72 hours. However, only one albino rabbit should be used first, if marked effects are expected. Furthermore, if it is thought that the substance could cause unreasonable pain, a local anesthetic should be used. The grading of the eye irritation is as shown in Appendix 2 (OECD, 1987).

Instrumental Examinations

Ophthalmoscopy

The ophthalmoscope is used in assessing effects of toxicants on various parts of the retina. The examination is generally intended to discover the existence of edema, hyperemia, or pallor; atrophy of the optic disk, pigmentation, or the state of the blood vessels. Changes in the vitreous humor, lens, aqueous humor, iris, and cornea can also be observed.

Visual Perimetry

Effect on the visual field can be readily determined in humans, but not in laboratory animals, except the nonhuman primates. Merigan (1979) described a procedure using macaque monkeys to demonstrate the loss of peripheral vision resulting from exposure to methyl mercury.

Other Procedures

Visual acuity and color vision are sensitive and useful indicators of effects on the visual system in humans. Procedures involving instrumentation, such as electro-oculography, and visual-evoked responses are also useful and can be incorporated in animal experimentation (Grant, 1980).

Histological and Biochemical Examinations

Light microscopy can usually pinpoint the site of action of toxicants, electron microscopy can demonstrate ultrastructural changes, and biochemical studies can reveal the mechanism of toxic effects. For example, with light microscopy, chloroquine has been observed to cause a thickening of the pigment epithelium, followed by migration of the pigment to the outer nuclear layer, and finally total atrophy of the photoreceptors (Meier-Ruge, 1968). Electron microscopy showed mitochondrial swelling and disorganization of the endoplasmic reticulum in the photoreceptor inner segment (Solze and McConnell, 1970). Biochemical studies revealed inhibition of many enzymatic reactions, especially those related to protein metabolism of the pigment epithelium.

In-Vitro Tests

Owing to humane concerns about the use of animals in eye irritation tests, a number of in-vitro tests have been developed. They involve the use of cells from isolated cornea and chorioallantoic membrane and measuring their uptake of dyes, such as neutral red, as an indicator of toxicity. Other proposed procedures include isolated rabbit eye and isolated chicken eye (Green, 1998). However, these tests apparently require much refinement and extensive validation.

EVALUATION

Eye irritation tests are widely used to assess the ocular irritancy of chemicals. In general, the albino rabbit is the animal of choice. Some intra-laboratory and inter-laboratory variations in the scores were noted in a collaborative study (Marzulli and Ruggles, 1973). Nevertheless, periodic collaborative studies tend to improve the reliability of the scores. The various modifications made on the Draize test also tend to reduce the variability of the results.

A large number of animal experimentations and clinical studies indicate that there is a fair correlation between humans and animals in their reactions to toxicants with respect to cataract formation and retinopathy (Grant, 1980; Potts, 1996).

REFERENCES

Axelsson U (1968). Glaucoma, miotic therapy and cataract. III. Visual loss due to lens changes in glaucoma eyes treated with paraoxon (Mintacol), echothiophate or pilocarpine. Acta Ophthalmol 46, 831.

CPSC (1988). Consumer product safety commission. Test for eye irritants. Code of federal regulations, Title 16. Federal Hazardous Substances Act Regulation, Part 1500.42.

Draize JH, Kelley EA (1952). Toxicity to eye mucosa of certain cosmetic preparations containing surface-active agents. Proc Sci Sect Toilet Goods Assoc 17, 1–4.

Gehring PJ (1971). The cataractogenic activity of chemical agents. CRC Crit Rev Toxicol 1, 93–118.

Grant WM (1980). The peripheral visual system as a target. In: Spencer BS, Schaumburg HH, eds. Experimental and Clinical Neurotoxicology. Baltimore, MD: Williams & Wilkins.

Green S (1998). Update on agency initiatives in alternative methods. In: Margulli FN, Maribach HI, eds. Dermatology Methods: The Laboratory Worker's Vade McCum. Philadelphia, PA: Taylor & Francis, 377–82.

Griffith JF, Nixon GA, Bruce RD, et al. (1980). Dose–response studies with chemical irritants in the albino rabbit eye as a basis for selecting optimum testing conditions for predicting hazard to the human eye. Toxicol Appl Pharmacol 55, 501–13.

Grimes P, Von Sallmann L (1966). Interference with cell proliferation and induction of polyploidy in rat lens epithelium during prolonged Myleran treatment. Exp Cell Res 62, 265–73.

Hackett RB, McDonald TO (1995). Assessing ocular irritation. In: Marzulli FN, Maibach HI, eds. Dermatotoxicology. Washington, DC.: Taylor & Francis.

Harrington DO (1976). The Visual Fields. St. Louis, MI: Mosby.

Harris JE, Gruber L (1972). Reversal of triparanol-induced cataracts in the rat. II. Exchange of 22Na, 42K, 86Rb in cataractous and clearing lenses. Invest Ophthalmol Vis Sci 11, 608–16.

Hayasaka S, Kodama T, Ohira A (2011). Retinal risks of high-dose ornithine supplements: a review. Br J Nutr 106, 801–11.

Heywood R (1982). Histopathological and laboratory assessment of visual dysfunction. Environ Health Perspect 44, 35–45.

Kinosita JH (1965). Cataracts in galactosemia. Invest Ophthalmol Vis Sci 4, 786–99.

Leong BKJ, Lund JE, Groehn JA, et al. (1987). Retinopathy from inhaling 4,4'-methylene-dianiline aerosols. Fundam Appl Toxicol 9, 645–58.

Marzulli FN, Ruggles DI (1973). Rabbit eye irritation test: collaborative study. J Am Assoc Anal Chem 56, 905–14.

Meier-Ruge M (1968). The pathophysiological morphology of the pigment epithelium and its importance for retinal structure and function. Med Prob Ophthalmol 8, 32–48.

Meier-Ruge W (1972). Drug-induced retinopathy. CRC Crit Rev Toxicol 1, 325–60.

Merigan WH (1979). Effects of toxicants on visual systems. Neurobehav Toxicol 1(Suppl. 1), 1522.

OECD (1987). OECD Guidelines for Testing of Chemicals. Paris: Organization for Economic Cooperation and Development.

OECD (2002). OECD guidelines for the testing of chemicals test no. 405. Acute Eye irritation/corrosion. Available from: http://www.oecd-ilibrary.org/environment/test-no-405-acute-eye-irritation-corrosion_9789264070646-en.

Ono S (1972). Presence of corticol-binding protein in the lens. Ophthalmic Res 3, 233–40.

Polyak S (1940). The Retina. Chicago, IL: University of Chicago Press.

Potts AM (1996). Toxic responses of the eye. In: Klaassen CD, ed. Casarett and Doull's Toxicology. New York, NY: McGraw-Hill.

Roberts JE (2011). Ultraviolet radiation as a risk factor for cataract and macular degeneration. Eye Contact Lens 37, 246–9.

Shore RE, Neriishi K, Nakashima E (2010). Epidemiological studies of cataract risk at low to moderate radiation doses: (not) seeing is believing. Radiat Res 174, 889–94.

Sippel TO (1966). Changes in water, protein and glutathione contents of the lens in the course of galactose cataract development in rats. Invest Ophthalmol Vis Sci 5, 568–75.

Solze DA, McConnell DG (1970). Ultrastructural changes in the rat photoreceptor inner segment during experimental chloroquine retinopathy. Ophthal Res 1, 140–8.

Vaughan D, Ashbury T (1983). General Ophthalmology, 10th edn. Los Altos, CA: Lange Medical Publications.

Woods DC, Contaxis I, Sweet D, et al. (1967). Response of rabbits to corticosteroids. I. Influence on growth, intraocular pressure and lens transparency. Am J Ophthalmol 63, 841–9.

Appendix 1   Cataractogenic Chemicals

Sugars (Glucose, Galactose, Xylose)	Tyrosine
Streptozotocin	2,4-Dinitrophenol and related compounds
Corticosteroids	
Naphthalene	Alkylating agents
Mimosine (leucenol)	Anticholinesterases
Methoxsalen	Chlorpromazine
Methionine sulfoximine	Triparanol
Polyriboinosinic acid	Dimethyl sulfoxide
Polyribocytidylic acid	2,4,6-Trinitrotoluene
Quietidine (1,4-bis(phenylisopropyl)-piperazine·2HCl)	Sympathomimetic drugs and morphine-like drugs
N-phenyl-β-hydrazinopropionitriles and related compounds	2,6-Dichloro-4-nitroaniline
	Iodoacetic acid
4 [3(7-Chloro-5,11-dihydrodibenz [b,e][1,4]-oxyazepin-5-YL)propyl]-1-piperazine ethanol dichloride	Mephenytoin
	Diquat
	Oral contraceptives
	Sulfaethoxypyridazine
	Thallium
	Paradichlorobenzene
	Heptachlor
	Desferal
	Thioacetamide

Appendix 2   Grading of Eye Irritation

Cornea	
No ulceration or opacity	0
Scattered or diffuse areas of opacity (other than slight dulling of normal luster), details of iris clearly visible	1
Easily discernible translucent area, details of iris slightly obscured	2
Necrotic area, no details of iris visible, size of pupil barely discernible	3
Opaque cornea, iris not discernible through the opacity	4
Iris	
Normal	0
Markedly deepened rugae, congestion, swelling, moderate circumcorneal heperemia, or injection; any of these or combination of any thereof, iris still reacting to light (sluggish reaction is positive)	1
No reaction to light, hemorrhage, gross destruction (any or all of these)	2
Conjunctiva redness (refers to palpebral and bulbar conjunctiva, cornea, and iris)	
Blood vessels normal	0
Some blood vessels definitely hyperemic (injected)	1
Diffuse, crimson color, individual vessels not easily discernible	2
Diffuse beefy red	3
Chemosis: lids and/or nictitating membranes	
No swelling	0
Any swelling above normal (includes nictating membranes)	1
Obvious swelling with partial eversion of lids	2
Swelling with lids about half closed	3
Swelling with lids more than half closed	4

Source: From OECD (1987) and OECD (2002).

17

Toxicology of the nervous system

INTRODUCTION

As a vital part of the body, the nervous system is shielded from toxicants in the blood by a unique protective mechanism, namely, the blood–brain barrier (BBB) and blood–nerve barrier (BNB). Nonetheless, it is susceptible to a variety of toxicants. For example, methyl mercury affects mainly the nervous system, although its concentration in the brain is comparable to that in most other tissues, and in fact it is much lower than that in the liver and kidneys.

The greater susceptibility may be attributed partly to the fact that neurons have a high metabolic rate, with little capacity for anaerobic metabolism. Furthermore, being electrically excitable, neurons tend to lose cell membrane integrity more readily. The great length of the axons is another reason for the nervous system being susceptible especially to toxic effects, because the cell body must supply its axon structurally and metabolically.

To facilitate the description of the various types of toxic effects and the procedures for their testing, the various parts of the nervous system are described.

Central and Peripheral Nervous System

The nervous system consists of two major parts: the central nervous system (CNS) and the peripheral nervous system (PNS). The CNS is comprised of the brain and the spinal cord, and the PNS covers the cranial and spinal nerves, which are either motor or sensory. The neurons of the sensory spinal nerves are located in the ganglia in the dorsal roots. In addition, the PNS also includes the sympathetic nerve system, which arises from neurons in the thoracic and lumbar region of the spinal cord, and the parasympathetic system, which stems from nerve fibers leaving the CNS via the cranial nerves and the sacral spinal roots.

Cells and Appendages

The principal cells in the nervous system are neurons, composed of perikarya, along with their dendrites and axons. These structures are responsible for the conduction of nerve impulses. The main supporting structure consists of various types of glial cells. Apart from a lack of conductivity, the glial cells differ from neurons in that the former, as most other types of cells, do reproduce, whereas the latter do not.

In the CNS the glial cells include astrocytes, oligodendrocytes (oligodendroglia), and microglia. Astrocytes help to maintain a proper microenvironment around the neurons and support the BBB. Oligodendroglia surrounds the axons in the CNS with a lipid-rich material, the myelin sheath, which provides electrical insulation. Microglia are basically macrophages that are located in the CNS. In the PNS the Schwann cells provide the myelin sheath, which wraps around the axon. The myelin sheath is interrupted by the nodes of Ranvier.

Neurotransmitters

Neurons are connected, via their axons, to other neurons at their dendrites or to the receptors in the glands or muscles. At nerve terminals, on excitation by an action potential, chemical neurotransmitters are released. The most common transmitters are acetylcholine and norepinephrine. However, there are several amine neurotransmitters in addition to norepinephrine, such as, dopamine, serotonin, and histamine. Furthermore, the following amino acids also act as neurotransmitters: 7-aminobutyric acid (GABA), glycine, glutamate, and aspartate. These transmitters are small molecules and act rapidly. They are synthesized in the presynaptic terminals. These neurotransmitters are presynthesized, stored in synaptic vesicles, and released upon excitation. Nitric oxide (NO), a recently discovered neurotransmitter, is different from the others in that, as a labile free radical, it is not presynthesized for storage in synaptic vesicles. It is synthesized, on demand, from l-arginine by NO synthase (Zhang and Snyder, 1995).

In addition to these small-molecule neurotransmitters, a large number of neuropeptides are slow-acting neurotransmitters/modulators. Some are released by the pituitary gland: ACTH, β-endorphin, growth hormone, thyrotropin, oxytocin, and vasopressin. A number of peptide transmitters act on gut and brain, for example, leucine enkephalin and methionine enkephalin.

Blood–Brain and Blood–Nerve Barriers

These barriers protect the nervous system from certain neurotoxicants. Differences in neurotoxicity sometimes can be explained on the basis of these barriers.

Blood–Brain Barrier

The endothelium in the brain is impermeable to substances of medium molecular weight, such as horseradish peroxidase (molecular weight: 40,000 Da; diameter: 5–6 nm), because the adjacent cells are tightly joined. Further, these cells have few micropinocytotic vesicles, which in capillaries of other tissues serve as an important transport mechanism across endothelial cells. Four major cellular elements such as endothelial cells (ECs), astrocyte end-feet, microglial cells, and pericytes play an important role in structural integrity and genesis of the BBB (Correale and Villa, 2009). However, highly lipid-soluble substances and the non-ionized fraction of a chemical are more permeable across the BBB. It is, therefore, similar to intact cell membranes in permeability.

The BBB is absent where the cells produce hormones or act as hormonal or chemoreceptors. Glutamate and a number of related compounds were shown to affect areas in the brain not protected by the BBB, such as the arcuate nucleus of the hypothalamus and the *area postrema* in various laboratory animals. These effects, while not observed in humans, are of interest because they may be used as tools in the study of such clinical conditions as Huntington's disease, drug-induced Parkinsonism, tardive dyskinesia, and sulfur amino acidopathies.

The BBB is effective in excluding many neurotoxicants, such as diphtheria, staphylococcus, and tetanus toxins. This is also true with doxorubicin, which affects the dorsal root ganglia but not the CNS. Mercury chloride has a small molecule but is hydrophilic and exists mainly in ionic form. Its concentration in the brain is minimal and so are its CNS effects. On the other hand, methyl mercury is lipophilic and thus readily crosses the BBB, thereby damaging the brain.

Blood–Nerve Barrier

Peripheral nerves are covered by two connective tissue sheaths, the perineurium and epineurium, and interlaced with the endoneurium. The BNB, also known as the blood–nerve interface, is nourished by the blood vessels in the endoneurium and supplemented by the lamellated cells of the perineural sheath. The BNB is not as effective as the BBB; therefore, the dorsal root ganglia are generally more susceptible than the neurons in the CNS to neurotoxicants. For example, doxorubicin affects neurons in the dorsal root ganglia but not those in the brain. Lead intoxication produces endothelial damage, increases permeability of blood–nerve interface, and causes demyelination as a primary pathological event (Mizisin and Weerasuriya, 2011).

NEUROTOXIC EFFECTS AND NEUROTOXICANTS

The effects may be classified according to the site of action. These include the neurons, the axons, the glial cells, and the vascular system. A toxicant, however, may affect more than one site. The following is a brief description of certain neurotoxic effects, along with the putative mode of action, grouped according to the site of action.

Figure 17.1 depicts damages to neurons, axons, and myelin sheath. *Neuronopathy* is represented by the damage to a second-order sensory neuron (4), which innervates corpuscle A, and a neuron in the dorsal root ganglion (3), which innervates corpuscle B. *Axonopathy* is represented by the damaged central axonal

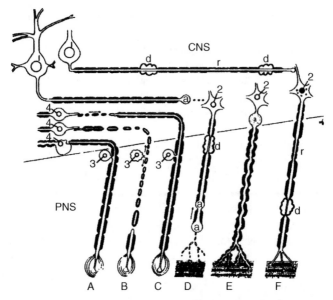

Figure 17.1   Cellular target sites of some neurotoxic chemicals illustrated by upper (1) and lower (2) motor neurons, dorsal root ganglion cells (3), and second-order sensory neurons (4) in the gracile nucleus of the medulla oblongata. The central nervous system (CNS) is represented above the sloping horizontal line and the peripheral nervous system (PNS) below. The peripheral receptors on fibers A–C are pacinian corpuscles. Fibers, D–F, innervate extrafusal muscle fibers: a, axonal degeneration; d, demyelination; r, remyelination of ventral root, and medulla oblongata. *Source*: Adapted from Spencer et al. (1980).

process of a sensory neuron, which innervates corpuscle C, and the axons of the lower motor neurons (2), which innervates muscle fibers D and E. *Myelinopathy* is shown along the axons of upper (1) and lower (2) motor neurons which innervates muscle fiber F.

Some neurotoxicants that induce these and other damages are described next.

Neuronopathy

Neurons, being dependent mainly on glucose as an energy source, are susceptible to anoxic and hypoglycemic conditions. A number of chemicals are well known for their anoxygenic effects in the brain. Barbiturates induce anoxia in the brain, especially in hippocampus and cerebellum. Permanent CNS damage even after barbiturate coma, however, is rare, possibly because of the reduced cell metabolism. On the other hand, prolonged exposure to carbon monoxide may induce permanent changes in the brain, arising from the development of a diffuse sclerosis of the white matter (leukoencephalopathy). Cyanide and azide inhibit cytochrome oxidase, thereby producing cytotoxic anoxia. Contamination of food products with tricresyl phosphate was shown to produce a delayed neuropathy related to the inhibition of "neuropathy target esterase" whereby there is damage to spinal nerves, the spinal cord, brain, and other tissues (Craig and Barth, 1999). This type of neuropathy also occurs following exposure to organophosphorous insecticides (Pope, 1999; see below).

The cell body of neurons may be affected directly by toxicants. Methyl mercury first produces focal loss of ribosomes and then disintegration and disappearance of the Nissl substances, especially in the small cells. These are followed by nuclear and perinuclear changes and finally by the loss of the entire neuron including its axon (Jacobs et al., 1977). The herbicide paraquat produces destruction of dopaminergic neurons via oxidative stress (Yang and Tiffany-Castiglioni, 2008). The paraquat-induced neuronal effects resemble the manifestations in Parkinson's disease. Doxorubicin (Adriamycin) affects neurons by intercalating with DNA, leading to a breakdown of the helical structures (Cho et al., 1980). This derangement inhibits the synthesis of RNA and neuronal protein. Since this drug does not cross the BBB, it can affect the neurons in the dorsal root ganglia (Fig. 17.1(B)) and autonomic ganglia, but not those in the CNS. On the other hand, methyl mercury does penetrate the BBB and thus damages the neurons in the CNS as well as those in the dorsal root ganglia.

Organotins are used as pesticides and as plasticizers. Upon entering the nervous system, they accumulate in the Golgi-like structures in the cell body. The cells then undergo swelling and necrosis (Bouldin et al., 1981).

Aluminum also penetrates the BBB and induces encephalopathy with neurofibrillar degeneration in cats and rabbits (DeBoni et al., 1976). Reviews in toxicology conclude that the use of aluminum cooking utensils and the use of various aluminum-containing food additives are safe (Soni et al., 2001; Krewski et al., 2007). Aluminum increases the permeability of BBB by changing its ultrastructure and the expression of occludin and F-actin, but zinc can protect the integrity of BBB and inhibit the decrease of tight junction protein occludin and F-actin expression in BBB in rats exposed to aluminum (Song et al., 2008).

Glutamate and related chemicals, in very large doses, are known to affect areas of the CNS devoid of BBB (see the section "Blood–Brain Barrier") and are considered as having neuroexcitatory and neurotoxic effects. The dendrites are the primary site of action. The perikarya are then affected, but the axons are spared (Fig. 17.1(A)). The toxicity may be mediated through NO (Dawson et al., 1991). Kainic acid is derived from a particular seaweed and it has been used in ascariasis; it is similar to glutamate but much more potent (Olney et al., 1974).

Alcohol in pregnant women may induce nervous system abnormalities in their offspring including abnormal neuronal migration and abnormal development of dendritic spines (Abel et al., 1983).

Axonopathy

Some axons are very long (up to 1 m), and the elements in the axons, such as neurofibrils, are synthesized not locally but in the cell body, and are transported along the axon. The axon may therefore be attacked either directly by toxicants or indirectly through damages to the cell body. Lesions may occur either in the proximal or in the distal sections of axons.

Proximal Axonopathy

β,β-Iminodiproprionitrile (IDPN) produces typical lesions of this type. IDPN has therefore been used as a model to study motor neuron diseases such as amyotrophic lateral sclerosis. The primary effect of IDPN is the impairment of slow axonal transport of neurofilaments, probably through aberrant phosphorylation of neurofilaments (Gold and Austin, 1991), while their synthesis is continued in the cell body. The accumulation of neurofilaments in the proximal axon causes it to enlarge and the distal axon to atrophy (Fig. 17.1(E)). The enlarged proximal axon in turn elicits local proliferation of the subpial astrocytic processes and extension of the processes filled with glial filaments along the proximal ventral root. The proximal swelling also stimulates splitting of myelin at the intraperiod line, formation of intramyelinic vacuoles, and ultimate demyelination. The Schwann cells in the demyelinated segment divide and remyelinate, and the repeated demyelination and remyelination give rise to "onion-bulb" formation (Griffin and Price, 1980).

Distal Axonopathy

Axons contain three types of neurofibrillary structures, namely, neurotubules, neurofilaments, and microfilaments. In addition, they contain mitochondria and smooth endoplasmic reticulum. These structures are especially susceptible to a variety of neurotoxicants. For example, thallium induces mitochondrial swelling and degeneration, and certain organophosphates and organic solvents cause derangement of the neurofibrillary structures, resulting in distal axonopathy.

An important type of distal axonopathy is produced by certain organophosphorus compounds such as tri-*o*-cresyl phosphate (TOCP), ethyl-4nitrophenyl phenylphosphonothioate (EPN), and leptophos. These compounds, besides inhibiting acetylcholinesterase, produce *delayed neuropathy*, which manifests mainly as paralysis of muscles. It affects especially long and large nerve fibers; hence the hind limbs are paralyzed before the forelimbs. TOCP has induced delayed neuropathy in 10,000 humans (see Appendix 2 of chap. 1). Although a number of other animals may also be affected, especially after repeated exposures, this toxicity is readily reproduced in hens, usually with a delay of 8–10 days after exposure. Because of the severity of delayed neurotoxicity, new organophosphorus chemicals are routinely tested for this potential hazard. OECD (1984) and EPA (1994) have published guidelines for such tests both after a single dose and after repeated administrations, using domestic hens. The condition is unrelated to acetylcholinesterase inhibition because potent inhibitors such as malathion, parathion, and carbaryl do not possess this toxic property. It is apparently associated with phosphorylation of the enzyme neuropathy target esterase (NTE; formerly known as neurotoxic esterase) (Abou-Donia, 1981; Johnson, 1990; Pope, 1999).

A different type of distal axonopathy is known to be produced by hexa-carbons such as *n*-hexane and methyl *n*-butyl ketone. These solvents produced toxic polyneuropathy among industrial workers, as has acrylamide (Exon 2006). Both produce marked neurofilament proliferation in axons, probably as a result of altered phosphorylation of certain proteins (Berti-Mattera et al., 1990). However, giant axonal swellings are common with hexacarbons (Fig. 17.1(D)), but are rare with acrylamide. Furthermore, sensory nerves are involved early with acrylamide but late with hexacarbons, which affect certain motor nerves first. Vincristine may produce accumulation of neurofibrils in the perikarya and axons. Vincristine disrupts the axonal neurotubules and neurofilaments, and blocks axoplasmic transport of these ultrastructures.

Clioquinol, a popular remedy and preventive drug for "travelers' diarrhea" in the 1960s and 1970s, induced disorders of the nervous system known as subacute myelo-optico-neuropathy in thousands of individuals (Appendix 2 of chap. 1). In humans and experimental animals, this compound produces central axonal degeneration of the dorsal root ganglion (Fig. 17.1(C)), as well as optic nerves (Worden et al., 1978).

Distal axonopathy has also been hypothesized as resulting from impairment of glycolytic enzyme activities in the axon (Spencer et al., 1979). These enzymes are responsible for the transport of neurofilaments, which are synthesized in the perikaryon and transported along the axon. Impairment of the activities of these enzymes would thus first affect the distal portion of the axon as well as the large, long nerve fibers, which have a greater energy demand on the perikarya. A second hypothesis postulates that the neurofilaments are directly affected by toxicants such as hexacarbons and acrylamide (Savolainen, 1977). Neurofilaments exposed to the toxicant for the longest period, namely, those located distally in long fibers, will be affected first.

Interference with Impulse Conduction

A number of toxicants act mainly on nerve membranes. These membranes normally maintain a negative resting potential. When stimulated, an action potential is generated. The resting and action potentials result from differences in the Na^+ and K^+ concentrations across the membrane, and their concentrations are maintained by the Na^+ channels. Tetrodotoxin, the toxic principle of puffer fish, has been shown to block the action potential by blocking the Na^+ channels. Saxitoxin, the toxic principle produced by the dinoflagellate *Gonyaulax* and taken up by the clam *Saxidomas giganteus*, also acts by blocking the sodium channels. Consumption of improperly cleaned puffer fish or contaminated clam can cause death through respiratory failure. DDT and pyrethroids are markedly different in chemical structure. However, their effects on the nervous systems are similar. They prolong the opening of the sodium channel, thereby initiating repetitive activity at the synapses and neuromuscular junctions (Narahashi, 1992).

Interference with Synaptic Transmission

Botulinum toxin, the most potent biologic toxin, is produced by *Clostridium botulinum*. Botulinum toxin induces the paralysis of muscles by impairing the release of acetylcholine from motor nerve endings. Black widow spider venom, on the other hand, induces an excessive release of acetylcholine and results in cramps and paralysis.

Tetanoplasmin, from the microbe *Clostridium tetani*, causes tetanus through its effect on the CNS. Tetanoplasmin blocks release of the inhibitory amino acid transmitters GABA and glycine, thereby producing spastic paralysis. The molecular weight of this proteinaceous dimer is about 150,000; therefore, it is too large to cross the BBB. However, it reaches the CNS by retrograde axonal transport (Schield et al., 1977).

Certain neurotoxins (e.g., anatoxin-S) may be produced by cyanobacteria in eutrophied lakes and ponds (chap. 23). These toxins interfere with the transmission of impulses from nerve terminals to muscles, thereby causing muscle paralysis (Carmicheal, 1994).

Acrylamide produces neurotoxicity by interfering with kinesin-related motor proteins in neurofilaments that are involved in fast antegrade transport of nerve signals between axons. Inhibition of these motor proteins and transaxonal transport of nerve growth factors result in impaired molecular transport from the cell body to distal axon, leading to the death of the nerve body. This is manifested as hind-limb splay, ataxia, and skeletal muscle weakness (Exon, 2006).

Glial Cells and Myelin

Myelinating Cells

Demyelination can result from injuries to myelinating cells (oligodendrocytes and Schwann cells). Neurotoxins of this type include lead, which affects Schwann cells possibly by interfering with their Ca^{2+} transport. Hypocholesterolemic agents such as triparanol, as expected, disrupt myelin sheath because of the high (70%) lipid content of myelin. However, they produce ultrastructural changes in oligodendrocytes before demyelination occurs. Diphtheria toxin demyelinates, possibly by affecting both the myelin and the myelinating cells. Triethyltin, ethidium bromide, and actinomycin are other examples of demyelinating toxins that act on the myelinating cells. The pesticide rotenone produces degeneration of the ganglion cell layer resulting in a neurodegenerative disorder associated with the destruction of the mitochondria (Zhang et al., 2006). This phenomenon is found in Leber's optic neuropathy and Parkinson's disease.

Myelin Sheath

Demyelination can also result from impacts on the myelin sheath. This type of effect generally involves a disruption of the membrane structure. Other modes of action include (*i*) inhibition of carbonic anhydrase or other enzymes involved in ion and water transport, (*ii*) inhibition of enzymes involved in oxidative phosphorylation, and (*iii*) chelation of metals. Neurotoxicants that act directly on the myelin sheath include triethyltin, lysolecithin, isoniazid, cyanate, hexachlorophene, and lead. Acetyl ethyl tetramethyl tetralin also causes myelinopathy through a complex mechanism (Fig. 17.1(F)).

Lead has been known for centuries as a neurotoxicant. Lead affects various parts of the nervous system, including myelin sheath. The PNS is affected before the CNS. In addition, lead affects motor nerves before the sensory, resulting in "wrist-drop" and "foot-drop." Its effects on the blood vessels are discussed next.

Blood Vessels and Edema

The permeability of the vascular system in the CNS and PNS may be increased by higher blood pressure or lower plasma osmolarity. It may also result from exposure to certain toxins. The greater permeability generally leads to an accumulation of fluids in the extracellular space. In addition, a number of neurotoxicants are known to induce cellular edema.

Extracellular Edema

Lead can damage the endothelial cells and cause extravasation of plasma in the brain, especially in the white matter, which has a greater compliance than the gray matter. The fact that suckling rats are more susceptible to lead has been attributed to the immaturity of the vascular system (Press, 1977). Lead has similar effects on the endoneurium, leading to increased endoneural fluid pressure and demyelination. Organic lead, such as tetraethyl lead, more readily penetrates the barriers and is therefore more toxic in this respect.

Mercury compounds can damage the endothelial cells and increase their permeability. Organic arsenicals produce edema and focal hemorrhages in the brain. Tellurium produces edema in the endoneurium. Chronic alcoholism is associated with endoneural edema.

Endoneural edema can also result from intramyelinic edema in hexachlorophene intoxication. Endoneural edema may also be associated with Wallerian degeneration due to mechanical injury.

Cellular Edema

Various parts of neurons may become edematous following exposure to toxicants. For example, 6-aminonicotinamide affects the perikaryon, cyanide and carbon monoxide affect the axon, and ouabain and methyl sulfoxime affect the presynaptic nerve endings.

Edema of astrocytes and oligodendrocytes may be produced by 6-aminonicotinamide. Ouabain can also affect astrocytes. Edema of Schwann cells may be induced by lead, which, as noted above, may also produce extracellular edema.

Triethyltin and isoniazid also produce edema of the myelin sheaths in the CNS. Hexachlorophene induces edema of the myelin sheaths both in the white matter of the brain and in the peripheral nerves.

TESTING PROCEDURES

Functional Observational Battery

A battery of observations, namely functional observational battery (FOB), has been devised to assess the neurotoxic effects (EPA, 1994; Kallman and Fowler, 1994). This is done in intact animals, usually rats or mice, and can be incorporated in other tests (chap. 6). These animals are exposed to the toxicant at two or three doses by an appropriate route. The duration of treatment and observation period vary from days to months according to the nature of the toxicant. The animals are observed for the following abnormalities:

(a)   Unusual body position, activity level, gait, etc.
(b)   Unusual behavior such as compulsive biting, self-mutilation, circling, and walking backward.
(c)   The presence of convulsions, tremors, lacrimation, red-colored tears, salivation, diarrhea, vocalization, etc.
(d)   Changes in sensory and motor functions (for details, see the following sections).

Neurologic Examinations

These examinations often provide an indication of the site of neurotoxicity. Most of these examinations can be performed in humans as well as in animals. The exceptions relate to the determination of *mental state* and many *sensory functions*, which can be more readily assessed in humans.

Cranial nerves I through XII have different functions, and their tests therefore vary. For example, tests of the acoustic and optic nerves involve the evaluation of responses to sound and light stimuli.

Motor examination includes inspection of muscles for weakness, atrophy, and fasciculation, which indicate dysfunction of the lower motor neuron, that is, the anterior horn cells, motor roots, and peripheral nerves. Spasticity is a sign of dysfunction of the upper motor neurons in the brain and their axons down to the spinal cord. Resting tremor is often associated with lesions in the basal ganglia or cerebellum. Intention tremor occurs during voluntary movement and is a manifestation of cerebellar disease.

Reflex examination includes deep tendon reflexes, the functioning of which involves the intrafusal receptors, dorsal root ganglia, anterior horn cells and their axons, neuromuscular junction, and muscle. Damage to any of these structures will cause these reflexes to be absent or hypoactive. On the other hand, when there is upper motor neuron dysfunction, these reflexes will be exaggerated.

The Babinski reflex is the most important superficial cutaneous reflex. Abnormal response is an indication of corticospinal dysfunction.

Gait abnormalities may also aid in locating the site of toxicity. For example, lower motor neuron disease causes a high-stepping gait. A scissoring, or stiff, gait indicates upper motor neuron lesion. Cerebellar dysfunction results in an ataxic or reeling gait.

Morphologic Examinations

Neurotoxicants may act on the CNS, the PNS, or both. They may induce lesions in the neuronal perikaryon or its axon, either proximally or distally, the myelinating cells or the myelin sheath itself, the astrocytes, or the endothelial cells. Morphologic examinations are, therefore, important in establishing the precise site of toxic lesions on an anatomic level. Examinations on cellular and ultrastructural levels often facilitate the differential diagnosis of the neuropathy.

Some of the commonly used techniques, along with a list of references, have been provided by Spencer et al. (1980). It is worth noting, however, that damage to endothelial cells can be demonstrated not only by signs of edema (fewer cells and nerve fiber per unit area) but also by increases in the pressure of the intracranial and endoneural fluids as well as by the penetration of tracer substances, such as horseradish peroxidase, through the endothelium.

Electrophysiological Examinations

Peripheral Nerves

A frequently used examination involves the measurement of *motor nerve* conduction velocity. This can be done on intact animals subjected to short-term or chronic exposure to neurotoxicants or on exposed nerves after local application of the toxicants. *Sensory nerve* conduction velocity and action potentials have also been measured in the study of neurotoxicity.

Electromyography

This procedure calls for the examination of the electrical activities of a muscle, at rest and when contracted, recorded with the aid of a needle electrode inserted into the muscle. Neurotoxicity may manifest as (*i*) abnormal insertional activity, (*ii*) occurrence of spontaneous electrical activity of a resting muscle, and (*iii*) interference pattern of electrical activity of motor units during voluntary muscle contraction (Goodgold and Eberstein, 1977).

BEHAVIORAL STUDIES: TESTING PROCEDURES

There is a large body of information on behavioral toxicology, resulting from a widespread feeling that behavior is a subtle and sensitive indicator of toxicity.

Table 17.1   Examples of Primary Level Neurobehavioral Tests for Rats or Mice

Neurobehavioral Function	Behavioral Test
Sensory	
Visual, olfactory, somatosensory, auditory	Localization
Pain	Tail flick
Orientation in space	Negative geotaxis
Motor	
Spontaneous activity	Activity in Automex
Muscular weakness	Forelimb grip; hind-limb extensor
Fatigability	Swim endurance
Tremor	Frequency of occurrence
Cognitive: Associative	
Learning and retention	One-way avoidance; step-through passive avoidance
Affective: Emotional	
Responsiveness	Startle to air puff; emergence in a novel environment
Physiological: Consummatory	
Thermoregulation	Body weight; food and water ingestion; core temperature

EPA (1994) has provided some guidelines on schedule-controlled operant behavior.*Source*: From Tilson et al. (1980).

However, this view has been questioned, for example, by Norton (1980), who stated: "Scientific data supporting this view are not only scanty but the available evidence often flatly contradicts this assumption." In the hope that improved testing procedures will increase the sensitivity and utility of this approach in neurotoxicology, this branch of neurotoxicology will undoubtedly grow. A few highlights of this subject are presented here.

The tests involve two types of responses: (*i*) unconditioned responses, which are either emitted (spontaneous) or elicited (reflex); (*ii*) conditioned responses, which may be considered as either "classic conditioning" (Pavlov) or operant conditioning (Skinner). The extent of the training required of the experimental animals and the neurobehavioral function to be assessed is also a useful criterion for the classification of the tests.

Simple Tests

Tilson et al. (1980) listed tests that require little or no prior training of the experimental animals (rats and mice) (Table 17.1).

More Involved Tests

The tests listed in Table 17.2 require extended or special training, frequent evaluation, and/or manipulation of motivational factors.

Table 17.2   Examples of Secondary Level Neurobehavioral Tests for Rats or Mice

Neurobehavioral Function	Behavioral Test
Sensory	
Visual, auditory, olfactory	Operant psychophysics
Gustatory	Taste discrimination
Somatosensory	T-maze discrimination
Orientation in space	T-maze discrimination
Pain	Operant titration
Motor	
Spontaneous activity	Diurnal cyclicity; patterning
Muscular strength	Operant response force
Tremor	Spectral analysis
Cognitive: Associative	
Learning and retention	Autoshaping; temporal discriminating; repeated acquisition
Affective: Emotional	
CNS excitability	Brain self-stimulation; aversion thresholds
Physiologic: Consummatory	
Thermoregulation	Diurnal patterning; cyclicity; preference

Source: From Tilson et al. (1980).

Procedures to Enhance Sensitivity

Because of the large functional reserve of the brain, focal damage may not result in any overt brain dysfunction. Such damage, however, may be demonstrated clinically with the use of *provocative* tests. These involve administering sodium amobarbital, raising body temperature, or lowering blood pH with the intravenous infusion of ammonium chloride (Lehrer, 1974).

Animals

Apart from rats and mice, other animals such as pigeons, cats, dogs, and monkeys are also commonly used, with testing procedures similar to those listed earlier.

EVALUATION

In view of the wide range of toxic effects on the nervous system, as outlined above, there is clearly a need for a battery of tests for the evaluation of neurotoxicants. It is also worth noting that the choice of animal species is critical in eliciting certain types of toxicity, such as delayed neurotoxicity. Furthermore, the nature of the toxicity on the nervous system, as on other organs, can vary according to the duration of exposure. For example, *n*-hexane and TOCP produce, after acute exposure, narcosis, but they induce axonopathy after repeated exposures.

The significance of a neurotoxic effect depends on its reversibility. In general, irreversible effects are more serious than reversible ones. The site of the effect also plays an important role. There are areas in the nervous system more critical to physiologic function than others. In addition, focal damage in areas with abundant functional reserve is likely to be less serious.

The behavioral effects are especially susceptible to endogenous and environmental variations. For example, Norton (1980) reported data to indicate a large variability of results both between animals of the same species and within the same animal at different times. It is therefore important to adhere to proper experimental procedures, such as sufficiently large number of animals, rigorously controlled experimental environment, and statistical analysis of results.

REFERENCES

Abel EJ, Jacobson S, Sherwin BJ (1983). In utero ethanol exposure: functional and structural brain damage. Neurobehav Toxicol Teratol 5, 139–46.

Abou-Donia MB (1981). Organophosphorus ester-induced delayed neurotoxicity. Annu Rev Pharmacol Toxicol 21, 511–48.

Berti-Mattera LN, Eichberg J, Schrama L, et al. (1990). Acrylamide administration alters protein phosphorylation and phospholipid metabolism in rat sciatic nerve. Toxicol Appl Pharmacol 103, 502–11.

Bouldin TW, Gaines ND, Bagvell CR, et al. (1981). Pathogenesis of trimethyltin neuronal toxicity. Am J Pathol 104, 237–49.

Carmicheal WW (1994). The toxins of cyanobacteria. Sci Am 270, 78–86.

Cho ES, Spencer PS, Jortner BS (1980). Doxorubicin. In: Spencer PS, Schaumberg HH, eds. Experimental and Clinical Neurotoxicology. Baltimore, MD: Williams & Wilkins, 440–55.

Correale J, Villa A (2009). Cellular elements of the blood-brain barrier. Neurochem Res 34. 2067–77.

Craig PH, Barth ML (1999). Evaluation of the hazards of industrial exposure to tricresyl phosphate: a review and interpretation of the literature. J Toxicol Environ Health B 2, 281–300.

Dawson VL, Dawson TM, London ED, et al. (1991). Nitric oxide mediates glutamate neurotoxicity in primary cortical culture. Proc Natl Acad Sci USA 88, 6368–71.

DeBoni U, Otros A, Scott JW, et al. (1976). Neurofibrillary degeneration induced by systemic aluminum. Acta Neuropathol 35, 285–94.

EPA (1994). Health Effects Testing Guidelines. Code Federal Refutations, Title 40, Part 798.

Exon JH (2006). A review of the toxicology of acrylamide. J Toxicol Environ Health B 9, 397–412.

Gold GB, Austin DR (1991). Regulation of aberrant neurofilament phosphorylation in neuronal perikarya. Brain Res 563, 151–62.

Goodgold J, Eberstein A (1977). Electrodiagnosis of Neuromuscular Diseases. Baltimore, MD: Williams & Wilkins.

Griffin JW, Price DL (1980). Proximal axonopathies induced by toxic chemicals. In: Spencer PS, and Schaumberg HH, eds. Experimental and Clinical Neurotoxicology. Baltimore, MD: Williams & Wilkins, 161–78.

Jacobs JM, Carmichael N, Cavanagh JB (1977). Ultrastructural studies in the nervous system of rabbits poisoned with methyl mercury. Toxicol Appl Pharmacol 39, 249–61.

Johnson MK (1990). Contemporary issues in toxicology. organophosphates and delayed neuropathy—Is NTE alive and well? Toxicol Appl Pharmacol 103, 385–99.

Kallman MJ, Fowler SC (1994). Assessment of chemically induced alterations in motor functions. In: Chang LW, ed. Principles of Neurotoxicology. New York, NY: Marcel Dekker, 373–96.

Krewski D, Yokel RA, Nieboer E, et al. (2007). Human health risk assessment for aluminium, aluminium oxide, and aluminium hydroxide. J Toxicol Environ Health B 10(Suppl. 1), 1–269.

Lehrer GM (1974). Measurement of minimal brain dysfunction. In: Xintaras C, Johnson BL, de Groot I, eds. Behavior Toxicology. Washington, DC: National Institute for Occupational Safety and Health.

Mizisin AP, Weerasuriya A (2011). Homeostatic regulation of the endoneurial microenvironment during development, aging and in response to trauma, disease and toxic insult. Acta Neuropathol 121, 291–312.

Narahashi T (1992). Nerve membrane Na^+ channels as targets of insecticides. Trends Pharmacol Sci 13, 236–41.

Norton S (1980). Behavioral toxicology: a critical appraisal. In: Witschi HR, ed. The Scientific Basis of Toxicity Assessment. Amsterdam, The Netherlands: Elsevier/ North Holland, 91–107.

OECD (1984). Delayed neurotoxicity of organophosphorus substances. In: Guidelines for Testing Chemicals. Paris, France: Organization for Economic Cooperation and Development.

Olney JW, Rhee V, Ho OL (1974). Kainic acid: a powerful neurotoxic analogue of glutamate. Brain Res 77, 507–12.

Pope CN (1999). Organophosphorous pesticides: do they all have the same mechanism of toxicity? J Toxicol Environ Health B 2, 161–81.

Press MF (1977). Lead encephalopathy in neonatal Long-Evans rats: morphologic studies. J Neuropathol Exp Neurol 36, 169–93.

Savolainen J (1977). Some aspects of the mechanism by which industrial solvents produce neurotoxic effects. Chem Biol Interact 18, 1–10.

Schield LK, Griffin JW, Drachman DB, et al. (1977). Retrograde axonal transport: a direct method for measurement of rate. Neurology 27, 393.

Song Y, Xue Y, Liu X, et al. (2008). Effects of acute exposure to aluminum on blood-brain barrier and the protection of zinc. Neurosci Lett 445, 42–6.

Soni MG, White SM, Flamm WG, et al. (2001). Safety evaluation of dietary aluminum. Reg Toxicol Pharmacol 33, 66–79.

Spencer PS, Bischoff MC, Schaumberg HH (1980). Neuropathological methods for the detection of neurotoxic disease. In: Spencer PS, Schaumberg HH, eds. Experimental and Clinical Neurotoxicology. Baltimore, MD: Williams & Wilkins, 743–57.

Spencer PS, Sabri MI, Schaumberg HH, et al. (1979). Does a defect in energy metabolism in the nerve fiber cause axonal degeneration in polyneuropathies? Ann Neurol 5, 501–7.

Tilson HA, Cabe PA, Burne TA (1980). Behavioral procedures for the assessment of neurotoxicity. In: Spencer PC, Schaumberg HH, eds. Experimental and Clinical Neurotoxicology. Baltimore, MD: Williams & Wilkins, 758–66.

Worden AN, Heywood R, Prentice DE, et al. (1978). Clioquinol toxicity in the dog. Toxicology 9, 227.

Yang W, Tiffany-Castiglioni E (2008). Paraquat-induced apoptosis in human neuroblastoma SH-SY5Y cells: involvement of p53 and mitochondria. J Toxicol Environ Health A 71, 289–99.

Zhang J, Snyder SH (1995). Nitric oxide in the nervous system. Am Rev Pharmacol Toxicol 35, 213–33.

Zhang X, Jones D, Gonzalez-Lima F (2006). Neurodegeneration produced by rotenone in the mouse retina: a potential model to investigate environmental pesticide contributions to neurodegenerative diseases. J Toxicol Environ Health A 69, 1681–97.

Appendix 1   Select Neurotoxicants Described in the Text

Acrylamide-A	*n*-Hexane-A
Actinomycin-M	IDPN-A
AETT-M	Kainic acid-N
Alcohol-N, T	Lead-MS
Alanosine-N	Leptophos-A
Aluminum-N	Lysolecithin-M
6-Aminonicotinamide-BV	Methyl *n*-butyl ketone-A
Anatoxin-C	Methyl mercury-N, BV
Arsenic-BV	Nicotine-C
Azide-N	Organotin-N
Barbiturate-N	Organic solvents-A
Botulinum toxin-C	Pyrethroids-C
Carbon monoxide-N	Saxitoxin-C
Clioquinol-A	Tellurium-BV, M
Cyanide-N, BV	Tetanoplasmin-C
DDT-C	Tetrodotoxin-C
Diphtheria toxin-M	Thallium-A
Doxorubicin-N	Triethyltin-M, BV
EPN-A	Triparanol-M
Ethidium bromide-M	TOCP-A
Glutamate-N	Vincristine-A
Hexachlorophene-M, BV	

Abbreviations: A, axonopathy; AETT, acetyl ethyl tetramethyl tetralin; BV, blood vessel and edema; C, conduction and transmission; M, myelinopathy; MS: multiple sites; N, neuropathy; T, teratogenicity.

18

Reproductive and cardiovascular systems

REPRODUCTIVE SYSTEM

Introduction

Reproductive Process and Organs

The reproductive process starts with gametogenesis. In the female animal, oogenesis involves the formation of primary oocytes from the primordial germ cells (oogonia) through mitosis. This development takes place during the fetal period and ceases at birth. Primary oocytes divide by meiosis to form secondary oocytes just before they are ovulated.

On the other hand, spermatogenesis starts with gonocytes during the fetal period, and these cells are transformed to spermatogonia after birth. Spermatogonia remain dormant until puberty, when proliferative activity begins again. Some of the spermatogonia multiply to form additional spermatogonia while others mature to spermatozoa. There are three intermediate stages. Spermatogonia divide by mitosis to form primary spermatocytes, which divide by meiosis to form secondary spermatocytes. These in turn divide to form spermatids. Finally, spermatids become spermatozoa by metamorphosis. The entire process is continuous, and the time required for spermatogonia to become spermatozoa is about 60 days (Fig. 18.1).

Fertilization requires not only functional ovum and spermatozoa but also effective delivery of the sperm and proper milieu. The conceptus, the fertilized ovum, is then implanted in the uterus and develops through embryonic and fetal stages. At the end of the gestational period, parturition takes place. The pups are suckled until weaning. They then grow and mature to start the reproductive process again, thus completing a reproductive cycle.

Other Cells and Organs

While gametocytes are the essential elements of the reproductive process, other cells and organs also play important roles.

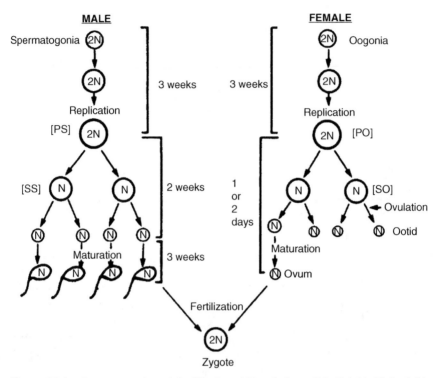

Figure 18.1 Gametogenesis and fertilization. *Abbreviations*: 2N, diploid; N, haploid; PO, primary oocyte; PS, primary spermatocyte; SO, secondary oocyte; SS, secondary spermatocyte. *Source*: From Brusick (1987).

In the male reproductive system, spermatogenesis takes place in the seminiferous tubules in the testis. In these tubules are the Sertoli cells, which extend from the basement membrane to the lumen of the seminiferous tubules and contain androgen-binding proteins (ABPs). The ABPs facilitate the movement of androgen to the spermatocytes for their development.

In addition, there are the Leydig cells, which are located in the interstitial tissue surrounding the seminiferous tubules. These cells are the main sites of synthesis of testosterone, which is essential not only for the development of the reproductive system but also for its proper functioning.

After leaving the testis, spermatozoa are stored in the epididymis to undergo changes in order to gain fertility capacity and for later delivery to the female reproductive system. In addition, the accessory organs, prostate, and seminal vesicle provide special nutrients and proper milieu for the sperm. These organs respond to the effect of testosterone, and hence their weights are indicators of the blood level of this hormone.

In the female reproductive system, the ova can be affected while they are in the ovaries. However, it is more often that the fertilized ova are affected either directly or indirectly through damages to the uterus.

Pharmacokinetics

Throughout the reproductive cycle, toxicants can act directly on the reproductive system or the conceptus, or indirectly via certain endocrine organs. Before chemicals act directly, they must reach the target organs in sufficiently high concentration. This concentration may be higher or lower than that in the blood. For example, with DDT, the concentration is almost 80-fold higher in the ovary than that in the plasma. A number of other substances were also shown to penetrate the oocyte, oviduct, uterine fluid, and blastocyst (Fabro, 1978).

Unlike the ovaries, the testis is protected by the blood–testis barrier (BTB) (Lee and Dixon, 1978). The BTB is a complex of a multicellular system composed of capillary endothelial cells, myoid cells, and membranes surrounding the seminiferous tubules and the tightly joined Sertoli cells in the tubules. This barrier, however, is less effective than the blood–brain barrier. The penetration rate of chemicals into the testis is governed by their molecular weights, their partition coefficients, and their ionic characteristics. The BTB is constituted of coexisting junctions between Sertoli cells near the basement membrane, which include tight junctions, basal ectoplasmic specializations, gap junctions, and desmosome-like junctions although the blood–brain barrier and the blood–retina barrier constitute tight junctions between endothelial cells (Su et al., 2011).

Testis contains both activating and detoxicating enzyme systems. These two enzyme systems, as noted in chapter 3, are capable of, respectively, increasing and decreasing the toxicities of chemicals. Furthermore, there is an efficient DNA repair mechanism in the premeiotic spermatogenic cells, but there is none in spermatids or in spermatozoa; mutations can therefore be induced by genotoxic substances on these cells.

TOXICANTS AND THEIR EFFECTS

The reproductive functions may be affected by toxicants through their effects on the reproductive system of either gender. In the male, the formation, development, storage, and delivery of spermatozoa may be adversely affected. The oocytes, in the females, are also susceptible to certain toxicants. In addition, the implantation of the fertilized ova as well as the growth and development of the conceptus may be affected. In both genders, some of the toxic effects are mediated through hormonal or nervous system activities.

Male Reproductive System

Many chemicals adversely affect spermatogenesis and produce testicular atrophy. These include food colors (e.g., Oil Yellow AB and Oil Yellow OB) (Allmark et al., 1955), pesticides (e.g., dibromochloropropane (DBCP)), plastics (phthalates), metals (e.g., arsenic, tin, lead, and cadmium), and organic solvents. A variety of other chemicals affect the testis, such as steroid hormones, alkylating agents, cyclohexylamine, and hexachlorophene.

In addition to reduced sperm count resulting from adverse effects on spermatogenesis, a toxicant may render spermatozoa defective, less mobile, or even dead. For example, both methyl methane sulfonate (MMS) and busulfan produce lethal mutations, but MMS affects spermatids and spermatozoa, whereas busulfan affects the pre-spermatogenic cells. These alkylating agents apparently attack the DNA of these cells with different repair mechanisms (Lee, 1983).

Spermatozoa may also be affected while being stored in epididymis. For example, the male antifertility agent α-chlorohydrin inhibits the fertilizing capacity of spermatozoa. Gossypol, another such agent that was extensively tried in China (Qian and Wang, 1984), probably acts through a similar mechanism.

The testis is hormonally regulated by the hypothalamus–pituitary–testis axis: follicle-stimulating hormone (FSH) is required in the initiation of spermatogenesis through the production of ABP in Sertoli cells, whereas luteinizing hormone (LH) acts on Leydig cells to synthesize testosterone. A toxicant may thus affect reproductive function via these endocrine hormones. An example is DBCP (dibromochloropropane), a fumigant used in agriculture, which induced among occupational workers azoospermia and oligospermia, along with elevated serum concentrations of LH and FSH (Miller et al., 1987).

Reproductive functions are also under the influence of the autonomic nervous system. Thus, the hypotensive drug losulazine, which acts by depleting norepinephrine, produces reversible infertility in male rats, probably through altered sexual behavior and ejaculatory disturbances (Mesfin et al., 1989). Guanethidine, another hypotensive drug, may produce or fail to induce pregnancy by interfering with seminal emission (Palmer, 1976).

Tumors may develop in the testis. For example, the herbicide linuron may induce Leydig cell tumors. The tumorigenesis is mediated through a sustained hypersecretion of LH (Cook et al., 1993). In contrast to rats, which are likely to develop Leydig cell tumors, testicular tumors are more likely to arise from germ cells in men. Cadmium has been reported to induce prostate cancer in men (Waalkes and Rehm, 1994).

Female Reproductive System

Oocytes may be damaged by chemotherapeutic agents such as nitrogen mustard and vinblastine, and polycyclic aromatic hydrocarbons such as 3-methylcholanthrene and benzo[a]pyrene. Prostaglandin synthetase inhibitors, for example, aspirin-like drugs, may block the release of ovulation. Oocytes before puberty are more resistant to the adverse effects of chemicals, evidently because they are dormant. Certain organochlorine pesticides such as methoxychlor, similar to estradiol, may increase the weight of the uterus (Eroschenko and Rourke, 1992).

Other reproductive functions may also be affected. Haloperidol prevents implantation. DDT and nicotine may affect the development and growth of the conceptus and thus lower the fetal weight (Fabro, 1978). Spironolactone may interfere with ovulation and implantation of the fertilized ovum; it may also retard the development of the sex organs of the offspring (Nagi and Virgo, 1982). Gossypol is also toxic in the female. It suppresses ovarian steroid hormone secretion, interrupts regular cyclicity and inhibits embryo implantation (Lin et al., 1994). There is a relationship between the extent of cigarette smoking and the onset of menopause; menopause is an indication of oocyte depletion (Miller et al., 1987). The toxic effects that are specifically related to the production of congenital anomalies are dealt with in chapter 9.

ROUTINE TESTING: MULTIGENERATION REPRODUCTION STUDIES

Animals and Doses

In general, rats are the animals of choice. A minimum of 20 females and 10 males are placed in each of three dose groups and a control group. OECD Guidelines (1995) recommend 10 animals of each gender. The doses are selected so that the high dose will produce some minimal toxic signs but will not result in a mortality of greater than 10%. The low dose will not induce any observable effect.

Prior to breeding, the animals are dosed for 10 weeks prior to mating. However, because of the difference in the time required for maturation of the gametes, the males are dosed for 70 days, the period of spermatogenesis, and the females are dosed for 14 days, the length of the development of the ova. Dosing of the females is continued through the gestation and lactation periods. The test chemical should be administered by a route that most closely resembles the human exposure condition.

To determine the potential effect of the chemical on the reproductive function of the offspring (F_1), a second generation offspring (F_2) is bred and reared to reproductive maturity.

Observations and Examinations

The adult animals are observed for the body weight, food consumption, general appearance, estrus cycle, and mating behavior. In addition, the fertility and nesting and nursing behaviors are also noted. Half of the maternal rats are sacrificed on day 13 of gestation for examination of corpora lutea, implantation, and resorption.

The other half of the pregnant rats is allowed to deliver their pups. The pups are examined for litter size, number of stillborn, gender distribution, and congenital anomalies. In addition, the viability and pup weight are recorded at birth, on day 4, and at weaning, and preferably also on day 12 or 14. Auditory and visual functions and behavior are also examined for subtle congenital defects.

An appropriate number of males and females are randomly selected from all generations and examined by gross necropsy and histopathology, especially with respect to the reproductive organs. In the males, weights and histopathology of the testes, epididymides, seminal vesicles, prostate, and pituitary often provide useful information on the site of action of the toxicant under test. Other indicators of the effects are the sperm count, and its motility and morphology, as well as the levels of certain hormones, especially testosterone, FSH, and TH. In the females, weights and histopathology of the vagina, uterus, oviduct, ovaries, and pituitary should be assessed along with the levels of the relevant hormones.

Additional details and references to the reproduction and fertility studies are provided in the test guidelines EPA (1994).

Evaluation

From these data, a number of disturbances of reproductive function can be deduced from the following indices:

1. Fertility index: the percentage of mating resulting in pregnancy.
2. Gestation index: the percentage of pregnancies resulting in the birth of live litters.
3. Viability index: the percentage of live pups that survive four days or longer.
4. Lactation index: the percentage of pups alive on day 4 that survive 21 days or longer.

Other indicators of effects include (*i*) mating index (the percentage of estrus cycles that had mating), (*ii*) male fertility index (the percentage of males exposed to fertile nonpregnant females that resulted in pregnancies), (*iii*) female fertility index (the percentage of females exposed to fertile males that resulted in pregnancies), and (*iv*) 12- or 14-day survival indices.

Multigeneration reproductive study can reveal a variety of toxic effects on the reproductive function as well as on the *conceptus*. Examples are indices of gestation, viability, and survival. However, nonspecific response (e.g., nonpregnancy) is common. It may follow unusual routes of administering the chemical, such as inhalation, topical application to the eye or nose, and parenteral administration. Excessive handling may also disturb the normal reproductive function. A number of other interfering factors are discussed by Palmer (1976).

The pathological examination may reveal suppression of spermatogenesis, advanced rates of follicle atresia, and ovulatory or meiotic failure.

OTHER TESTS

The effects revealed in multigeneration reproduction studies outlined above may result from paternal, maternal, or fetal exposure. Thus, additional tests are often conducted to establish the cause of the effect. A few such tests are outlined here.

Pathological examinations are useful in identifying a variety of toxic effects. The weight of testis is a simple but sensitive index of testicular damages. The extent and nature of such damages can often be assessed microscopically. The weights of prostate and seminal vesicle are often correlated with levels of testosterone. Similarly, a gross and microscopic analysis of *semen* is useful in epidemiological and animal studies. The sperm count and the motility, survival, and morphology of the spermatozoa often provide information about toxic effects on the testis (Eliasson,

1978). As noted above, certain toxicants affect the reproductive function through disturbances of *hormones*, especially testosterone, estrogens, FSH, and LH. Assays of their levels may indicate the mode of action of the toxicant.

The *perfused male reproductive tracts* have been shown to be useful models in studying the effects of chemicals on the secretion and accumulation of androgens (Bardin et al., 1978).

Certain *biomarkers* have been used in a variety of tests for disorders of the reproductive system. For example, DNA probes have been used to detect gene mutation and excessive deletions and translocations in meiotic, and postmeiotic germ cells as well as Sertoli and Leydig cells in the testis (Hecht, 1987).

CARDIOVASCULAR SYSTEM

General Considerations

The cardiovascular system is composed of two parts: the heart and the blood vessels. The heart is a vital organ in the body. Although it is not a common target organ, it can be damaged by a variety of chemicals. They act either directly on the myocardium or indirectly through the nervous system or blood vessels. A list of such chemicals, as compiled by Van Stee (1980), is reproduced in Table 18.1.

Table 18.1   Cardiotoxic Drugs and Chemicals

Cardiomyopathy	
Allylamine	Adrenergic agonists
Furazolidone	Methysergide
Ethanol	Vasodilators
Cobalt	
Interference with nucleic acid metabolism and protein synthesis	
Antineoplastic drugs	
Electrophysiological Mechanisms	
Cardiotonic drugs	Local anesthetics
Phenytoin (diphenylhydantoin)	Emetine
Tricyclic antidepressants	Chlordimeform
Clofibrate	Contrast media
Lithium	Antimalarial drugs
Propylene glycol	Calcium antagonists
Nonspecific Myocardial Depression	
Lipid-soluble, organic compounds	Antimicrobial antibiotics
Myocardial depressant factor	Carbromide, carbromal
Involvement with lipid metabolism	
High cholesterol diet	Brominated vegetable oils
Rapeseed oil	
Miscellaneous	
Phenothiazines	

Source: From Van Stee (1980).

The heart is mainly composed of myocardial cells, each measuring about $15 \times 80\,\mu m$. Unlike skeletal muscle cells, each of which is innervated, only some of the heart muscle cells are innervated. However, these cells are joined, at their ends, to each other by the nexus. It has low resistance and thus allows a rapid transmission of electrical stimulus from one cell to the next. These characteristics are essential to the programmed sequence of contraction of different parts of the heart.

The myocardium is different from skeletal muscles also in that there is less contractile material (50% vs. 80%) but much more mitochondrial material (35% vs. 2%). Mitochondria evidently play an important role in the cardiac contractility and are a common subcellular target of cardiotoxicity.

Myocardial contraction involves the liberation of energy from oxidative metabolism, conservation of the energy by adenosine triphosphate and creatine phosphate, and utilization of the energy by contractile proteins. The most vulnerable mechanisms include the utilization of energy and intracellular movement of calcium ion, which is involved in the contractility of myocardium as well as regulating enzyme activities, transduction of hormonal information, etc.

The vascular system consists of arteries, arterioles, capillaries, venules, and veins. A toxicant may affect any of these vessels; the seriousness of the effect depends on the physiological role of the organ that is supplied by the affected blood vessel.

TOXIC EFFECTS ON THE HEART

Cardiomyopathy

The usual toxic effects of cobalt are polycythemia, goiter, and signs of gastrointestinal irritation such as vomiting and diarrhea. However, its inclusion in beer as a foam stabilizer produced a number of serious and fatal cases of cardiomyopathy. Subsequent studies showed that there is also intramitochondrial accumulation of calcium. The toxicity of cobalt on the heart was greatly enhanced by malnutrition, especially the deficiency of certain amino acids. Among the heavy beer drinkers, this condition existed because of the large caloric intake of beer. It was also noted that cobalt ions depressed oxygen uptake and interfered with cardiac energy metabolism in the tricarboxylic acid cycle, as thiamine deficiency dose (Grice, 1972). As noted above, Ca^{2+} plays a vital role in various functions of myocardium. Cobalt may reduce the available myocardial Ca^{2+} by complexing with macromolecules and may also be antagonistic to endogenous Ca^{2+}.

Adrenergic β-receptor agonists, isoproterenol in particular, and vasodilating antihypertensive drugs, such as hydralazine, are capable of inducing myocardial necrosis. The former chemicals have direct adrenergic effects, whereas the antihypertensive drugs exert adrenergic effects via the induced hypotension. These effects produce an augmented transmembrane calcium influx, which in turn causes an increase in the rate and force of contraction. This, along with the concomitant hypotension, results in cardiac hypoxia. The hypoxia and the calcium deposits in the mitochondria produce disintegration of organelles and sarcolemma (Balazs et al., 1981).

Interference with Nucleic Acid Synthesis

The anthracycline antibiotics, doxorubicin and daunorubicin, are effective antineoplastic drugs. However, they produce hypotension, tachycardia, and arrhythmias acutely. More prolonged administration produces degeneration and atrophy of cardiac muscle cells and interstitial edema and fibrosis. The likely mode of action is the binding of these antibiotics to mitochondrial and nuclear DNA, which in turn interferes with the synthesis of RNA and protein. This effect on the heart is important because the half-life of the contractile proteins is short (12 weeks). Other possible mechanisms of action include peroxidation of membrane lipids and hypotension resulting from the release of cytokines (Van Stee, 1980). The mechanism of doxorubicin cardiotoxicity is particularly involved in apoptosis mediated by calcium overload and iron-catalyzed formation of free radicals while the anticancer mode of action is due to the inhibition of topoisomerase II (Bernard et al., 2011). Doxorubicin, containing quinones in chemical structure, increases reactive oxygen species (ROS) generation in primary cultures of cardiomyocytes in a time- and concentration-dependent manner (Fu et al., 2010).

Arrhythmias

A number of fluorocarbons are capable of producing cardiac arrhythmias. This effect is mediated by a sensitization of the heart to epinephrine, depression of contractility, reduction of coronary blood flow, and reflex increase in sympathetic and vagal impulses to the heart following irritation of mucosa in the respiratory tract (Aviado, 1978).

Tricyclic antidepressants can also induce cardiac arrhythmias. These effects are likely the result of imbalances within the autonomic regulatory system of the heart. Propylene glycol, a common solvent, can convert ventricular tachycardia induced by deslanoside into ventricular fibrillation (Keller et al., 1992).

Myocardial Depression

A number of lipid-soluble organic compounds, such as general anesthetics, depress cardiac contractility. The probable mechanism of action is a nonspecific expansion of various cellular membranes by the insertion of chemically indifferent molecules in the hydrophobic regions of integral proteins and membrane phospholipids.

Antibiotics, such as amphotericin B, chloramphenicol, streptomycin, and tetracycline, produce hypotension through depression of cardiac contractility. The mechanism of action appears to be related to an inhibition of Ca^{2+} bound to superficial membrane sites (Keller et al., 1992).

Miscellaneous

Rapeseed oil, a common cooking oil in many parts of the world, produces accumulation of lipid globules in heart muscles in rats. This effect was attributed to the high content of erucic acid in rapeseed oil. Brominated vegetable oils, used in adjusting the density of flavoring oils and in enhancing cloudy stability in beverages, induce biochemical and morphological changes in cardiac myofibrils. The coloring Brown FK also produces severe morphological changes in the heart muscles (Grice, 1972).

TOXIC EFFECTS ON BLOOD VESSELS

Increased Capillary Permeability

Lead, mercury, and several other toxicants damage endothelial cells of capillaries in the brain. This effect will result in brain edema and an impairment of the blood–brain barrier (chap. 16). Inhalation of irritating gas induces pulmonary edema (chap. 11). Recently, multiwalled carbon nanotubes used in electronics, automotive, and aerospace industries and medical devices were found to increase cell permeability in endothelial cells.

Endothelial Damage

Monocrotaline, a plant toxin, may produce pulmonary vascular damage. This chemical, after ingestion, is bioactivated in the liver, but sufficient amounts of the active metabolites leave the liver and produce cross-linking of DNA in the endothelial cells of the pulmonary vasculature. This effect may damage the repairing capability of the endothelial cells leading to thrombosis and progressive pulmonary hypertension (Boor et al., 1995; Schultze and Roth, 1998). Arsenic has been suggested as the cause of the *black-foot* disease, a result of peripheral endarteritis (Lin et al., 1998)

Vasoconstriction and Vasodilatation

Ingestion of ergot alkaloids (fungal contaminants in certain foods) may produce gangrene resulting from vasoconstriction. A clinical syndrome known as "black-foot disease" is endemic in certain areas in South America and Taiwan. It has been attributed to vasoconstriction following consumption of drinking water with high levels of arsenic (chap. 23). Exposure to pure oxygen over a prolonged period may result in blindness, especially among premature infants, evidently because of the associated vasoconstriction in the eye.

Occupational workers exposed to nitroglycerin on work days have been reported to have died suddenly of heart attack on weekends. Apparently, the continued exposure to a coronary dilator has rendered the workers accustomed to a low level of coronary flow, and the sudden cessation of exposure to the coronary dilator precipitated coronary insufficiency.

The musculature of the coronary artery may be damaged by large doses of certain hypotensive drugs such as minoxidil and hydralazine. The lesion may be a result of exaggerated pharmacodynamic changes (Boor et al., 1995).

Others

Degenerative Changes

Atherosclerosis is a complex degenerative disease affecting mainly large blood vessels such as the coronary and carotid arteries. Narrowing of these arteries may result in heart attacks and strokes, respectively. While the etiology of atherosclerosis is complex, certain toxicants may aggravate the pathological condition. Carbon monoxide may increase the permeability of capillaries surrounding these arteries and promote the degenerative process (Yang et al., 1998). Exposure to air pollutants has resulted in an increased frequency of hospital admissions for cardiovascular disease, congestive heart failure, and higher mortality (Chung et al., 2005; Dominic et al., 2005; Yang (2008). CS_2 produces damage to the endothelium. Ramos et al. (1994) observed that certain allylamines and aromatic hydrocarbons may contribute to the development of atherosclerosis. These toxicants may act through nitric oxide and endothelin on the smooth muscle and endothelium of arteries, and induce vascular lesions, which may contribute to the development of atherosclerosis.

Fibrosis

Cadmium and lead may affect blood vessels in the kidney producing renal fibrosis. The impairment of blood supply may interfere with the "nonexcretory functions" of the kidney (chap. 14), and indirectly produce hypertension.

Hypersensitivity Reaction

Gold salts, penicillin, sulfonamides, and a number of other toxicants may induce vasculitis or exacerbate preexisting polyarteritis. The condition usually affects small vessels and is associated with the infiltration of eosinophils and mononuclear cells indicating an involvement of the immune system.

Tumors

Tumors of blood vessels may result from certain toxicants. For example, vinyl chloride was reported to produce hemangiosarcoma in the liver in humans and animals (chap. 7); hemangioendothelioma was shown to result from exposure to thorium dioxide.

TESTING PROCEDURES

Cardiovascular toxicity can be studied in intact normal animals, in animals with specific pathological conditions such as hypertension or diabetes mellitus, or in isolated hearts and blood vessels.

Normal Animals

Various examinations for cardiovascular toxicity can be performed on animals in conventional toxicity studies. These include blood pressure, heart rate, and electro-cardiography. The rate of blood flow is a useful indicator of the functions of the cardiovascular systems, and can be measured using, among others, pulsed Doppler flow meter (Haywood et al., 1981). The status of the arterioles, capillaries, and venules can be studied either at a specific site of organism (e.g., conjunctiva and retina) or through microvascular chamber which can be chronically placed on a laboratory animal (Smith et al., 1994). Functional tests, such as swimming until exhaustion, have been suggested. At necropsy, the organ weight is often deter-mined. Gross, light, and, in particular, electron microscopic examinations are valu-able. Biochemical studies of the myocardium and of the blood are also useful.

Animals with Pathological Conditions

The hearts of rabbits fed a diet containing 2% cholesterol become atherosclerotic. These hearts are more susceptible to myocardial ischemia (Lee et al., 1978). Other models, such as infarcted myocardium, cardiomyopathic hamster, obesity, and drug interaction models, have been briefly described and referenced by Van Stee (1980).

Isolated Heart

The isolated, perfused heart is a common model for studying the effects of drugs on the strength and rate of heart contractions and the rate of coronary flow. It was also used to detect the cardiac effects of toxicants. For example, Toy et al. (1976) showed that certain halogenated alkanes depressed the peak left ventricular pres-sure as well as the rate of increase of that pressure. The isolated atrium and cul-tured heart cells have also been used in the study of cardiotoxicity (Adams et al., 1978; Sperelakis, 1978).

Evaluation

The cardiovascular toxicity of chemicals is not readily detected in conventional toxicity studies. For example, the toxic effects of cobalt and the anthracycline anti-biotics on the heart were reproduced in animal experiments only after they were detected in humans first. Negative results, therefore, do not necessarily exclude potential cardiotoxicity.

To demonstrate such toxicity, specific testing procedures may be required. These procedures usually mimic the clinical conditions. For example, intermittent administration of the anthracycline antibiotics was necessary to elicit cardiotoxicity; presumably continuous treatment caused the animals to die from other toxic effects before heart lesions developed. The toxicity of adrenergic β-receptor agonists is best detected in acute studies; the effects of prolonged treatment may be masked by tolerance development. The effect of cobalt on the heart is more readily revealed when the animals are on a protein- and vitamin-deficient diet (Balazs and Ferrans, 1978).

REFERENCES

Adams HR, Parker JL, Durrett LR (1978). Cardiac toxicities of antibiotics. Environ Health Perspect 26, 217–231.

Allmark MG, Grice HC, Lu FC (1955). Chronic toxicity studies on food colors: Observations on the toxicity of FD&C Yellow No. 3 (Oil Yellow AB) and FD&C Yellow No. 4 (Oil Yellow OB) in rats. J Pharm Pharmacol 7, 591–603.

Aviado DM (1978). Effects of fluorocarbons, chlorinated solvents, and inosine on the cardiopulmonary system. Environ Health Perspect 26, 207–216.

Balazs T, Ferrans VJ (1978). Cardiac lesions induced by chemicals. Environ Health Perspect 26, 181–191.

Balazs T, Ferrans VJ, El-Hage A, et al. (1981). Study of the mechanism of hydralazine-induced myocardial necrosis in the rat. Toxicol Appl Pharmacol 59, 524–534.

Bardin CW, Baker HWG, Jefferson LS, et al. (1978). Methods for perfusing male reproductive tract: Models for studying drugs and hormone metabolism. Environ Health Perspect 24, 51–59.

Bernard Y, Ribeiro N, Thuaud F, et al. (2011). Flavaglines alleviate doxorubicin cardiotoxicity: Implication of Hsp27. PLoS One 6, e25302.

Boor PJ, Gotlieb AI, Joseph EC, et al. (1995). Chemical-induced vasculature injury. Toxicol Appl Pharmacol 132, 177–195.

Brusick D (1987). Principles of Genetic Toxicology, 2nd edn. New York, NY: Plenum Press.

Chung CC, Tsai SS, Ho SC, et al. (2005). Air pollution and hospital admissions for cardiovascular disease in Taipei. Environ Res 98, 130–139.

Cook JC, Mullin LS, Frame SR, et al. (1993). Investigation of a mechanism for Leydig cell tumorigenesis by linuron. Toxicol Appl Pharmacol 119, 195–204.

Dominic F, McDermott A, Daniels M, et al. (2005). Revised analysis of the national morbidity, mortality and air pollution study: Mortality among residents of 90 cities. J Toxicol Environ Health A 68, 1071–1092.

Eliasson R (1978). Semen analysis. Environ Health Perspect 24, 81–85.

EPA (1994). Health Effects Test Guidelines. Washington, DC.: U.S. Environmental Protection Agency.

Eroschenko VP, Rourke AW (1992). Stimulating influences of the technical grade methoxychlor and estradiol on protein synthesis in the uterus of the immature mouse. J Occup Med Toxicol 1, 307–315.

Fabro S (1978). Penetration of chemicals into the oocyte, uterine fluid and preimplantation blastocyst. Environ Health Persp 24, 25–29.

Fu Z, Guo J, Jing L, et al. (2010). Enhanced toxicity and ROS generation by doxorubicin in primary cultures of cardiomyocytes from neonatal metallothionein-I/II null mice. Toxicol In Vitro 24, 1584–1591.

Grice HC (1972). The changing role of pathology in modern safety evaluation. CRC Crit Rev Toxicol 1, 119–152.

Haywood JR, Shaffer RA, Fink GD, et al. (1981). Regional blood flow measurements with pulsed Doppler flowmeter in conscious rat. Am J Physiol 241, 14273–14278.

Hecht NB (1987). Detecting the effects of toxic agents on spermatogenesis using DNA probes. Environ Health Perspect 74, 31–40.

Keller RS, Parker JL, Adams HR (1992). Cardiovascular toxicity of antibacterial antibiotics. In: Costa D, ed. Cardiovascular Toxicology. New York, NY: Raven Press, 165–195.

Lee IP (1983). Adaptive biochemical repair response toward germ cell DNA damage. Am J Ind Med 4, 135–147.

Lee IP, Dixon RL (1978). Factors influencing reproduction and genetic toxic effects on male gonads. Environ Health Perspect 24, 117–127.

Lee RJ, Zaidi IH, Baky SH (1978). Pathophysiology of the atherosclerotic rabbit. Environ Health Perspect 26, 225–231.

Lin T-H, Huang Y-L, Wang M-Y (1998). Arsenic species in drinking water, hair, fingernails and urine of patient's with blackfoot disease. J Toxicol Environ Health A 53, 85–93.

Lin YC, Coskun S, Sanbuissho A (1994). Effects of gossypol on in vitro bovine oocyte maturation and steroidogenesis in bovine granulosa cells. Theriogenology 41, 1601–1611.

Mesfin GM, Morris DF, Seaman WJ, et al. (1989). Testicular lesions in rats treated with a sympatholytic hypotensive agent (losulazine). J Am Coll Toxicol 8, 525–538.

Miller RK, Kellogg CK, Saltzman RA (1987). Reproductive and perinatal toxicology. In: Haley TJ, Berndt WO, eds. Handbook of Toxicology. Washington, DC.: Hemisphere, 195–309.

Nagi S, Virgo BB (1982). The effects of spironolactone on reproductive functions in female rats and mice. Toxicol Appl Pharmacol 66, 221–228.

OECD (1995). OECD guidelines for testing of chemicals: Reproduction/developmental toxicity screening test. Paris, France: Organization of Economic Development.

Palmer AK (1976). Assessment of current test procedures. Environ Health Perspect 18, 97–104.

Qian S, Wang Z (1984). Gossypol: A potential antifertility agent for males. Annu Rev Pharmacol Toxicol 24, 329–360.

Ramos KS, Bowes RC, Ou XL, et al. (1994). Responses of vascular smooth cells to toxic insult: Cellular and molecular perspectives for environmental toxicants. J Toxicol Environ Health 43, 419–440.

Schultze AE, Roth RA (1998). Monocrotaline pulmonary hypertension—The monocrotaline model and involvement of the hemostatic system. J Toxicol Environ Health B 1, 271–346.

Smith TL, Koman LA, Mosberg AT (1994). Cardiovascular physiology and methods for toxicology. In: Hayes AW, ed. Principles and Methods of Toxicology. New York, NY: Raven Press.

Sperelakis N (1978). Cultured heart cell reaggregate model for studying cardiac toxicology. Environ Health Perspect 26, 243–267.

Su L, Mruk DD, Cheng CY (2011). Drug transporters, the blood-testis barrier, and spermatogenesis. J Endocrinol 208, 207–223.

Toy PA, Van Stee EW, Harris AM, et al. (1976). The effects of three halogenated alkanes on excitation and contraction in the isolated, perfused rabbit heart. Toxicol Appl Pharmacol 38, 7–17.

Van Stee EW (1980). Myocardial toxicity. In: Witschi HR, ed. The Scientific Basis of Toxicity Assessment. New York, NY: Elsevier/North Holland.

Waalkes MP, Rehm S (1994). Cadmium and prostate cancer. J Toxicol Environ Health 43, 251–269.

Yang CY (2008). Air pollution and hospital; admissions for congestive heart failure in a subtropical city: Taipei, Taiwan. J Toxicol Environ Health A 71, 1085–1090.

Yang W, Jennison BL, Omaye ST (1998). Cardiovascular disease hospitalization and ambient levels of carbon monoxide. J Toxicol Environ Health A 55, 185–196.

19

Toxicology of the endocrine system

INTRODUCTION

Endocrine system is highly complex, which regulates numerous bodily functions and development. The main function of the endocrine system is to maintain homeostasis, which it achieves using hormones synthesized and secreted from glands, such as the hypothalamus, pituitary (luteinizing hormone, follicle-stimulating hormone, etc.), pineal (melatonin), pancreas (insulin), and sex organs [ovaries (estrogens and progestins) and testes (androgens)], thyroid, parathyroid, and adrenal glands (corticosteroids). Hormones are generally classified as lipid derivatives (e.g., eicosanoids/steroids), peptides, and amines, which are synthesized from arachidonic acid/cholesterol, proteins, and amino acids (e.g., tyrosine, tryptophan), respectively. Disruption of the endocrine system by endocrine-disrupting chemicals (EDCs) can produce developmental toxicity, reproductive toxicity, carcinogenicity, mutagenicity, neurotoxicity, and immunotoxicity (Choi et al., 2004). In addition, EDCs have been reported to act as obesogens and to be associated with diabetes (Baillie-Hamilton, 2002; Thayer et al., 2012). Since the publication of Rachel Carson's book *Silent Spring*, there has been a great deal of concern over EDCs and much attention has been paid to these chemicals.

ENDOCRINE-DISRUPTING CHEMICALS

EDCs (also called endocrine disruptors) are defined as chemicals that are structurally similar to hormones, which interfere with the synthesis, secretion, transport, metabolism, and binding action of natural endogenous hormones (EPA, 1998). Initially concern focused on chemicals with estrogen-like activities, but it has become increasingly apparent that EDCs may mimic or interfere with the actions of all endocrine hormones including androgens, thyroid, adrenal, and pituitary hormones (Colborn et al., 1993; DeRosa et al., 1998; Whitehead and Rice, 2006). Furthermore, one single EDC may have multiple hormonal effects, including

Table 19.1   Preliminary List of Chemicals with Endocrine Disrupting Effects by Animal Study

Type	Chemicals	
Industrial chemicals	Bisphenol A, phthalate esters, p-nonylphenol, octylphenol, polychlorinated biphenyls, pentachlorophenol, styrene, 2,3,7, 8-TCDD, tributyltin chloride	
Pesticides	Herbicides	Alachlor, amitrole, atrazine, 2,4-D, metribuzin, nitrofen, 2,4,5-T, trifluralin
	Insecticides	Beta-BHC, gamma-BHC (lindane), carbaryl, chlordane, *p,p′*-DDD, *p,p′*-DDE, *p,p′*-DDT, dicofol, dieldrin, endosulfan, heptachlor, heptachlor epoxide, methomyl, methoxychlor, mirex, trans-nonachlor, oxychlordane, parathion, pyrethroids (synthetic), toxaphene
	Nematocides	Aldicarb, 1,2-dibromo-3-chloropropane
Heavy metals	Cadmium, lead, mercury, arsenic	
Pharmaceuticals	Diethylstilbestrol, tamoxifen, raloxifene, flutamide, finasteride	
Plant and fungal agents	Zearalenone, coumestrol, genistein, daidzein	

Abbreviations: DDT, dichlorodiphenyltrichloroethane; TCDD, tetrachlorodibenzo-p-dioxin. *Source*: From Choi et al., 2004.

estrogenic/anti-estrogenic, androgenic/anti-androgenic, or thyroid/anti-thyroid effects (McKinney and Waller, 1998). EDCs are present both in the environment and in foods, and may originate from pesticides, combustion products, plasticizers, detergents, or heavy metals (Table 19.1).

CLASSIFICATION OF ENDOCRINE DISRUPTORS

Humans are exposed to various environmental chemicals with endocrine-disrupting activity during daily life, because EDCs are found in low quantities in a variety of consumer products. EDCs that are commonly found in the environment include herbicides, fungicides, insecticides, and industrial/commercial agents such as bisphenol A (BPA), alkylphenol, phthalates, polychlorinated biphenyls (PCBs), and other chlorinated compounds. Accordingly, various EDCs, such as, PCBs, 2,3,7,8-tetrachlorodibenzo-p-dioxin, dichloro-diphenyl trichloroethane (DDT), BPA, polybrominated diphenyl ethers (PBDEs), and a variety of phthalate esters (PEs), are commonly detected in human blood and urine. These chemicals are classified as estrogenic/anti-estrogenic, androgenic/antiandrogenic chemicals, or those that affect thyroid hormone functions (Choi et al., 2004) (Fig. 19.1). It is also possible that these compounds affect other important hormones like insulin.

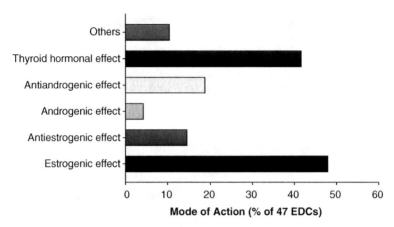

Figure 19.1 Hormone-modulating effects of the 48 endocrine disrupting chemicals (EDCs) classified by Centers for Disease Control and Prevention. Some EDCs have multiple hormone-modulating effects, but counted once.

Alkylphenol Polyethoxylates

Alkylphenol polyethoxylates (APEs) are used as nonionic surfactants in industrial and household cleaning agents, in the manufacture of paints and plastics, in pesticide formulations, and in the manufacture of rubber goods (Giger et al., 1984). APEs released into sewage are metabolized by microbes in sewage sludge to alkylphenolic compounds (APs). These compounds are relatively stable and have been detected in surface water, sediments, and in fish fat (Klecka et al., 2010). Several experimental studies demonstrated that APs possess some estrogenic activity (Munkittrick et al., 1998).

Although the mechanisms are unclear, octylphenol (OP) was found to suppress testicular function significantly in adult male rats. In particular, it reduced testes size, lowered testosterone concentrations, and decreased spermatogenesis (Blake and Boockfor, 1997). OP was also reported to be toxic to aquatic animals and exert adverse effects on murine splenocytes (Nair-Menon et al., 1996). Of the APs tested for estrogenicity, OP was found to be approximately 1000-fold less potent than 17β–estradiol (E2) in vitro (White et al., 1994).

Bisphenol A

BPA is a major component in epoxy and polycarbonate (PC) resins, which are widely used as ingredients in protective coatings on food containers and as adhesives in packaging products (Howe and Borodinsky, 1998). PC is widely used in the manufacture of plastic, and BPA accounts for about 63% of the total consumption of PC (Chemical Profile, 1999). Brotons et al. (1995) first demonstrated estrogenic activity in components extracted from canned foodstuffs and identified BPA from the inner coating as an estrogenic material. Krishnan et al. (1993) first reported BPA release from PC flasks and coated food cans (10–20 g/can) during autoclaving. BPA has since been detected at concentrations ranging from 4 to 23 g/can in both extracted foods and water from autoclaved cans (Perez et al., 1998). In addition, BPA has also been used as a sealant in dentistry and found in saliva (90–931 g) collected from subjects one hour after dental therapy (Olea et al., 1996). Based on the results of studies of the migration of BPA from packing into food, the European Union (EU) initially established a specific migration limit for BPA of 3 mg/kg of food in 2002 and later amended this to 0.6 mg/kg in 2004. The maximal acceptable dose for BPA established by the Environmental Protection Agency (EPA) is 50 g/kg of body weight per day (EPA, 1997).

BPA has been evaluated as a weak estrogenic agent in uterotrophic assays using immature or ovariectomized animals. The ability of BPA to induce uterotrophic activity varies among species, strains, and routes of exposure, and between immature and ovariectomized animals. Gould et al. (1998) found that BPA (150 mg/kg/day) orally administered to immature Sprague-Dawley female rats did not induce any uterotrophic response, but did find uterine progesterone levels significantly increased. Coldham et al. (1997) showed that a subcutaneous injection of 320 mg/kg/day BPA was inactive in an immature mouse uterotrophic assays, and in a recent study, no uterotrophic response to BPA was observed in immature mice following BPA administration at 100 mg/kg/day subcutaneously, but BPA at 1000 mg/kg/day did induce a positive uterotrophic response (Mehmood et al., 2000). Although it is controversial, overall, it is considered that BPA does not pose a significant health risk to humans, including newborns and babies (Willhite et al., 2008; Hengstler et al., 2011).

Phthalate Esters

PEs are found in some soft toys, flooring, medical equipment, cosmetics, and air fresheners. Di(2-ethylhexyl) phthalate (DEHP) is the most abundant phthalate in the environment and mono-(2-ethylhexyl) phthalate is its primary metabolite, which correlates with DEHP in toxicokinetics study (Koo and Lee, 2007). Other important phthalates include di(n-butyl) phthalate, diethyl phthalate, butyl-benzyl phthalate, and di(n-octyl) phthalate. PEs are of potential health concern, because they are suspected to modulate the endocrine systems of animals and some investigators implicated these chemicals with increase in male reproductive system disorders observed in man (Kim et al., 2004; Swan, 2006). In particular, PE exposure might exert significant adverse effects on the reproductive systems of infants (Kaiser, 2005).

In 2002, the U.S. Food and Drug Administration (FDA) released a report that cautioned against polyvinyl chloride (PVC) devices containing DEHP. However, DEHP is widely used as a plasticizer in the manufacture of various plastics such as PVC and for the manufacture of many medical devices. This widespread use leads to significant exposure through contaminated foods, food packaging materials, and medical products (Koo and Lee, 2004; Silva et al., 2005). Based on these results, California, Korea, Europe, and Japan banned manufacturers from using some phthalates in children's toys. However, risk assessments have shown that human exposure levels to PEs generally do not exceed safe limits (Koo and Lee, 2005).

Polybrominated Diphenyl Ethers

PBDEs are found in fire retardants, in the plastic cases of televisions and computers, and in electronic items, carpets, lighting, bedding, clothing, car components, foam cushions, and other textile materials. Commercial PBDE products are predominantly the penta-, octa- and decabromodiphenyl ethers. Today, the consumption of decabromodiphenyl ether (deca-BDE) accounts for over 80% of the PBDEs produced, whereas pentabromodiphenyl ether (penta-BDE) and octabromodiphenyl ether (octa-BDE) products constitute about 12% and 6%, respectively (de Wit, 2002). PBDEs have been found in indoor and outdoor air (Wilford et al., 2004), and dust samples (Stapleton et al., 2005).

PBDEs are being increasingly detected in human milk, tissue, and serum samples (Mazdai et al., 2003), and the most prevalent PBDE congeners in human samples are PBDE-47 and PBDE-99. Therefore, the widespread uses of PBDEs and their increasing levels in the environment have increased concerns about possible adverse effects on human health. PBDEs are structurally similar to PCBs and exert similar neurotoxic effects. PBDEs have the potential to disrupt thyroid hormone balance and may contribute to a variety of neurological and developmental defects, including low intelligence and learning disabilities.

However, another report suggests that there was no correlation between serum thyroxin (T4) and total PBDE concentrations (Kim et al., 2012). Nonetheless, many of the most common PBDEs were banned by the EU in 2006.

Other Suspected Endocrine Disruptors

Other suspected EDCs include xenoestrogens, such as, DDT and its metabolites (o,p'-DDT or p,p'-DDE), which bind to estrogen receptor (ER). The fungicide procymidone binds to the androgen receptor (AR) and acts as a competitive inhibitor of androgen (Gray et al., 1999). Furthermore, environmental contaminants, such as some polycyclic aromatic hydrocarbons (PAHs) (Vinggaard et al., 2000) and PCBs (Schrader and Cooke, 2003), have been shown to act as anti-androgens in vitro, but the mode of action of these compounds has not been determined. An environmental contaminant of uncertain origin, tris-(4-chlorophenyl)-methanol has also been found to be a potent AR antagonist. Other examples of suspected EDCs are vinclozolin, zearalenone, dioxins, furans, phenols, and several pesticides, such as pyrethroid, carbamate, and organochlorine insecticides and their derivatives.

MOLECULAR MECHANISMS OF ENDOCRINE DISRUPTION

EDCs have been reported to interfere with the production, release, transport, metabolism, binding, actions, and eliminations of the natural hormones responsible for maintaining homeostasis and regulating body development. While the contributions of these activities to cancer risk have not been clearly defined, data from several sources collectively indicate that studies of EDC action should take into consideration the cellular environment and genetic, and possibly epigenetic changes. The effects of xenobiotics on the development of several human cancers were identified several decades ago. Although the mechanisms of EDC-related cancer have not been fully elucidated, possible modes of action include, alterations of metabolic activation, interactions between endogenous hormones, growth factors, and the perturbations of transcription pathways. We will now further discuss the mechanisms of carcinogenesis underlying the actions of EDCs.

Free Radical Production

As previously described (Choi et al., 2004), EDCs may have a wide-ranging variety of endocrine-disrupting effects, including developmental disorders, carcinogenicity, mutagenicity, immunotoxicity, and neurotoxicity. Choi and Lee (2004) demonstrated that about 94% of the 48 EDCs classified by the Centers for Disease Control and Prevention generate free radicals and that this might represent a common toxic mechanism underlying the effects of EDCs (Fig. 19.2).

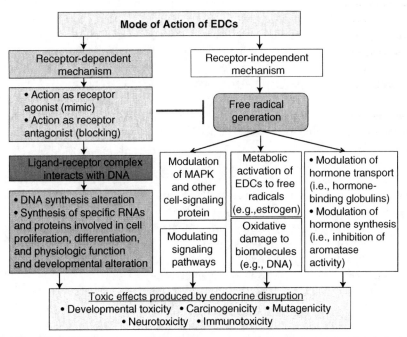

Figure 19.2 The mode of action of endocrine disruptors during cancer development and toxicities.

Later, it was also postulated that oxidative stress induced by EDCs is a common mechanism of carcinogenesis (Keri et al., 2007)..

Nuclear Receptor–Mediated Carcinogenicity

Exposure to EDCs may increase the risk of cancer in hormone-dependent organs (prostatic, breast, testicular, and endometrial cancer). On the other hand, a number of EDCs, including *o, p'*-DDT, PCB, pesticides, and heavy metals, act as initiators and/or promoters of carcinogenesis (Yusof and Edwards, 1990). EDCs may play important roles in the development of human cancer via interactions with estrogens, growth factors (and their receptors), transduction signaling pathways, oncogene activation, or tumor suppressor gene inactivation (Janosek et al., 2006). The first receptor-mediated mechanism involves the activation of responsive elements on DNA, which results in the increased expression of target genes. Alternatively, inter-actions between compounds and receptors might negatively affect receptor binding to responsive elements on DNA, and thus suppress receptor action.

The nuclear receptor superfamily is a large group of receptors that regulate a wide range of physiological functions, including cell growth and proliferation, cellular differentiation, the maintenance of homeostasis, and other toxicological processes (Janosek et al., 2006). This family of structurally related ligand-inducible transcription factors includes ER, AR, thyroid hormone receptor (TR), and retinoid receptors (retinoic acid receptor and retinoid X receptor), and other molecules known as orphan receptors. After binding of a specific ligand, the struc-tural conformation of the receptor is changed and the receptor translocates into the nucleus, binds to the corresponding responsive element on DNA, and triggers gene expression. Further, cross-talk exists between these receptors, for example between peroxisome proliferator-activated receptors and ER, TR, and retinoic acid receptor, and this modulates gene regulation (Corton and Lapinskas, 2005). However, the complexity of cross-talk within endocrine signaling pathways is not clearly understood, and therefore, evidence linking exposure to EDCs with adverse human health effects is lacking.

ERs may directly regulate various genes, including those encoding hormones, proteases, angiogenesis promoters (e.g., vascular endothelial growth factor), cell survival proteins (e.g., Bcl-2 and Bax) and cell proliferation proteins (e.g., cyclin D and CDKs). In addition, ERs may affect transcription without directly binding to DNA by associating with other transcription factors, such as, activator protein-1 (AP-1) or specificity protein 1 (Sp1). In addition, the develop-ment of tumors in reproductive organs often depends on the actions of sex hormones, but the mechanisms involved are unclear.

Many compounds have been shown to produce adverse effects at multiple levels of thyroid signaling in vitro and in vivo (Langer, 1998). Ryu et al. (2007) demonstrated that thyroid hormone receptor-α1 (TR-α1) mRNA levels are increased by chronic DBP exposure in rats. In addition, Rao et al.(2003) postu-lated that the TR directly affects both the development of prepubertal testes and the regulation of follicle-stimulating hormone receptor and luteinizing hormone receptor gene expression, which may further modulate the effects of gonadotropins on testis functions. Furthermore, Ryu et al. (2007) showed that TR-1 protein and mRNA levels are expressed at significantly higher levels in the testes of DBP-exposed rats, which indicates that TR-α1 may be an essential mediator of the adverse effects of DBP and contribute to DBP-induced dysgenesis of testicular growth and development. Barlow and Foster (2003) have demonstrated that exposure to anti-androgens interrupts the action of androgen at the receptor level, which suggests that the downregulation of testicular AR during the early development stages alters androgen-mediated testis development and growth.

EPIGENETIC REGULATION OF TRANSGENERATIONAL DISEASES

The binding of EDCs to endogenous hormone receptors alters hormone signaling, and thus, influences the normal endocrine system (McKinney and Waller, 1998). In particular, exposure to estrogenic chemicals during embryonic or postnatal development may produce transgenerational abnormalities in male reproductive tissues, including testes, seminal vesicles, and prostate (Anway and Skinner, 2008) and increase the risk of tumor development (Ho et al., 2006a). The possible involvement of epigenetic mechanisms in endocrine disruption helps explain the transgenerational effects of some EDCs. Early studies showed that treatment with diethylstilbestrol during pregnancy resulted in vaginal adenocarcinoma in female offspring in humans (Herbst et al., 1971) and mice (McLachlan et al., 1980). It now appears that these transgenerational phenotypes are in part involved in the epigenetic reprogramming of male germline cells. Thus, epigenomic alterations seem to provide a mechanism for transgenerational changes in imprinting genes. For example, exposure to the fungicide vinclozolin during embryonic gonadal sex determination alters the epigenetic programming of the male germline to induce altered DNA methylation patterns in various genes (Birnbaum and Fenton, 2003). Ho et al. (2006b) demonstrated that exposure of rats to low doses of estradiol or BPA during the neonatal developmental period increased susceptibility to precancerous prostatic lesions in aged animals and sensitized the prostate gland in adult-induced hormonal carcinogenesis. Further, these findings support the existence of a correlation between fetal exposure to EDCs and cancer development (Birnbaum and Fenton, 2003).

The epigenetic mechanism for endocrine disruption induced by EDCs involves altered DNA methylation in the germ-line that appears to transmit transgenerational adult-onset diseases such as spermatogenic defects, prostate disease, kidney disease, and cancer (Anway and Skinner, 2008). These epigenetic changes are brought about by mechanisms involving DNA methylation, histone modifications, and non-coding RNAs in the regulations of gene expression patterns. Epigenetic mechanisms are essential for normal development and differentiation, but can be misdirected, which leads to disease, most notably cancer. Indeed, mounting evidence indicates that environmental exposure to EDCs, particularly during early development can induce epigenetic changes that may be transmitted in subsequent generations or serve as the basis for diseases that develop later in life. Methylation profiles can be used as molecular markers to distinguish subtypes of cancers and potentially as predictors of disease outcome and treatment response. The role of epigenetics in diagnosis and treatment are likely to increase as mechanisms leading to the transcriptional silencing of genes involved in human cancer are revealed.

Emerging evidence suggests that epigenetic programming has the potential to affect protein function much later in life and potentially across generations, which adds a layer of complexity to the impact of early life exposure to EDCs on endocrine homeostasis across life span and into subsequent generations. The multifactorial nature of endocrine-related disorders must also be considered when designing studies and selecting appropriate animal models for mechanistic studies.

ADVERSE EFFECTS OF ENDOCRINE DISRUPTORS

Numerous investigations indicate that EDCs pose a threat to wildlife, animals, and humans. Ever since the harmful impact of EDCs on wildlife was described by Rachel Carson in her book *Silent Spring*, their influences on various animals and humans have been continuously reported. The main harmful impact of EDCs is to produce abnormal conditions within the body by mimicking hormones at the molecular level.

Wildlife Species

Many researchers have observed the harmful impacts of EDCs on species such as shellfish, reptiles, fish, birds, and mammals. The following is a summary of impacts on wildlife species reported to date.

Shellfish: The most representative harmful impact on wildlife species is imposex that occurs among gastropods such as turban shells or sea snails, whereby a female becomes a male due to the superimposition of a male sex organ on its body. This ecological phenomenon can produce drastic population decreases because it produces female sterility. Imposex was first discovered in female sea snails that inhabited Plymouth, England in 1969, and subsequently, it was found that such phenomenon resulted from sea water contamination by organotin compounds such as tributyltin (Birchenough et al., 2002).

Birds: A reproductive disorder produced by DDT is well established in birds. The mechanism responsible was a lack of eggshell calcification, which resulted in a failure to hatch (Rattner et al., 1984). This phenomenon mostly affects birds further up the food chain such as sea gulls, cormorants, herons, pelicans, falcons, and eagles. In the case of sea gulls, abnormal female–female pairing and multiple egg-laying have been observed. Decreases in sexual intercourse frequency, indifference to the opposite sex, mating between the same sex, a decrease in newborns, and reductions in immune function have also been reported.

Fish: In Japan, while confirming sexual imbalance among carp due to reduced numbers of males in some streams, it was found that the sexual imbalance was associated with relatively high levels of APEs. Many reports have been issued on the impacts of substances like APEs, which are the degradation products of synthetic detergents or nonionic surfactants. Discoveries reported in various parts of England of fish with ambiguous gender identities also seem to be related to APEs (Rice et al., 2003). When these APEs were injected into tanks containing rainbow trout, researchers found that testicular development was hindered. In the same experiment, it was found that vitellogenin, which is normally produced only in the liver of females, was produced in males. In addition, observations of abnormal reproductive ability and male immaturity were reported in Coho (silver) salmon inhabiting Lake Erie (Leatherland et al., 1982).

Reptiles and Amphibians: The representative case for reptiles was reported in Lake Apopka, Florida, where the population of alligators was reduced by 50% after accidental DDT leakage. This contamination produced male alligators to become females and male sex organ shrinkage (Semenza et al., 1997). In the case of red-eared sliders, PCB exposure was found to reduce successful egg hatching, and led to the majority of eggs to give rise to females (Moss et al., 2009). In addition, many reports on frogs showed that exposure to dioxins, heavy metals, or dibenzofurans reduced the hatching rates and increased the mutations (Fort et al., 2004).

Mammals: Like other animals, various reports have been issued on the harmful impacts by EDCs on mammals. For example, marked reductions in otter counts, a high death rate of minke whale infants, a population decrease among polar bears, and mass mortality of striped dolphins in the Mediterranean sea have been reported to be related to EDCs (Sonne et al., 2009). The harmful impacts frequently reported in mammals are population decreases, male sex organ disorders, and immune system disorders, which are now also issues of concern in man.

Humans

EDCs probably exert harmful effects on humans, but supporting evidence is limited. In Taiwan, growth delay, attention deficit hyperactivity disorder, and undersized penises during puberty were observed in children whose mothers used cooking oil contaminated with PCBs (Yu et al., 2000). A mother who had been exposed to synthetic estrogen was found to have a daughter with a rare type of vaginal cancer and her son possessed a malformed penis (Mericskay et al., 2005). Among the children of women whose diets contained fish from the Great Lakes when young, the proportion of children with a small brain size at birth with developmental disabilities was relatively large (Seegal, 1999). In Danish men, sperm counts fell from 113 million/mL to 66 million/mL (Carlsen et al., 1992). In French men, counts fell from 89 million/mL in 1976 to 60 million/mL and sperm motility decreased (Auger et al., 1995). In Japan, it was found that the average sperm count of a man in his 20s living in the Tokyo suburbs was 46 million/mL, which was only a half that of a man in his 40s (84 million/mL). Researchers proposed that estrogen might be a possible cause. In the United States, it was concluded that women exposed to DDT or PCBs are at the risk of developing breast cancer (Wolff and Toniolo, 1995). Taken together, reducing sperm counts; increasing numbers of breast, prostate, and testicular cancers, and sterility; malformations; attention deficit hyperactivity disorder; and learning disorders in children might be related to exposure to EDCs. However, unambiguous evidence is needed.

EVALUATION OF ENDOCRINE DISRUPTORS

The Organization for Economic Cooperation and Development (OECD) and the U.S. EPA approved various in-vitro and in-vivo assays for EDCs. In particular, the U.S. EPA Office of Chemical Safety and Pollution Prevention introduced EDC testing methods in Test Guideline Series 890. Detailed information on these test methods can be found at: http://www.epa.gov/endo/. On the other hand, OECD test guidelines for EDCs and test details are available and are briefly summarized here (OECD, 2012).

In-Vitro Assays

Androgen Receptor Binding Assay

The AR binding assay is an in-vitro screening assay that checks whether the test substance has the potential to interact with AR. The assay uses AR isolated from rat (Sprague Dawley) ventral prostate. This screening assay measures the receptor-binding affinity of a test substance by evaluating its ability to substitute bound reference androgen, usually 5α-dihydrotestosterone or R1881 (a synthetic androgen). The AR binding assay (a radioligand binding assay) consists of two saturation-binding and competitive-binding experiments (EPA, 2009a).

Estrogen Receptor Binding Assay

This assay is an in-vitro screening assay that checks whether the test substance has the potential to interact with ER. This screening assay uses ER prepared from rat (Sprague Dawley) uterine cytosol, and evaluates the ability of the test substance to substitute 17β-estradiol, an endogenous hormone. This assay is a competitive inhibition assay against radiolabeled estradiol that binds to rat ER, and consists of two saturation binding and competitive binding experiments (EPA, 2009b).

Estrogen Receptor Transcriptional Activation Assay

The estrogen receptor transcriptional activation assay is an in-vitro screening assay that determines whether a test substance binds to and activates ER (EPA, 2011a). After incubating human cervical tumor from a human estrogen receptor-alpha (hERα)-HeLa-9903 cell line with a test substance, this assay is based on the measurement of luciferase activity using a luminometer after lysing cells and adding luciferin substrate.

Aromatase (Human Recombinant) Assay

The aromatase assay is an in-vitro screening assay used to determine whether the test substance inhibits the catalytic activity of cytochrome P450 enzyme aromatase (also known as CYP19)(EPA, 2011b). This assay measures aromatase activity by using liquid scintillation counting sample tritiated water (^3H_2O) released when [^3H] ASDN is converted into estrone.

Steroidogenesis Assay

This assay uses human adrenocortical carcinoma H295R cell line to measure cell viability and the levels of relevant hormones (testosterone and estradiol).

In-Vivo Assay

Amphibian Metamorphosis Assay

Amphibian metamorphosis assay is an in-vivo screening assay used to determine whether the test substance interferes with the normal function of the hypothalamus–pituitary–thyroid axis (OECD, 2009). The assay is conducted using a negative (clean water) control after exposing Nieuwkoop–Faber stage 51 African clawed frog (Xenopus laevis) tadpoles to the test substance at three different concentrations (at least) for 21 days. Observational endpoints are hind limb length , snout-to-vent length, developmental stage, body weight, thyroid histopathology, and daily observations of mortality and clinical signs. This experimental method is important because it is the only assay capable of detecting thyroid activity in animals undergoing morphological development.

Fish Short-Term Reproduction Assay

Fish short-term reproduction assay is an in-vivo screening assay used to determine whether the test substance interferes with the normal structure and function of the hypothalamic–pituitary–gonadal axis. The assay is conducted using a negative control by exposing sexually mature male and female fathead minnow (*Pimephales promelas*) to the test substance at least three different concentrations for 21 days. The observational endpoints are survival (mortality), fecundity, fertilization success, gonado-somatic index, gonad histology, plasma vitellogenin, sex steroid levels, secondary sex characteristics, and other clinical signs.

Female Pubertal Assay

This is an in-vivo screening assay used to determine whether the test substance interacts with the endocrine system during pubertal development and affects thyroid function in juvenile/peripubertal female rats. The assay is conducted by administering the test substance daily by oral gavage to Sprague-Dawley male rats from post-natal day (PND) 22 to PND 42. Observational endpoints include daily body weight, vaginal opening, organ weights, histology (including colloid area and follicular cell height in thyroid), hormones [total serum thyroxine (T4), serum thyroid-stimulating hormone], estrous cyclicity, and clinical serum chemistry.

Male Pubertal Assay

This is an *in-vivo* screening assay used to determine whether the test substance interacts with the endocrine system during pubertal development and affects thyroid function in intact juvenile/peripubertal male rats. The assay is conducted by administering the test substance daily by oral gavage to Sprague-Dawley male rats from PND 23 to PND 53. Observational endpoints include daily body weight, preputial separation, reproductive system organ weight, histology (including colloid area and follicular cell height in thyroid), hormones (total serum testosterone, total serum thyroxine (T4), serum thyroid-stimulating hormone), and clinical serum chemistry.

Uterotrophic Assay

The uterotrophic assay is an in-vivo screening test used to determine whether the test substance shows the physiological activity expected of an estrogen agonist (e.g., 17β-estradiol), as determined by an increase in uterine weight (EPA, 2009d). Young adult female rats (Sprague-Dawley and Wistar strains are preferred) after ovariectomy with adequate time for uterine tissues to regress are used as test animals. The test substance is administered daily for a minimum of three consecutive days. The recommended reference estrogen agonist is 17α-ethynyl estradiol (at 0.3 μg/kg/day subcutaneous or 1.0 μg/kg/day by oral gavage) for positive control, and distilled water for negative control. Twenty-four hours after the last administration, test animals are autopsied, and uterus weights measured. For test substances, it is recommended that the agonist component be administered at least at two doses (a high dose at or just below the maximum tolerated dose but not exceeding the dose limit (1000 mg/kg/day).

Hershberger Assay

The Hershberger assay is a short-term in-vivo screening test that uses accessory tissues of the male reproductive tract to determine the androgenic or antiandrogenic activity of the test substance (Hershberger et al., 1953; EPA, 2009c). The five androgen-dependent tissues examined are ventral prostate, seminal vesicle (plus fluids and coagulating glands), levator ani plus bulbocavernosus, paired Cowper's glands, and glans penis. This assay is based on the weight changes of these five androgen-dependent tissues in castrated-peripubertal male rats (Sprague-Dawley and Wistar strains are recommended, not Fischer 344). The reference androgen agonist used is testosterone propionate (at 0.2 or 0.4 mg/kg/day subcutaneous), and the reference androgen antagonist is flutamide (3 mg/kg/day) for positive control. For test substances, it is recommended that the androgen agonist component be administered at least at two doses (a high dose at or just below the maximum tolerated dose but not exceeding the dose limit (1000 mg/kg/day), and the androgen antagonist component be administered at least three doses.

Test Guideline 407

OECD Test Guideline 407 (TG407) originally was a repeated-dose 28-day oral toxicity study in rodents, but recently a draft that updated parameters on endocrine effects was proposed. The major updated contents were concerning the estrous cycle, sexual maturity, sex organ observation, and relevant hormone measurements. Details of this experimental method can be found at: http://www. oecd.org/dataoecd/.

REFERENCES

Anway MD, Skinner MK (2008). Epigenetic programming of the germ line: effects of endocrine disruptors on the development of transgenerational disease. Reprod Biomed Online 16, 23–5.

Auger J, Kunstmann JM, Czyglik F, et al. (1995). Decline in semen quality among fertile men in Paris during the past 20 years. New Engl J Med 332, 281–5.

Baillie-Hamilton PF (2002). Chemical toxins: a hypothesis to explain the global obesity epidemic. J Altern Complement Med 8, 185–92.

Barlow NJ, Foster PMD (2003). Pathogenesis of male reproductive tract lesions from gestation through adulthood following in utero exposure to di(n-butyl) phthalate. Toxicol Pathol 31, 397–410.

Birnbaum LS, Fenton SE (2003). Cancer and developmental exposure to endocrine disruptors. Environ Health Perspect 111, 389–94.

Birchenough AC, Barnes N, Evans SM, et al. (2002). A review and assessment of tributyltin contamination in the North Sea, based on surveys of butyltin tissue burdens and imposex/intersex in four species of neogastropods. Mar Pollut Bull 44, 534–43.

Blake CA, Boockfor FR (1997) Chronic administration of the environmental pollutant 4-tert-octylphenol to adult male rats interferes with the secretion of luteinizing hormone, follicle-stimulating hormone, prolactin, and testosterone. Biol Reprod 57, 255–66.

Brotons JA, Olea-Serrano MF, Villalobos M, et al. (1995). Xenoestrogens released from lacquer coatings in food cans. Environ Health Perspect 103, 608–12.

Carlsen E, Giwercman A, Keiding N, et al. (1992). Evidence for decreasing quality of semen during past 50 years [see comments], BMJ 305, 609–13.

Chemical Profile (1999). ChemoExpo profile archives "Bisphenol-A". Available from: http://www. fobchemicals.com

Choi SM, Lee BM (2004). An alternative mode of action of endocrine-disrupting chemicals and chemoprevention. J Toxicol Environ Health, Part B 7, 451–63.

Choi SM, Yoo SD, Lee BM (2004) Toxicological characteristics of endocrine-disrupting chemicals: developmental toxicity, carcinogenicity, and mutagenicity. J Toxicol Environ Health, Part B 7, 1–24.

Colborn T, vom Saal FS, Soto AM (1993). Developmental effects of endocrine-disrupting chemicals in wildlife and humans. Environ Health Perspect 101, 378–84.

Coldham NG, Dave M, Sivapathasundaram S, et al., (1997). Elevation of a recombinant yeast cell estrogen screening assay. Environ Health Perspect 105, 734–42.

Corton JC, Lapinskas PJ (2005). Peroxisome proliferator-activated receptors: mediators of phthalate ester-induced effects in the male reproductive tract? Toxicol Sci 83, 4–17.

DeRosa, C., Richter, P., Pohl, H. et al (1998) Environmental exposures that affect the endocrine system: public health implications. J. Toxicol. Environ. Health B 1: 3–26.

de Wit CA (2002). An overview of brominated flame retardants in the environment. Chemosphere 46, 583–624.

EPA (1997) U.S. Environmental Protection Agency "Integrated Risk Information System" on-line.

EPA (1998). Research Plan for Endocrine Disruptors. EPA/600/R-98/087. Washington, DC:U.S. Environmental Protection Agency, Office of Research and Development. Available from: http://www.epa.gov/scipoly/oscpendo/ docs/edstac/exesum14.pdf

EPA (2009a) Endocrine disruptor screening program test guidelines OPPTS 890.1150: Androgen receptor binding (rat prostate cytosol). EPA 640-C-09-003. Washington DC.

EPA (2009b) Endocrine disruptor screening program test guidelines OPPTS 890.1250: Estrogen receptor binding (rat uterine cytosol). EPA 740-C-09-005. Washington DC.

EPA (2009c) Endocrine disruptor screening program test guidelines OPPTS 890.1400: Hershberger Bioassay. EPA 740-C-09-008. Washington DC.

EPA (2009d) Endocrine disruptor screening program test guidelines OPPTS 890.1600: Uterotrophic Assay. EPA 740-C-09-0010. Washington DC.

EPA (2011a). Estrogen Receptor Transcriptional Activation (Human Cell Line – Hela-9903)

Standard Evaluation Procedure (SEP). Available from: http://www.epa.gov/endo/pubs/ toresources/seps/Final_890.1300_ERTA_SEP_9.15.11.pdf.

EPA (2011b). Aromatase Assay (Human Recombinant) OCSPP Guideline 890.1200 Standard Evaluation Procedure (SEP).

Endocrine Disruptor Screening Program. U.S. Environmental Protection Agency Washington, DC. Available from: http://www.epa.gov/endo/pubs/toresources/seps/Final_890.1200_Aromatase_Assay_SEP_%208.1.11.pdf

Fort DJ, Thomas JH, Rogers RL, et al. (2004). Evaluation of the developmental and reproductive toxicity of methoxychlor using an anuran (Xenopus tropicalis) chronic exposure model. Toxicol Sci 81, 443–53.

Giger W, Brunner PH, Schaffner C (1984). 4-Nonylphenol in sewage sludge: accumulation of toxic metabolites from nonionic surfactants. Science 225, 623–5.

Gould JC, Leonard LS, Maness SC, et al. (1998). Bisphenol A interacts with the estrogen receptor alpha in a distinct manner from estradiol. Mol Cell Endocrinol 142, 203–14.

Gray LE Jr, Wolf C, Lambright C, et al. (1999). Administration of potentially antiandrogenic pesticides (procymidone, linuron, iprodione, chlozolinate, p,p'-DDE, and ketoconazole) and toxic substances (dibutyl- and diethylhexyl phthalate, PCB 169, and ethane dimethane sulphonate) during sexual differentiation produces diverse profiles of reproductive malformations in the male rat. Toxicol Ind Health 15, 94–118.

Hengstler JG, Foth H, Gebel T, et al. (2011). Critical evaluation of key evidence on the human health hazards of exposure to bisphenol A. Crit Rev Toxicol 41, 263–91.

Herbst AL, Ulfelder H, Poskanzer DC (1971). Adenocarcinoma of the vagina. Association of maternal stilbstrol therapy with tumor appearance in young women. New Eng J Med 284, 878–81.

Hershberger L, Shipley E, Meyer R (1953). Myotrophic activity of 19-nortestosterone and other steroids determined by modified levator ani muscle method. Proc Soc Exp Biol Med 83, 175–80.

Ho SM, Leung YK, Chung I (2006a). Estrogens and antiestrogens as etiological factors and therapeutics for prostate cancer. Ann New York Acad Sci 1089, 177–93.

Ho SM, Tang WY, Belmonte de Frausto J, et al. (2006b). Developmental exposure to estradiol and bisphenol A increases susceptibility to prostate carcinogenesis and epigenetically regulates phosphodiesterase type 4 variant 4. Cancer Res 66, 5624–32.

Howe SR, Borodinsky L (1998). Potential exposure to bisphenol A from food-contact use of polycarbonate resins. Food Addit Contam 15, 370–5.

Janosek J, Hilscherová K, Bláha L, et al. (2006). Environmental xenobiotics and nuclear receptors--interactions, effects and in vitro assessment. Toxicol In Vitro 20, 18–37.

Kaiser J (2005). Toxicology. panel finds no proof that phthalates harm infant reproductive systems. Science 310, 422

Keri RA, Ho SM, Hunt PA, et al. (2007). An evaluation of evidence for the carcinogenic activity of bisphenol A. Reprod Toxicol 24, 240–52.

Kim HS, Kim TS, Shin JH, et al. (2004). Neonatal exposure to di(n-butyl) phthalate (DBP) alters male reproductive-tract development. J Toxicol Environ Health 67, 2045–60.

Kim TH, Bang du Y, Lim HJ, et al. (2012). Comparisons of polybrominated diphenyl ethers levels in paired South Korean cord blood, maternal blood, and breast milk samples. Chemosphere 87, 97–104.

Klecka G, Persoon C, Currie R (2010). Chemicals of emerging concern in the Great Lakes Basin: an analysis of environmental exposures. Rev Environ Contam Toxicol. 207, 1–93.

Koo HJ, Lee BM (2004). Estimated exposure to phthalates in cosmetics and risk assessment. J Toxicol Environ Health Part A 67, 1901–14.

Koo HJ, Lee BM (2005). Human monitoring of phthalates and risk assessment. J Toxicol Environ Health 68, 1379–92.

Koo HJ, Lee BM (2007) Toxicokinetic relationship between di(2-ethylhexyl) phthalate (DEHP) and mono(2-ethylhexyl) phthalate in rats. J Toxicol Environ Health Part A 70, 383–7.

Krishnan AV, Stathis P, Permuth SF, et al. (1993). Bisphenol-A: an estrogenic substance is released from polycarbonate flasks during autoclaving. Endocrinology 132, 2279–86.

Langer P (1998). Mini review: polychlorinated biphenyls and the thyroid gland. Endocrine Regul 32, 193–203.

Leatherland JF, Copeland P, Sumpter JP, et al. (1982). Hormonal control of gonadal maturation and development of secondary sexual characteristics in coho salmon, oncorhynchus kisutch, from lakes ontario, erie, and michigan. Gen Comp Endocrinol 48, 196–204.

Mazdai A, Dodder NG, Abernathy MP, et al. (2003). Polybrominated diphenyl ethers in maternal and fetal blood samples. Environ Health Perspect 111, 1249–52.

McKinney, J.D., Waller, C.L. (1998) Molecular determinants of hormone mimicry: halogenated aromatic hydrocarbon environmental agents. J Toxixicol. Environ. Health B 1: 27–58.

McLachlan JA, Newbold RR, Bullock BC (1980) Long-term effects on the female mouse genital tract associated with prenatal exposure to diethylstilbestrol. Cancer Res 40, 3988–99.

Mehmood Z, Smith AG, Tucker MJ, et al. (2000). The development of methods for assessing the in vivo oestrogen-like effects of xenobiotics in CD-1 mice. Food Chem Toxicol 38, 493–501.

Mericskay M, Carta L, Sassoon D (2005). Diethylstilbestrol exposure in utero: a paradigm for mechanisms leading to adult disease. Birth Defects Res Part A Clin Mol Teratol 73, 133–5.

Moss S, Keller JM, Richards S, et al. (2009). Concentrations of persistent organic pollutants in plasma from two species of turtle from the Tennessee River Gorge. Chemosphere 76, 194–204.

Munkittrick KR, McMaster ME, McCarthy LH, et al. (1998). An overview of recent studies on the potential of pulp-mill effluents to alter reproductive parameters in fish. J Toxicol Environ Health Part B 1, 347–71.

Nair-Menon JU, Campbell GT, Blake CA (1996) Toxic effects of octylphenol on cultured rat and murine splenocytes. Toxicol Appl Pharmacol 139, 437–44.

OECD (2009). Guideline for the Testing of Chemicals: The Amphibian Metamorphosis Assay. Test Guideline 231, Adopted 7 September 2009. Organisation for Economic Co-operation and Development: Washington Center. Available from: www.oecd-wash.org.

OECD (2012). Endocrine Disrupter Testing and Assessment. Available from: http://www.oecd.org/document/62/0,2340,en_2649_34377_2348606_1_1_1_1,00.html

Olea N, Pulgar R, Pérez P, et al. (1996). Estrogenicity of resin-based composites and sealants used in dentistry. Environ Health Perspect 104, 298–305.

Perez P, Pulgar R, Olea-Serrano F, et al. (1998). The estrogenicity of bisphenol A-related diphenylalkanes with various substituents at the central carbon and the hydroxy groups. Environ Health Perspect 106, 167–74.

Rao JN, Liang JY, Chakraborti P, et al. (2003). Effect of thyroid hormone on the development and gene expression of hormone receptors in rat testes in vivo. J Endocrinol Invest 26, 435–43.

Rattner BA, Eroschenko VP, Fox GA, et al. (1984). Avian endocrine responses to environmental pollutants. J Exp Zool 232, 683–9.

Rice CP, Schmitz-Afonso I, Loyo-Rosales JE, et al. (2003). Alkylphenol and alkylphenol-ethoxylates in carp, water, and sediment from the Cuyahoga River, Ohio. Environ Sci Technol 37, 3747–54.

Ryu JY, Lee BM, Kacew S, Kim HS (2007). Identification of differentially expressed genes in the testis of Sprague-Dawley rats treated with di(n-butyl) phthalate. Toxicology 234, 103–12.

Schrader TJ, Cooke GM (2003) Effects of Aroclors and individual PCB congeners on activation of the human androgen receptor in vitro. Reprod Toxicol 17, 15–23.

Seegal RF (1999). Are PCBs the major neurotoxicant in Great Lakes salmon? Environ Res 80(2 Pt 2), S38–45.

Semenza JC, Tolbert PE, Rubin CH, et al. (1997). Reproductive toxins and alligator abnormalities at Lake Apopka, Florida. Environ Health Perspect 105, 1030–2.

Silva MJ, Reidy JA, Samandar E, et al. (2005). Detection of phthalate metabolites in human saliva. Arch Toxicol 79, 647–52.

Sonne C, Wolkers H, Leifsson PS, et al. (2009). Chronic dietary exposure to environmental organochlorine contaminants induces thyroid gland lesions in Arctic foxes (Vulpes lagopus). Environ Res 109, 702–11.

Stapleton HM, Dodder NG, Offenberg JH, et al. (2005). Polybrominated diphenyl ethers in house dust and clothes dryer lint. Environ Sci Technol 39, 925–31.

Swan SH (2006). Prenatal phthalate exposure and anogenital distance in male infants. Environ Health Perspect 114, A88–9.

Thayer KA, Heindel JJ, Bucher JR, et al. (2012). Role of environmental chemicals in diabetes and obesity: a national toxicology program workshop report. Environ Health Perspect 120, 779–89.

Vinggaard AM, Hnida C, Larsen JC (2000). Environmental polycyclic aromatic hydrocarbons affect androgen receptor activation in vitro. Toxicology 145, 173–83.

Whitehead SA, Rice S (2006) Endocrine-disrupting chemicals as modulators of sex steroid synthesis. Best Pract Res Clin Endocrinol Metabol 20, 45–61.

White R, Jobling S, Hoare SA, et al. (1994). Environmentally persistent alkylphenolic compounds are estrogenic. Endocrinology 135, 175–82.

Wilford BH, Harner T., Zhu J et al. (2004). Passive sampling survey of polybrominated diphenyl ether flame retardants in indoor and outdoor air in Ottawa, Canada: implications for sources and exposure. Environl Sci Technol 38, 5312–18.

Willhite, C.C., Ball, G.L., McLellan, C.J. (2008). Derivation of a bisphenol A oral refernce dose (RfD) and drinking water equivalent concentration. J Toxicol. Environ. Health B 11, 69–146.

Wolff MS, Toniolo PG (1995). Environmental organochlorine exposure as a potential etiologic factor in breast cancer. Environ Health Perspect 103(Suppl 7), 141–5.

Yu ML, Guo YL, Hsu CC, et al. (2000). Menstruation and reproduction in women with polychlorinated biphenyl (PCB) poisoning: long-term follow-up interviews of the women from the Taiwan Yucheng cohort. Int J Epidemiol 29, 672–7.

Yusof YA, Edwards AM (1990). Stimulation of DNA synthesis in primary rat hepatocyte cultures by liver tumor promoters: interactions with other growth factors. Carcinogenesis 11, 761–70.

20

Food additives and contaminants

INTRODUCTION

As the global population increases, there has been a growing demand for more food. Various physical means and chemical substances have been developed and utilized to increase food supply. However, the increased efficiency of farming has reduced the number of farmers. In addition, with industrialization and urbanization, many more people are living away from the farmland. These social changes have resulted in an ever-increasing demand for processed foods that can be transported from the farm to the city and that will retain their nutritive value and organoleptic properties. These demands have been met largely by the addition of chemicals known as food additives. These chemicals serve a variety of technological functions as described in the section, "Functional Groups of Direct Food Additives".

Legal Definition of Food Additives

The following definition has been adopted by the Codex Alimentarius Commission, an intergovernmental agency consisting of more than 150 nations (FAO/WHO, 1994).

A *food additive* is any substance not normally consumed as a food by itself and not normally used as a typical ingredient of the food, whether or not it has nutritive value. The intentional addition of this to food, for a technological (including organoleptic) purpose, in the manufacture, processing, preparation, treatment, packing, packaging, transport, or holding of such food, results or is reasonably expected to result (directly or indirectly) in it or its byproducts becoming a component of, or otherwise, affecting the characteristics of such foods. The term does not include "contaminants" or substances added to food for maintaining or improving nutritional qualities.

The U.S. legal definition appearing in the U.S. Federal Food, Drug, and Cosmetic Act, as amended in October 1976 (1979), is different from the above in several aspects. The U.S. legislation excludes color additives and those substances that are to be added to food, but are defined as "generally recognized as safe

(GRAS)." On the other hand, the U.S. legislation considers nutritional supplements and irradiated foods as food additives.

Classification of Food Additives and Contaminants

Functional Groups of Direct Food Additives

A number of chemicals are added to food to increase its shelf life, to render food more amenable to mass production, or to enhance its consumer appeal with respect to color, flavor, texture, and convenience. These chemicals are grouped according to their technological functions. Detailed listing of various groups of food additives and their uses is given in a Codex document (FAO/WHO, 1994). The major functional groups and some examples are listed in Appendix 1.

Indirect (Unintentional) Food Additives

The substances described above are intentionally added to foods for specific technological purposes. Consequently they are considered "direct" or "intentional" food additives. However, a number of substances may become part of the foods, as a result of their use during the production, processing, or storage of the foods. These include antibiotics and anabolic agents used during the raising of farm animals, residues from the food processing machinery, and migrants from packaging materials. In recent years, the genetic modification of crops has yielded greater production of food products, with a similar nutritive value; however, the consequences with respect to human health still remain unresolved. The genetically modified food may not be able to be metabolized by humans or may produce byproducts that individuals cannot handle and subsequently produce toxic reactions. GMF plays a crucial role in increasing the food supply, but one needs to be aware of the potential adverse effects.

Food Contaminants

These substances are present in foods as a result of environmental pollution or faulty handling of the food. In other words, they serve no useful purpose either in the final food product or in its processing. Examples are mercury in fish harvested from contaminated fish farms, and mycotoxins found in improperly stored nuts and grains. Thus, they differ from both direct and indirect food additives.

International Aspects

Food, raw and processed, is commonly traded internationally. The additives and contaminants (and residues of pesticides) must be considered acceptable for the protection of the health of consumers. However, food that is considered acceptable by the exporting country may not be considered acceptable by the importing country. This was the case with beef from Canada after the outbreak of the "Mad Cow Disease," which was controlled by eradication of all infected animals, yet the importing countries still did not accept Canadian cattle.

In an attempt to reduce such disputes, the World Health Organization (WHO) and the Food and Agriculture Organization of the United Nations (FAO), at the request of the governments, established mechanisms to provide independent toxicological evaluation. The mechanisms created were the Joint FAO/WHO Expert Committee on Food Additives and Contaminants (JECFA) and the Joint FAO/WHO Meeting of Experts on Pesticide Residues (JMPR). Members of these committees were selected from a panel of internationally known experts, acting independently.

Since their inception in the early 1960s, they have been convened annually. During these meetings, they have evaluated and re-evaluated many food additives, contaminants, and pesticide residues. Acceptable daily intakes (ADIs) are allocated to those chemicals that the toxicological data so indicates. The ADIs are used by regulatory agencies in some countries.

More importantly, the ADIs are used by the Joint FAO/WHO Food Standard Program and the Codex Alimentarius Commission to establish international food standards. There are more than 150 nations that are members of the commission. Some details on the relationship among the national food regulatory agencies, national research facilities, and the Codex Alimentarius Commission are given in chapter 27. A comprehensive review of this subject is provided in a review (Lu, 1988).

TOXICOLOGICAL TESTING AND EVALUATION

Categories of Data Required

As these chemicals are added to foods to be consumed by large numbers of people, they are in general extensively tested and strictly evaluated. Furthermore, because of their low toxicity, precise LD_{50}s are, as a rule, not required. The studies required by JECFA are categorized as follows:

1. Biochemical, including absorption, distribution, elimination (and storage), biotransformation, and effects on enzymes and other biochemical parameters
2. Acute toxicity
3. Short-term toxicity
4. Chronic toxicity
5. Reproductive toxicity
6. Mutagenicity
7. Carcinogenicity
8. Teratogenicity (developmental)
9. Clinical observations in humans

Extent of Testing

The JECFA considers, as a general rule, that the types of biological data listed above are required for proper evaluation of food additives. However, for certain groups of additives, depending on their chemical nature, source, and usage, much less data are required. These include:

1. Components of food and closely related chemicals including vitamins
2. Certain enzymes used in food processing
3. Certain food colors
4. Certain metals (e.g., copper, iron, and zinc)

Detailed descriptions of the types of additives and the required data are given in several WHO reports (WHO, 1974, 1982a, 1986). These descriptions are summarized in a review article (Lu, 1988).

The U.S. Food and Drug Administration established a set of criteria to determine the "level of concern," (LOC), which in turn dictated the extent of testing required (FDA, 1982). The LOC was determined by the chemical structure of the additive and concentration in food. Additives are placed in three categories according to their chemical structure: A, B, and C. Additives of low probable toxicity are assigned to category A. This category comprises nine types of chemicals, such as, simple aliphatic, noncyclic hydrocarbons with no unsaturation; sugars and polysaccharides; fats and fatty acids; and endogenous inorganic salts of alkali metals (Na and K) and alkaline earth metals (Mg and Ca). Additives with functional groups of high probable toxicity are assigned to category C. Additives of intermediate or unknown probable toxicity are assigned to category B.

Evaluation

As described in chapter 27, the toxicological evaluation of food additives follows the procedure of determining the adequacy of data, establishing an appropriate no-observed effect level, and selecting a proper safety factor to obtain the acceptable daily intake. This procedure is generally adopted by many national regulatory agencies, including the U.S. Food and Drug Administration, as well as the international organizations WHO and FAO. The toxicological basis for drafting the provisions for food additives in the International Food Standards is provided by the JECFA. The interrelationship between the various national and international bodies is described in a review article (Lu, 1988).

Generally Recognized as Safe

As noted above, the U.S. legislation considers certain chemicals to be "generally recognized as safe." This was done originally in 1958, and that list included more than 600 direct additives, with a variety of technological functions, and some 2000 indirect additives. Since then, the list of direct additives has been expanded, mainly by the addition of more than 1000 flavoring ingredients proposed by the

Flavor and Extract Manufacturers' Association. GRAS substances are evaluated by the Select Committee on GRAS Substances.

On the basis of new toxicological information, the safety of a number of substances on the list has since been questioned. The most notable was the suspected carcinogenicity of the artificial sweetener cyclamate. As a result, the FDA, in 1970, asked the Life Sciences Research Office of the Federation of American Societies for Experimental Biology to evaluate the safety of all the substances on the GRAS list. A Select Committee on GRAS Substances was formed and issued many reports containing its conclusion and summaries of the available information on 468 substances. A detailed account of the study by the committee is given by Carr (1987).

ADDITIVES OF TOXICOLOGICAL CONCERN

Some 600 intentional food additives are being added to a variety of our foods. The toxicity of most of these additives has been evaluated according to the prevailing procedure and considered to be "safe." However, the use of some additives has been restricted, suspended, or requires label declaration, because of toxicological concern.

Carcinogenicity

The safety of *saccharin,* for example, has been questioned because of its reported carcinogenicity. In fact, the first study that revealed increased bladder tumors in rats involved the dosing of the animals with a combination of saccharin and cyclamate in a ratio of 1:9. Saccharin has been found to be excreted as such and is nonmutagenic in most test systems. However, a large-scale experiment carried out in a Canadian Government Laboratory showed that rats that fed on a diet with 7.5% saccharin developed bladder tumors (Arnold et al., 1977). The significance of this finding is somewhat doubtful because of the excessively high dosage and because the tumors occurred mainly among the male rats of the second generation. A recent epidemiological study suggests that artificial sweeteners including consumption of saccharin and aspartame may not be associated with cancer risk in Italy (Bosetti et al., 2009), whereas, increased cases of urinary tract tumors were observed in a case-control study in Argentina (Andreatta et al., 2008).

Cyclamates were considered innocuous and were used widely in foods and beverages for many years. However, doubt was cast on their safety because of the discovery that they were metabolized to cyclohexylamine by intestinal flora in animals and humans, which appears to be more toxic (Classen et al., 1968). Its use as a food additive was suspended in 1969, when it was discovered that a mixture of saccharin and cyclamate increased the incidence of bladder tumors in rats (Price et al., 1970). Subsequent studies on cyclamate showed no carcinogenicity, and the short-term mutagenicity tests yielded no consistent results. This was also true of cyclohexylamine. Summaries of the reports are included in two publications

(IARC, 1980; WHO, 1982a). Its use has been restored in a number of countries, although it is still not permitted for use as an additive in the United States.

Nitrates and *nitrites* are useful preservatives and they impart a special color and flavor to treated meat such as ham and corned beef. However, they can form, with certain amines, a variety of nitrosamines, many of which are potent carcinogens. However, nitrates and nitrites are valuable in controlling toxin-forming microorganisms such as *Clostridium botulinum*. In addition, some of the epidemiological and clinical studies demonstrate that nitrates and nitrites of plant origin may play essential physiological roles in supporting cardiovascular health and gastrointestinal immune function (Hord et al., 2009). Furthermore, nitrites occur in the body, notably in the saliva, and it has been demonstrated that nitrosation of certain amines can occur in the stomach.

For these reasons, the use of these preservatives has not been suspended, but the amount used has been reduced. On the other hand, the preservative *diethyl pyrocarbonate* (DEPC) presents a distinctly different picture. It has been used in a variety of beverages, but its use has been suspended. This decision was based on the finding that DEPC may combine with the ammonium ion in beverages to form urethane, a wide-spectrum carcinogen in all animal species tested, and on the fact that its use is not indispensable.

Butylated hydroxyanisole (BHA) and *butylated hydroxytoluene* (BHT) are widely used antioxidants and have been investigated in several long-term studies without revealing any serious adverse effects. However, Ito et al. (1983) reported that BHA, at very high dietary levels, induced hyperplasia and tumors in the forestomach of rats. As the tumors were only found in the forestomach, the relevance of this finding in terms of human health hazard was questioned. Additional studies using species without a forestomach were performed. The results were negative in dogs, and the increased mitotic rate in the esophagus of pigs was questionable (WHO, 1989). Olsen et al. (1983) reported an increase in hepatocellular adenoma and carcinoma. However, several other studies yielded negative results. Furthermore, other studies on these antioxidants produced cancer-protective effects (Prochaska et al., 1985). In spite of these conflicting results, BHA and BHT are still being used.

Hypersensitivity Reactions

A number of food additives are known to induce hypersensitivity reactions in susceptible individuals. As they affect only a small proportion of the general population, and because their effects are usually mild and transitory, most regulatory agencies consider label declaration as a sufficient method to provide warning to these individuals. The following are the more commonly known ones.

Tartrazine, a widely used yellow color in a variety of processed foods, has been known to induce allergic reactions, especially among those who are allergic to aspirin (Juhlin, 1980).

Sulfur dioxide and related chemicals, such as bisulfites and metabisulfites, are used as preservatives in processed foods as well as salads. In the latter case, these chemicals help to preserve the freshness of the vegetables. As it is difficult to provide warning labels, such use has been discouraged.

Monosodium glutamate (MSG) has been used as a flavor enhancer for many decades in China and Japan. No untoward effects have been reported. However, a "Chinese restaurant syndrome" has been reported (Schaumberg et al., 1969). It usually appears after the individual has consumed a special Chinese soup, which contains relatively large amounts of MSG. The hypersensitivity reaction consists of a burning sensation, tingling in the face and neck, tightness in the chest, and so on. On account of these findings, it is now possible, in many restaurants, to order soups and other dishes specifying "no MSG." For additional details, see Kenney (1986) and Jinap and Hajeb (2010). The fact that adverse reactions to MSG have not been observed in the Far East is evidently related to the custom of consuming the soup as the last course, that is, on a full stomach, thereby delaying the absorption of this chemical and preventing a dramatic rise in blood level.

Other Adverse Effects

In addition to carcinogenicity and hypersensitivity reactions, the discovery of other adverse effects has prompted regulatory decisions or additional investigations. The examples are, heart lesions in laboratory animals associated with brominated vegetable oils (BVO), a suspending agent in certain beverages, and liver lesions associated with Orange RN and Ponceau 2R, which were responsible for the suspension of their use. Other effects such as red blood cell damage (Orange RN), storage in tissues (BVO), and testicular atrophy (cyclohexylamine from cyclamate) were contributing factors to the toxicological decisions on these additives (see Lu, 1979a).

INDIRECT ADDITIVES AND CONTAMINANTS

Apart from direct food additives, there are a large number of indirect additives and some contaminants that pose toxicological problems and require different control measures. The problems are highlighted as follows.

Indirect Food Additives

The most important of these chemicals are: (i) The constituents of the packaging material, which may migrate into the food that is in contact with them, and (ii) animal drug residues that are commonly used in raising food-producing animals.

Packaging Materials

A number of substances may migrate from food containers, wrappers, and the like, to the food that is packaged in them. Most of the chemicals that might migrate from the conventional types of packaging materials, such as paper and wood, had been considered safe and included in the FDA's GRAS list. More recently, however, the packaging items are generally made of polymeric materials. The polymers per se are generally inert, but the components, the monomers, which are present to some extent, residual reactants, intermediates, manufacturing aids, solvents, and plastic additives, as well as the products of side reaction and chemical degradation by-products may migrate into the food that is in contact with them. Some of these chemicals have been shown to be toxic.

Vinyl chloride has been shown to be a human carcinogen at high levels of exposure, and acrylonitrile is a probable human carcinogen. Both are carcinogenic in a number of animal species (chap. 7). Currently, bisphenol A, which is widely used in the linings of metal cans and feeding bottles, was found to be an endocrine-disrupting chemical in animals, in very high quantities (Wilhite et al., 2008). The release of phthalates from food packaging has raised concerns, due to the estrogenic effects of these compounds in animals. Administration of phthalates in very high concentrations is known to produce testicular dysfunction in rats (Kim et al., 2004). However, no human data showing an abnormal reproductive function in humans are available, as the concentration of phthalates or bisphenol A released is exceedingly small and not environmentally realistic. Thus, because of the exceedingly low levels of exposure from migration to food, these chemicals continue to be used and provisionally approved. The difficulty one faces is that the adverse responses reported are due to the concentration, but when there is interpolation to risk, the concentration cannot be attained by humans.

Animal Drug Residues in Human Food

There are essentially three types of drugs used in food-producing animals that may leave residues in human food, such as meat, milk, and eggs. The drugs not only present a problem related to the parent chemicals, but it is also necessary to consider their metabolites, which are produced as a result of the metabolic processes, including bioactivation in the animals, which may possess different toxic properties (Hayes and Borzelleca, 1982).

Therapeutic drugs, such as the anthelmintic agents febantel, fenbendazole, and oxfendazole, are generally used in individual animals for specific disease and only over short periods. Therefore, they do not pose a widespread health concern. On the other hand, tranquilizing agents such as chlorpromazine and propylpromazine are used shortly before slaughter, and hence, leave residues in the meat. Their use is therefore not allowed (WHO, 1995).

Antibiotics such as benzyl penicillin and oxytetracycline are usually incorporated in the animal feeds to prevent outbreaks of bacterial diseases and to promote growth. The residue levels are generally extremely low and not expected to induce toxic effects. These antibiotics can result in resistance in humans, which is a concern.

Anabolic agents are growth-promoting substances and are implanted subcutaneously in a part of the animal that is usually not eaten, such as the ear.

Their residue levels in the meat are low enough to be essentially devoid of general toxic effects, except carcinogenicity. A carcinogen may be effective at extremely low-dose levels. Diethylstilbestrol (DES) is no longer used as a growth promoter, because of the discovery that tumors of genital organs have developed in the offspring of mothers who had taken DES in large doses during pregnancy, for medical purposes.

The anabolic agents in use may be considered either "endogenous" or "exogenous." The former includes estradiol, progesterone, and testosterone. The latter includes porcine somatotropin, and trenbolone acetate. Trenbolone has been shown to be teratogenic and immunotoxic in the avian species (Quinn et al., 2007). The "endogenous" anabolic agents are considered indistinguishable from the endogenous hormones, and the "erogenous" hormones leave very low levels of residues. Acceptable daily intakes have been allocated to their residues (WHO, 2000a).

CONTAMINANTS

There are three main types of food contaminants: mycotoxins, heavy metals, and synthetic chemicals. They contaminate food because of growing or harvesting from contaminated soil or water, improper handling, and accidental release from industrial sources.

Mycotoxins

Aflatoxins, produced by the mold *Aspergillus flavus*, occur in nuts and grains, especially when these commodities are stored in a humid and warm climate. These toxins exist as mixtures of aflatoxins B_1, B_2, G_1, and G_2. Among these aflatoxins, B_1 is the most potent carcinogen in most species of animals, especially the rat. In one experiment, rats fed on a diet containing 1 ppb of aflatoxin B_1 had hyperplastic nodules and carcinoma of the liver (Wogan et al., 1974). Aflatoxins G_1 and M_1 (a metabolite of B_1 occurring in milk) are also carcinogenic, but much less potent. Positive correlation was noted between aflatoxin intake and liver cancer incidence in certain regions in Africa and Thailand (IARC, 1976). Lu (2003) has provided a more extensive review on aflatoxins. As noted in chapter 3, aflatoxin is bioactivated to aflatoxin-8,9-epoxide, which may covalently bind to DNA, and thus initiate carcinogenesis.

A number of other mycotoxins also occur in foods. Deoxynivalenol occurs commonly in cereal-based foods. Deoxynivalenol was shown to produce gastrointestinal disturbances, immune dysfunction, and anorexia (Pestka and Smolinki, 2005). Ochratoxin A is present in dairy products, chocolate, beer, coffee, wine, poultry, and pork. Ochratoxin A produces Balkan endemic nephropathy as well as cancer (Clark and Snedeker, 2006). Their characteristics are summarized in Table 20.1. Additional information on these and other mycotoxins may be found in two WHO publications (1990, 2000b).

Table 20.1 Source, Occurrence, and Toxicity of Certain Mycotoxins

Mycotoxin	Source	Occurrence	Toxic Effects
Aflatoxins	*Aspergillus*	Nuts, grains	Liver cancer
Ergot	*Claviceps purpurea*	Grains, especially rye	Ergotism (spasm, cramps, dry gangrene)
Fumonisin B$_1$	*Fusarium*	Maize	Esophageal cancer
Ochratoxins	*Aspergillus* *Penicillium*	Grains	Nephropathy Cancer
Trichothecenes	*Fusarium* *trichoderma*	Grains	Vomiting, diarrhea, skin inflammation, multiple hemorrhage
Zearalenone	*Fusarium*	Grains	Estrogenic effects

Source: From WHO (1990, 2000b).

Table 20.2 Source, Occurrence, and Toxicity of Certain Neurotoxins in Marine Animals

Toxins	Source	Occurrence	Toxic Effects
Botulinum toxin	*Clostridium botulinum*	Improperly canned food	Impairing ACh release
Ciquatoxin	Blue-green algae	Large coastal fishes	Various effects on nervous and G.I. systems
Domoic acid	*Pseudonitzschia multiseries and Pseudonitzschia australis*	Mussels, seaweed, and red algae	Memory loss, seizure, and gastroenteritis
Saxitoxin	*Gonyolax*	Clams	Blocking of nerve conduction
Tetrodotoxin	Uncertain	Puffer fish	Blocking of nerve conduction

Neurotoxins

Certain toxins are found in marine animals that are used as food (Table 20.2). The notable ones are saxitoxin, which may be present in clams, and tetradotoxin, which is found in puffer fish, especially in its ovaries. An important and extremely toxic substance is the botulinum toxin. It is produced by the bacteria *C. botulinum* in improperly canned food. The major toxic effects of these toxins are on the nervous system. Descriptions of these effects are provided in chapter 17. Another toxin (ciguatoxin) is occasionally present in large coastal fishes, in certain geographical areas, notably the Caribbean Sea. In addition to the nervous system, it often produces toxic effects on the GI system.

Metals

The toxic properties of a number of metals are described in chapter 21, but human exposure via food is highlighted in this section. Among the metals that have produced the most concern are mercury, lead, cadmium, and arsenic.

A number of acute and chronic poisoning episodes have resulted from improper application or consumption of alkyl *mercury* compounds used as fungicides to preserve seed grains. Others followed consumption of fish contaminated with methyl mercury. The compound can be formed via bioactivation (aided by microorganisms in the mud) of mercury discharged from factories (e.g., in Minamata and Niigata, Japan; Appendix 2 of chap. 1). On account of the biomagnification factor along the food chain, large carnivorous fishes generally contain much higher levels of methyl mercury (WHO, 1976; Bayen et al., 2005).

Lead has been used as a fuel additive, in lead batteries, paints, and so on. Humans are exposed to this metal via air, water, and food. According to one analysis, daily intakes from these media amount to 15, 20, and 140 µg, respectively (NRC Canada, 1973). One unusual source of lead intake is improperly fired ceramic foodware, which may release large amounts of lead from the glaze, and which has produced a number of poisonings. This fact has prompted the promulgation of limits in the extent of release of lead from various types of foodware (WHO, 1979). The estimated intake of lead from ceramic ware would be in the range of 30–80 µg/day if all the wares in use released this metal to the legal limit (Lu, 1979b). Among certain populations, ceramic foodware still constitutes an important source of lead (Rojas-Lopez et al., 1994).

Cadmium is used as a pigment and occurs in the environment, especially through the refining of zinc ores, which contain varying concentrations of cadmium. It enters the food chain through pollution of soil and water. The Itai-Itai disease in Japan has been attributed to chronic exposure to cadmium, through long-term ingestion of contaminated rice. It may also be leached from decorated ceramic foodware.

Arsenic contamination is primarily attributed to the smelting and mining industries. It enters the food chain through pollution of soil and water. Arsenic poisoning results in black foot disease (peripheral vascular disorder), hyperkeratotic lesions on the skin leading to cancer, as well as liver cancer (Bernstam and Nriagu, 2000).

Certain Organic Compounds

Among these chemicals are *organochlorine insecticides*, which have been widely used. Their use has been discontinued because of their persistence in the environment. However, they are still present in foods, in trace amounts. Others include *polychlorinated biphenyls* (PCB), which are used in electrical capacitors and transformers, as plasticizers and heat exchangers, and in paper manufacturing. Through leakage and discharge of waste, they enter the environment. On account of their persistence and biomagnification properties, they enter the food chain.

Table 20.3   Action Levels for Certain Food Contaminants

Contaminants	Commodity	Action Level
Aflatoxin	Nuts	20 ppb
	Foods and feeds	20 ppb
	Milk[a]	0.5 ppb
Aldrin and dieldrin	Various foods	0.02–0.3 ppm
Cadmium, in leaching solution from ceramic ware	Flat ware	0.5 μμg/mL
	Small hollowware	0.5 μg/mL
	Large hollowware	0.25 μg/mL
Lead, in leaching solution from ceramic ware	Flatware	3.0 μg/mL
	Small hollowware	2.0 μg/mL
	Large hollowware	1.0 μg/mL
Mercury	Fish, shellfish, crustaceans	1.0 ppm
	Wheat	1.0 ppm
Polychlorinated biphenyls	Red meat (fat basis)	3 ppm

[a]Aflatoxin M1.*Source*: From FDA (2000).

These chemicals have attracted much attention because of the episode of consumption of a batch of rice oil contaminated with PCB through a leak in a heat exchanger, in 1968. Thousands of consumers in Japan were affected (Appendix 2 of chap. 1). The main sign of toxicity was chloracne, although there were many other symptoms and signs (chap 1). Similarly, an inadvertent addition of *polybrominated biphenyls* (PBB) to cattle feed, in Michigan, resulted in the contamination of a large amount of beef and milk. In addition, some polybrominated flame retardants used in electronics, furniture, and the like, resulted in the contamination of various foods, including fruits, vegetables, and baby food.

The "action levels" for these and other contaminants have been established by the U.S. FDA, to control their levels in food and feed. Some of them are listed in Table 20.3.

REFERENCES

Andreatta MM, Muñoz SE, Lantieri MJ, et al. (2008). Artificial sweetener consumption and urinary tract tumors in Cordoba, Argentina. Prev Med 47, 136–9.

Arnold DL, Moodie CA, Stavric D, et al. (1977). Canadian saccharin study. Science 197,320.

Bayen S, Koroleva E, Lee HK, et al. (2005). Persistent organic pollutants and heavy metals in typical seafoods consumed in Singapore. J Toxicol Environ Health A 68, 151–66.

Bernstam L, Nriagu J (2000). Molecular aspects of arsenic stress. J Toxicol Environ Health B 3, 293–322.

Bosetti C, Gallus S, Talamini R, et al. (2009). Artificial sweeteners and the risk of gastric, pancreatic, and endometrial cancers in Italy. Cancer Epidemiol Biomarkers Prev 18, 2235–8.

Carr CJ (1987). Food additives: a benefit/risk dilemma. In: Haley TJ, Berndt WO, eds. Handbook of Toxicology. Washington, DC.: Hemisphere.

Clark HA, Snedeker SM (2006). Ochratoxin A: its cancer risk and potential for exposure. J Toxicol Environ Health B 9, 265–96.

Classen HG, Marquardt P, Spath M (1968). Sympathomimetic effects of cyclohexylamine. Arzneimittel Forsch 18, 590–4.

FAO/WHO (1994). Food Additives. Codex Alimentarius, vol. XIV. Rome: Food Agriculture Organization of the United Nations.

FDA (1982). Toxicological principles for the safety assessment of direct additives and color additives used in food. US. Food and Drug Administration. Springfield, VA: National Technical Information Service, PB 83–170696.

FDA (2000). Action levels for poisonous or deleterious substances in human food and animal feed. Washington, DC.: Food and Drug Administration.

Hayes JR, Borzelleca JF (1982). Biodisposition of xenobiotics in animals. In: Beitz DC, Hanson R, eds. Animal Products in Human Nutrition. New York, NY: Academic Press, 225–59.

Hord NG, Tang Y, Bryan NS. (2009). Food sources of nitrates and nitrites: the physiologic context for potential health benefits. Am J Clin Nutr 90, 1–10.

IARC (1976). Evaluation of Carcinogenic Risk of Chemicals to Man, vol. 10. Some Naturally Occurring Substances. Lyon, France: International Agency for Research on Cancer.

IARC (1980). Evaluation of the Carcinogenic Risk of Chemicals to Humans, vol. 22. Some Non-Nutritive Sweetening Agents. Lyon, France: International Agency for Research on Cancer.

Ito N, Fukushima S, Hagiwara A, et al. (1983). Carcinogenicity of butylated hydroxyanisole in F344 rats. J Natl Cancer Inst 70, 343–52.

Jinap S, Hajeb P. (2010). Glutamate. its applications in food and contribution to health. Appetite 55, 1–10.

Juhlin L (1980). Incidence of intolerance to food additives. Int J Dermatol 19, 548–51.

Kenney RA (1986). The Chinese restaurant syndrome: an anecdote revisited. Food Chem Toxicol 24, 351–4.

Kim HS, Kim TS, Shin JH, et al. (2004). Neonatal exposure to di(n-butyl)phthalate alters male reproductive tract development. J Toxicol Environ Health A 67, 2045–60.

Lu FC (1979a). The safety of food additives: the dynamics of the issue. In: Deichmann WB, ed. Toxicology and Occupational Medicine. New York, NY: Elsevier/North Holland.

Lu FC (1979b). Review of Total Intake of Lead from All Sources. WHO: HCS/CER/79.5. Geneva, Switzerland: World Health Organization.

Lu FC (1988). Acceptable daily intake: Inception, evolution and application. Reg Toxicol Pharmacol 8, 45–60.

Lu FC (2003). Assessment of safety/risk vs. public health: aflatoxins and hepacarcinoma. Environ Health and Prev Med 7, 235–8.

NRC Canada (1973). Lead in the Canadian environment. NRCC No. 13682. Ottawa: National Research Council of Canada.

Olsen P, Bille N, Meyer O (1983). Hepatocellular neoplasms in rats induced by butylated hydroxytoluene (BHT). Acta Pharmacol Toxicol 54, 433–4.

Pestka JJ, Smolinski AT (2005). Deoxynivalenol: toxicology and potential effects on humans. J Toxicol Environ Health B 8, 39–69.

Price JM, Biava CG, Oser BL, et al. (1970). Bladder tumors in rats fed cyclohexylamine or high doses of a mixture of cyclamate and saccharin. Science 167, 1131–2.

Prochaska HJ, DeLong MJ, Talalay P (1985). On the mechanisms of induction of cancer-protective enzymes: a unifying proposal. Proc Natl Acad Sci USA 82, 8232–6.

Quinn MJ, McKernan M, Lavoie ET, et al. (2007). Immunotoxicity of trenbolone acetate in Japanese quail. J Toxicol Environ Health A 70, 88–93.

Rojas-Lopez M, Santos-Burgoa C, Rios C, et al. (1994). Use of lead-glazed ceramics is the main factor associated to high lead in blood levels in two Mexican rural communities. J Toxicol Environ Health 42, 45–52.

Schaumberg HH, Byck R, Gerstl R, et al. (1969). Monosodium glutamate: its pharmacology and role in the Chinese restaurant syndrome. Science 163, 826.

U.S. Federal Food, Drug, and Cosmetic Act, As Amended (1979). Washington, DC.: US. Government Printing Office.

WHO (1974). Toxicological Evaluation of Certain Food Additives with a Review of General Principles and of Specifications (17th Report). Tech Rep Ser 539. Geneva, Switzerland: World Health Organization.

WHO (1976). Mercury. Environmental Health Criteria 1. Geneva, Switzerland: World Health Organization.

WHO (1979). Ceramic Foodware Safety. Report of a Meeting of Experts. HCS/79.7. Geneva, Switzerland: World Health Organization.

WHO (1982a). Evaluation of Certain Food Additives and Contaminants (26th Report). Tech Rep Ser 683. Geneva, Switzerland: World Health Organization.

WHO (1986). Evaluation of Certain Food Additives and Contaminants (29th Report). Tech Rep Ser 733. Geneva, Switzerland: World Health Organization.

WHO (1989). Evaluation of Certain Food Additives and Contaminants. WHO Food Additives Series 24. Geneva, Switzerland: World Health Organization.

WHO (1990). Selected Mycotoxins: Ochratoxins, Trichothecene, Ergot Environ Health Criteria No. 105. Geneva, Switzerland: World Health Organization.

WHO (1995). Evaluation of Certain Veterinary Drug Residues in Food (38th Report). Tech Rep Ser 815. Geneva, Switzerland: World Health Organization.

WHO (2000a). Toxicological Evaluation of Certain Veterinary Drug Residues in Food. Food Additives Series No. 43. Geneva, Switzerland: World Health Organization.

WHO (2000b). Fumonisin B1. Environ Health Criteria No. 219. Geneva, Switzerland:World Health Organization.

Wilhite CC, Ball GL, McLellan CJ (2008). Derivation of a bisphenol A oral reference dose and drinking water equivalent concentration. J Toxicol Environ Health B 11, 69–145.

Wogan GN, Paglialunga S, Newberne PM (1974). Carcinogenic effects of low dietary levels of anatoxin B in rats. Food Cosmet Toxicol 12, 681–5.

Appendix 1   Major Functional Groups of Direct Food Additives

1. Preservatives are added to prolong the shelf life of foods by preventing or inhibiting microbial growth. Examples are benzoic acid, propionic acid, and sorbic acid, their salts, nitrates and nitrites, and sulfur dioxide and related compounds.
2. Antioxidants are added to oils to prevent them from becoming rancid, which is a result of oxidative changes. Some are added to fruits and vegetables to prevent enzymatic browning. The commonly used ones include butylated hydroxyanisole, butylated hydroxytoluene, various gallates, ascorbic acid and its salts, and α-tocopherol.
3. Emulsifying, stabilizing, and thickening agents are added to improve the homogeneity, stability, and "body" of a variety of food products. These include mono- and diglycerides, sucrose esters of fatty acids, lecithin, salts of various types of phosphates, modified starches, calcium gluconate, calcium citrate, agar, alginic acid and its salts, various vegetable gums, and cellulose derivatives.
4. Colors are used to enhance the visual appeal of food products. Some of these substances are derived from natural colors, such as carotene, chlorophyll, and cochineal. Others are synthetic, such as allura red, amaranth, azorubine, indigotine, and tartrazine.
5. Flavors and flavor enhancers. The flavors constitute the largest group of food additives. However, they are used, in general, at very low levels in foods. Some are synthetic (mainly esters, aldehydes, and ketones) and others are derived from natural sources (such as oleoresins, plant extracts, and essential oils). Flavor enhancers, such as monosodium glutamate, enhance the flavor of the food to which it is added.
6. Artificial sweeteners have a strong sweet taste, but have little or no caloric value. They are therefore useful for diabetics and for those who wish to enjoy the sweet taste without increasing the caloric intake. The notable ones are the cyclamates, saccharin, and aspartame.
7. Nutrients include vitamins, minerals, and essential amino acids. As noted above, national regulations in most countries, contrary to those of the United States, do not consider these as food additives. However, a food additive used for a technological reason may incidentally have certain nutritional values. For example, riboflavin may be used as a color, but it is also a vitamin.
8. Miscellaneous groups. These include (a) acidity regulators (acids and bases), which are used to adjust the pH of beverages and canned fruits and vegetables; (b) anticaking agents, which are added to salt, sugar, etc., to maintain their free-flowing property; (c) antifoaming agents, which are added to liquids to prevent foaming; (d) flour treatment agents, which are added to flour to improve its baking qualities; (e) glazing agents; (f) propellants; and (g) raising agents.

21

Toxicity of pesticides

INTRODUCTION

Value of Pesticides

Pesticides are substances that kill or control *pests*. There are various types of pests. The most common are insects. Some of them serve as vectors for diseases. The most important vector-borne diseases, malaria and onchocerciasis ("river blindness"), are transmitted to humans by mosquitoes and black flies. Both diseases are debilitating and affect millions of people in the tropical and subtropical regions. Other vector-borne diseases include filariasis, yellow fever, rickettsial pox, viral encephalitis, typhus, and bubonic plague. Insecticides have helped control these diseases.

Insects are also detrimental to various *plants* and their products. Insecticides are, therefore, widely used to protect the farmer's products. Although most of the insecticides currently in use are synthetic chemicals, a number of natural substances have been used by farmers for a long time. These substances include nicotine from tobacco, pyrethrum from flowers of a species of chrysanthemum, and various compounds of lead, copper, and arsenic.

Besides insects, *weeds* constitute a very important nuisance to the farmer. Before the introduction of herbicides, farmers used to spend much time to remove the weeds manually, a very time-consuming and backbreaking task. Other pesticides have also been developed to control other pests such as *fungi*, *rodents*, and others. The great variety of agricultural uses and chemical categories may be seen from a recent compilation of the 230 pesticides that have been evaluated and reevaluated by the WHO Expert Committee on Pesticide Residues since 1965 (Lu, 1995).

A number of *household pesticide* products are also available to control household nuisance pests, such as flies and mosquitoes.

Adverse Effects of Pesticides

These may involve human health and/or the environment. The most dramatic of such effects on humans are the accidental acute poisonings. Several major outbreaks of poisoning with methyl and ethyl mercury compounds and hexachlorobenzene as fungicides and with parathion, an organophosphorus insecticide, have occurred in several parts of the world involving thousands of individuals and hundreds of deaths. A few examples are listed in Appendix 2 of chapter 1. Individual cases of acute poisoning have usually resulted from ingestion of large quantities of pesticides accidentally or with suicidal intent.

Occupational exposure to pesticides may involve workers engaged in the manufacturing, formulating, and application of pesticides. The pesticides enter the body generally through the respiratory tract and by dermal absorption, but small amounts may enter the gastrointestinal tract through the use of contaminated hands and utensils; this route of exposure is the most frequent in cases of accidental child ingestion of household products. This type of poisoning is more likely to happen with pesticides that are more toxic acutely. The major public health concern, however, is the ingestion of pesticide residues in foods, as this may involve large populations, especially children over long periods of time (Infante-Rivard and Weichenthal, 2007; Wigle et al., 2008).

In addition to these human health hazards, pesticides may have a serious impact on the *environment*. Apart from large-scale accidental release to the environment, only minimal levels are found in various environmental media. However, the levels are likely to be higher with pesticides that are persistent and/or have a propensity for biomagnification. In the latter case, the concentration of a pesticide increases as it moves through the trophic chain. The organism with a high concentration may be adversely affected. For example, the bald eagle was nearly extinct because of its fragile egg shells, which is a toxic effect of high levels of dichlorodiphenyltrichloroethane (DDT) bioaccumulated through the contaminated food chain of the bird. Daily intake of seafoods in Singapore was found to contain excessive amounts of DDT and heptachlor as a result of biomagnification, and risk of cancer might be significantly higher as a consequence in this population (Bayen et al., 2005). Such environmental pollution may also affect human health by virtue of the contaminated soil and water, which then results in the production of contaminated human food and drinking water.

CATEGORIES OF PESTICIDES

Pesticides are usually grouped according to their uses and their chemical nature. The major groups are as follows.

Insecticides

As noted above, this is the largest group of pesticides and consists of a number of different chemical subgroups.

Organophosphorous Insecticides

These are esters of phosphoric acid or thiophosphoric acid, represented by dichlorvos and parathion, respectively. They act by inhibiting acetylcholinesterase (AChE), resulting in an accumulation of acetylcholine (ACh) (Pope, 1999). The excess ACh induces a variety of symptoms and signs. The severity of the symptoms and signs is more or less correlated with the extent of the inhibition of AChE in blood, but the precise relationship varies depending on the compound (Clegg and van Gemert, 1999).

In addition to parathion and dichlorvos, other pesticides in this group include parathion-methyl, azinphos-methyl (Guthion), chlorfenvinphos, diazinon, dimethoate, disulfoton (Di-Syston), malathion, mevinphos, and trichlorfon (Dipterex). Their toxicities vary over a wide range (Appendix 1).

Carbamate Insecticides

These are esters of *N*-methylcarbamic acid. They also act by inhibiting AChE. However, their effects on the enzyme are much more readily reversible than those of the organophosphorous (OP) insecticides. Insecticides of this class include carbaryl (Sevin), aldicarb (Temik), carbofuran, methomyl, and propoxur (Baygon). In addition, with carbamates, signs of toxicity appear more promptly and, for many of them, there is a greater range from the doses that cause minor toxic effects to those that are lethal. For this reason, on an acute basis, the carbamates are considered safer than the OP insecticides. The OP insecticides are currently banned from use in most industrialized countries. Table 1 of chapter 20 also lists their toxicities.

Organochlorine Insecticides

These include the chlorinated ethane derivatives, the cyclodienes, and the hexachlorocyclohexanes. Some of these chemicals (e.g., DDT) were introduced in the 1940s and were widely used in agricultural and health programs. This was because of their relatively low acute toxicity and their persistence, which reduced the need for repeated applications. However, the persistence has later been recognized as a liability rather than an asset.

Both DDT and methoxychlor are chlorinated ethane derivatives, but methoxychlor is much less toxic and less persistent than DDT. The cyclodiene insecticide endrin is extremely toxic; aldrin and dieldrin are somewhat less toxic; and chlordane, heptachlor, and mirex even less toxic. Lindane is the gamma isomer of hexachlorocyclohexane (HCH) that is in use. It is highly toxic but less cumulative. Consequently, lindane is used much more widely than HCH, especially for hair lice in children. Organochlorine (OC) insecticides are less water soluble than OP or carbamate insecticides and more persistent in the environment.

Botanical and Other Insecticides

These include nicotine from tobacco. It is extremely toxic acutely and acts on the nervous system. Pyrethrum is obtained from the flowers of *Chrysanthemum cinerariaefolium*. An enzyme inhibitor, piperonyl butoxide, is often used in combination with this insecticide as a synergist. Pyrethrum has a low toxicity in mammals but is allergenic to sensitive individuals, producing contact dermatitis and is also a neurotoxicant. The major active principles in pyrethrum are pyrethrin I and II. The former, pyrethrin I, acts on the central nervous system and the latter on the peripheral nervous system. Both are synthesized and more stable than pyrethrum. Rotenone is extracted from the roots of the plant *Derris elliptica*. It also has a low toxicity in mammals but is more toxic to insects and fish. Many microorganisms are known to be pathogenic to insects. The ones being used are *Bacillus thuringiensis* and certain insect baculoviruses, not known to be pathogenic to humans.

Herbicides

There are several types of herbicides. Some retard the growth of weeds by inhibiting photosynthesis, respiration, cell division, or synthesis of protein or lipids. Others act as growth stimulants thereby disturbing the normal growth (Ecobichon, 1998).

Chlorophenoxy compounds are exemplified by 2,4-dichlorophenoxyacetic acid (2,4-D) and 2,4,5-trichlorophenoxyacetic acid (2,4,5-T). They act in plants as growth hormones. Their toxicities in animals are relatively low. However, chloracne, the main toxic effect of 2,4,5-T in humans, seems attributable to the contaminant 2,3,7,8-tetrachlorobenzo-*p*-dioxin .

Bipyridyl herbicides, such as paraquat and diquat, have been widely used. They exert their toxicity via the formation of free radicals. The toxicity of paraquat is characterized by its pulmonary effects not only after exposure via inhalation but also by the oral route, as noted in chapter 12. Oral paraquat ingestion and death occur frequently in individuals committed to suicide.

Other herbicides include dinitro-*o*-cresol, amitrole, the carbamates propham and chloropropham, and a number of other chemicals.

Fungicides

Mercury compounds such as methyl and ethyl mercury are very effective fungicides and had been widely used to preserve seed grains. However, several tragic accidents, involving numerous deaths and permanent neurological damage, occurred with their use (Appendix 2 of chap. 1). This fact has deterred their further use.

Dicarboximides include the dimethyl thiocarbamates (ferbam, thiram, and ziram) and the ethylene bisdithiocarbamates (maneb, nabam, and zineb). These compounds have relatively low acute toxicity and have hence been widely used in agriculture. However, there is concern about their carcinogenic potential.

Phthalimide derivatives such as captan and folpet have very low acute and chronic toxicity. However, captan was found to reduce body weight of pups of treated rats and folpet-induced keratosis of the gastrointestinal (GI) tract (FAO, 1990).

Substituted aromatics such as pentachlorophenol (PCP) have been widely used as wood preservatives. PCP increases metabolic rate through uncoupling of oxidative phosphorylation. It has a low LD_{50} but its technical grade is more toxic, indicating greater toxicity of its contaminants. Pentachloro nitrobenzene (PCNB) has been used as a fungicide in treating soil. It is somewhat less toxic acutely than PCP, but may be carcinogenic.

Other fungicides include certain *N*-heterocyclic compounds such as benomyl and thiobendazole. These chemicals have very low toxicity and have been widely used in agriculture. Hexachlorobenzene has been used as a seed treatment agent but has caused mass poisoning (Appendix 2 of chap. 1).

Rodenticides

Warfarin is an anticoagulant by acting as an antimetabolite to vitamin K, thereby inhibiting the formation of prothrombin. It has been widely used because its toxicity is observed only after repeated ingestion, a circumstance unlikely to occur among children and pets.

Thioureas such as α-naphthyl thiourea are extremely toxic to rats but only moderately toxic to humans. Their main toxicity is pulmonary edema and pleural effusion.

Sodium fluoroacetate ("1080") and fluoroacetamide ("1081") are extremely toxic and their use has hence been restricted to licensed personnel. They exert toxic effect through blockage of the citric acid cycle as described in chapter 4 under "Lethal Synthesis."

Other rodenticides include botanical products such as the alkaloid strychnine, a potent CNS stimulant, and red squill, which contain the glycosides scillaren A and scillaren B. These glycosides, similar to digitalis, have cardiotonic and central emetic effects. Because of the latter effect, these substances are relatively nontoxic to most mammals but are potent poisons to rats, which do not vomit. Inorganic rodenticides include zinc phosphide, thallium sulfate, arsenic trioxide, and elemental phosphorus, acting through different mechanisms.

Fumigants

As the name implies, this group of pesticides includes a number of gases, liquids that readily vaporize, and solids that release gases by chemical reactions. In the gaseous form, they permeate storage areas and soil to control insects, rodents, and soil nematodes. Many fumigants, such as acrylonitrile, chloropicrin, and ethylene dibromide, are reactive chemicals and are also used widely in the chemical industry; some of them will be described in chapter 26.

TOXICOLOGICAL PROPERTIES

Toxicity on the Nervous System

The OC insecticides stimulate the nervous system and induce paresthesia, susceptibility to stimulation, irritability, disturbed equilibrium, tremor, and convulsions. The precise mode of action is not known. However, some of these chemicals, such as aldrin, dieldrin, and lindane, induce facilitation and hyperexcitation at synaptic and neuromuscular junctions, resulting in repetitive discharge in central, sensory, and motor neurons. DDT may exert its toxic effect in the nervous system by adversely affecting the axon membrane (Doherty, 1979; Narahashi, 1980).

The OP and carbamate insecticides inhibit AChE (Pope, 1999). Normally, the neurotransmitter ACh is released at the synapses. Once the nerve impulse is transmitted, the released ACh is hydrolyzed to acetic acid and choline by AChE at the site. Upon exposure to OP and carbamate insecticides, AChE is inhibited, resulting in an accumulation of ACh. The accumulated ACh in the CNS will induce tremor, incoordination, convulsions (Clegg and van Gemert, 1999). In the autonomic nervous system AChE inhibition produces diarrhea, involuntary urination, bronchoconstriction, miosis, etc. Acetylcholine accumulation at the neuromuscular junction will lead to contraction of the muscles, followed by weakness, loss of reflexes, and paralysis. The inhibition of AChE induced by carbamates is readily reversible, whereas that following exposure to OP compounds is generally less readily so. In fact, certain OP compounds, such as diisopropyl fluorophosphate (DFP), produce irreversible inhibition; recovery only follows synthesis of new AChE.

Several OP compounds, including DFP, tri-*o*-cresyl phosphate (TOCP), leptophos, mipafox, and trichlorofon, cause a "delayed neurotoxicity."

As noted above, pyrethrin I and II act on different parts of the nervous system.

Interactions

The most notable type of interaction is the *potentiation* observed between certain OP insecticides. Frawley and coworkers (1957) reported marked potentiation of the toxicity of the *o*-ethyl-*o*-(4-nitrophenyl) phenyl phosphonothioate and malathion. Combinations of a number of OP insecticides have since been tested. Some showed additive effects, others were less than additive, and still others were synergistic. The most pronounced potentiation (about 100-fold increase) was observed between malathion and TOCP. The mechanism of the potentiation was attributed to the inhibition of enzymes, such as carboxyl esterase and amidases, which are responsible for the detoxication of certain OP compounds such as malathion and its more toxic metabolite malaoxon (Murphy, 1969).

Carcinogenicity

The OP insecticides, in general, in adults are not carcinogenic, with the exception of compounds that contain halogens such as tetrachlorvinphos. These chemicals possess the properties of OC insecticides (see the next paragraph). However, it is worth noting that children are a more susceptible subpopulation. There is epidemiological evidence of increased frequency of cancer in children exposed to OP insecticides (Infante-Rivard and Weichenthal, 2007; Wigle et al., 2008). The carbamate insecticides per se are not carcinogenic either. However, carbaryl was shown to form, in the presence of nitrous acid, nitrosocarbaryl, which is known to be carcinogenic. A number of other pesticides are also nitrosatable under extreme conditions, and their products are carcinogenic and mutagenic (IARC, 1983). However, because of the unrealistic conditions required for such nitrosation to take place, the health concern arising from this type of reaction is questionable.

On the other hand, the OC insecticides tested were all found to induce hepatoma in mice (IARC, 1983). The pesticide that aroused most controversy has been DDT. It did not produce carcinogenicity in rats, hamsters, and several other mammalian species. Furthermore, epidemiological findings are essentially negative, and so are the short-term mutagenesis tests. For these reasons the WHO Expert Committee on Pesticide Residues reaffirmed in 1984 the acceptable daily intake (ADI) for DDT and several other OC insecticides. A comprehensive review of the toxicological data and their interpretations on DDT was provided by Coulston (1985). Nevertheless, its use has been restricted or suspended in several nations based partly on this potential health hazard and partly on its ecological impact. It is worth noting that in certain underdeveloped countries DDT must be applied in order to counteract malaria development. The only pesticide on which there is some epidemiological evidence of carcinogenicity is hexachlorocyclohexane (Wang et al., 1988).

The fumigants ethylene dibromide and 1,2-dibromo-3-chloropropane were found to produce highly malignant squamous cell carcinoma in the stomach of rats and mice (IARC, 1977). However, their use has not been restricted or suspended, because the fumigated foods, upon aeration, contain negligible residue levels.

Amitrole (aminotriazole), a herbicide, produces thyroid tumors apparently through an indirect mechanism (Steinhoff et al., 1983). Thyroid peroxidase normally oxidizes iodine to an oxidized form, which then conjugates with tyrosine to form thyroxine (T4). Amitrole inhibits this enzyme, thus lowering T4 levels. This lowered level, through a biofeedback mechanism, stimulates pituitary gland to release more thyroid-stimulating hormone (TSH). TSH in turn stimulates thyroid gland to become hyperplastic and eventually to form tumors. Amitrole is thus a "secondary carcinogen." Similarly, the ethylene bisdithiocarbamate fumigants (mancozeb, maneb, nabam, and zineb) were also reported to produce thyroid tumors. This action is evidently mediated through the major breakdown and metabolic product ethylene thiourea. In general, many of endocrine-disrupting chemicals (EDCs) are pesticides and their major toxicities include carcinogenicity, developmental toxicity, mutagenicity, immunotoxicity, and neurotoxicity (Choi et al., 2004).

Teratogenicity and Its Effects on Reproductive Functions

In the late 1960s, several articles appeared reporting a variety of teratogenic and reproductive effects of carbaryl in dogs. Summaries of these reports have been included in a monograph (WHO, 1970). A comprehensive study in rats, given carbaryl in the diet at doses of 100 or 200 mg/kg showed no effect on various reproductive functions and no teratogenic effects. Some effects were observed in rats given carbaryl by gavage (Weil et al., 1972). The authors attributed the effects in rats to the gavage method of administering the pesticide and the effects in the dog to its routes of biotransformation of carbaryl being different from those in humans and several other species.

Other pesticides reported as having teratogenic effects include the dithio-carbamate fungicides. Such effects are likely due, at least partly, to their break-down product ETU (WHO, 1974). In addition, abamectin, dinocap, glyphosate, and procymidone induced cleft palate, defects in the neural tube, renal defects, and hypospadia, respectively (Lu, 1995). An extensive, comprehensive review of pesticides and developmental outcomes including fetal death, intrauterine growth retardation, preterm birth, and birth defects is provided by Weselak et al. (2007). In chicken embryos, the simultaneous administration of 2,4-D containing herbi-cide and cadmium or copper produced higher embryo mortality as well as devel-opmental anomalies than individual administration (Juhász et al., 2006).

Other Adverse Effects

Certain *renal* effects of carbaryl were reported in a group of human volunteers ingesting carbaryl at a daily dose of 0.12 mg/kg for six weeks. There was an increase in the ratio of urinary amino acid nitrogen to creatinine, compared with those taking placebo. This was interpreted as an indication of a decrease in the ability of the proximal convoluted tubules to reabsorb amino acids. This effect was not observed in individuals taking carbaryl at 0.06 mg/kg daily (Wills et al., 1968).

Paraquat produces *pulmonary* edema, hemorrhage, and fibrosis (Smith and Heath, 1976) following either inhalation or ingestion, but the closely related her-bicide diquat does not (see also chap. 12). However, both the chemicals are toxic to cultured lung cells. As paraquat is retained in the lung and diquat is not, it is evident that the difference between those two herbicides in their pulmonary toxic-ity is related to the special affinity of paraquat for certain pulmonary cells (type II cells). In addition, paraquat produces Parkinson's disease (PD)-like lesions in certain strains of rodents and may increase the risk of developing PD in humans (Berry et al., 2010).

Hypersensitivity reactions to pyrethrum have been reported. The most com-mon form is contact dermatitis (Vial et al., 1996). This type of reaction is not serious in the general population but may have serious consequences in immuno-compromised individuals such as AIDS patients with non-Hodgkin's lymphoma, lupus erythematosus, or rheumatoid arthritis. Asthma has also been reported. Ana-phylactic reactions are rare (Hayes, 1982).

Organochlorine insecticides, such as DDT, chlordecone, and mirex, are hepatotoxic, inducing *liver* enlargement and centrolobular necrosis. They are also inducers of microsomal mono-oxygenases, thereby affecting the toxicity of other chemicals.

A number of OP, carbamate, and OC insecticides, the dithiocarbamate fungi-cides, and herbicides alter various *immune functions* (Vial et al., 1996). For example, malathion, methyl parathion, carbaryl, DDT, paraquat, and diquat have been shown to depress antibody formation, impair leukocyte phagocytosis, and reduce the germinal centers in spleen, thymus, and lymph nodes (Koller, 1979; Street, 1981).

Bioaccumulation and Biomagnification

These properties per se do not necessarily represent adverse biological effects. They are generally associated with substances that are lipophilic and resistant to breakdown. The OC pesticides in general are more persistent in the environment and tend to be stored in the fat depot. However, the bioaccumulation is more marked with some chemicals than others. For example, DDT is stored in the body fat for a much longer time than methoxychlor. The half-lives of these insecticides in rats are 6–12 months and 12 weeks, respectively.

Their persistence in the environment may create ecological problems. DDT and related chemicals in the environment enhance the metabolism of estrogens in birds. In the egg-laying and nestling cycle of certain birds, this disturbance of hormones adversely affects reproduction and survival of the young (Peakall, 1970). There is evidence that the estrogenic actions of DDT are responsible for the development of breast cancer and disorders of male reproductive functions (Roy et al., 1997).

Biomagnification is the result of bioaccumulation in the organism alone or in conjunction with persistence in the environment. For example, DDT is lipophilic, and thus occurs in the fat portion of body fluids including milk. While a mother's daily intake of DDT may be 0.5 µg/kg, her breast-fed baby's daily DDT intake be 11.2 µg/kg. This magnification results from the fact that DDT is stored in the human body at 10- to 20-fold chronic daily intake level and the baby consumes essentially only the milk. Furthermore, the caloric intake per kilogram body weight is higher in babies compared with that in adults. The significance of the much greater intake of DDT by babies is not clear, because of the relatively short duration of this greater level of intake and the remarkable insensitivity of the young versus the adult (Lu et al., 1965).

The biomagnification is even more marked in carnivorous animals. DDT and methyl mercury can accumulate through a series of plankton, small fish, large fish, and birds, and result in a magnification of the concentration amounting to several hundred-fold (Woodwell, 1967). The decision to suspend the use of DDT was partly based on its adverse ecological impact, as noted earlier.

TESTING, EVALUATION, AND CONTROL

Categories of Data Required

Various categories of data are required in the evaluation of pesticides. The basic data required are essentially the same as those listed for food additives (see chap. 18). However, a number of specific toxicological problems have been encountered with pesticides as outlined in the preceding section. The additional studies for certain pesticides include the following.

LD50 and Short-Term Toxicity

Because of the greater acute toxicity of most pesticides, the LD_{50} is usually determined more precisely. Furthermore, in view of the fact that certain occupational workers such as manufacturers, formulators, and applicators may be exposed through the skin and respiratory tract, the dermal LD_{50} and the LC_{50} by inhalation are generally required to be found out. As occupational workers are likely to be exposed for some length of time, the toxicity of repeated exposure through dermal and inhalation is generally ascertained (see chaps. 12 and 15).

Delayed Neurotoxicity (Peripheral Axonopathy)

This type of toxicity has been observed with a number of OP insecticides. The appropriate test is performed on new chemicals of this group to exclude this potential hazard (see chap. 17).

Interaction

Marked interaction exists between certain pairs of OP insecticides. The potential health hazard is assessed using LD_{50}s of the individual chemicals alone and in combination.

Toxicological Evaluation

The assessment of an ADI involves assessing the database for completeness and relevance, determining a no-observed-adverse-effect level (NOAEL) in terms of mg/kg body weight, and selecting an appropriate safety factor to extrapolate to an ADI for humans, also in terms of mg/kg body weight. A list of the ADIs of the 230 pesticides that have been evaluated and re-evaluated by the WHO Expert Committee on Pesticide Residues since 1965, along with the NOAELs, safety factors, and critical effects is included in a review article (Lu, 1995).

While all pesticides are toxic, they vary in the nature and magnitude of toxicity. Certain pesticides have an inherent potential for specific toxic effects. The presence of such properties must be assessed by conducting appropriate tests, before determining a NOAEL. The size of the safety factor will depend on a number of factors, as discussed in chapter 26.

Standards

Tolerances

To protect the health of the consumer, standards are formulated. The standards, in the form of "tolerances" (also known as "maximum residue limits") are established.

The standards provide maximum permitted levels in each food commodity in which the pesticide may leave residues following its use. A pesticide may be used during any one or more stages of the preplanting, growth, harvesting, handling, and storage of the food crop.

Dietary Intakes

Several procedures are used to ensure that the total intake of each pesticide from its residues in all food commodities does not exceed its ADI. One procedure involves chemical analysis of the residue levels in food represented in the "total diet" and the calculation of the "dietary intake" of each pesticide by adding the products of the residue levels and the per capita consumption of each of these foods. The latest survey by the U.S. Food and Drug Administration (FDA) shows that the dietary intakes of all the pesticides analyzed were considerably lower than the corresponding ADIs (FDA, 1987).

The other procedure, which is much simpler, involves calculating the "potential daily intake" and comparing it with the corresponding ADI. The former figure is obtained by adding the products of the tolerance levels in each of the foods and the per capita consumption of these foods. Evidently the potential daily intake represents an overestimation. First, a pesticide is not necessarily used in all the food commodities in which there are tolerances. Furthermore, in a vast majority of the cases, the actual residue levels are much lower than the tolerances. Nevertheless, this procedure offers distinct advantages. Apart from a few industrialized countries, figures for dietary intakes of pesticides are not available; for them the potential daily intakes provide a ready yardstick for assessing the health hazards to the consumer posed by the dietary intake of pesticides. The overestimation may also compensate for differences in dietary habits in different parts of the world and for variations in the levels of pesticide residues in certain foods. According to actual analysis, the residue levels may, although infrequently, exceed the tolerances (see also chap. 27).

Apart from assessing the potential hazard of pesticides, the dietary intake figures, obtained by analysis or calculation, are also used in assessing, and possibly in recommending the modification of the agricultural use of these chemicals. Where the residue levels appear too high, they may be lowered, for example, by a reduction of the rate of application or by an increase of the interval between the last application and harvesting of the food crop.

GULF WAR SYNDROME

Between August 1990 and April 1991 there were over 750,000 military personnel from United States, Canada, and United Kingdom who participated in the air, sea, and ground war in the Persian Gulf region. During this war, service personnel were concurrently exposed to certain biological, chemical, and psychological environments. In particular among some veterans, there was an increased frequency of chronic symptoms including headache, loss of memory, fatigue, muscle and joint pain, ataxia, skin rash, respiratory difficulties, and GI tract disturbances. Potential exposure was to fumes and smoke from the following: military operations, oil-well fires, diesel exhaust, toxic paints, pesticides, fire sand, depleted uranium, chemo-prophylactic agents, and multiple immunizations. The variety of symptoms reported by veterans make it unlikely that a single etiological cause was responsible for producing the Gulf War illnesses.

It was suggested by the news media that chemical interactions among pyridostigmine bromide (PB), permethrin, and *N,N*-diethyl-*m*-toluamide (DEET) might contribute to Gulf War illnesses. This reported mixture served to protect the military personnel against insect-borne diseases. Furthermore, PB protected against potential nerve gas attack. However, heavy use of DEET by 1–5% of the Persian Gulf War veterans (7000–35,000 persons) may be related to the unexpected increase in the number of complaints of some of the veterans, which included fatigue, joint pain, ataxia, and rash (Institute of Medicine, 1995). Other complaints reported by "heavy users" of DEET were stumbling, weakness, and muscle cramps. The fact that these complaints occurred with excess frequency within this subpopulation can be deemed that exposure to contaminants in the Persian Gulf was responsible for this illness. A comprehensive toxicological assessment of Gulf War veterans has been carried out and some of pesticides are described here (Brown, 2006).

Pyridostigmine bromide (PB) is a quaternary ammonium carbamate that has been approved by the FDA as a treatment for myasthenia gravis and the reversal of nondepolarizing neuromuscular blocking agents. PB was used in the Gulf War at a dose of one 30 mg tablet every 8 hours (90 mg/day). PB was taken for about two weeks at the start of the air war in mid-January and again at the start of the ground war in mid-February. The majority of service members in the theater of operations took some PB during these periods. Toxicity from an overdose of PB results from the accumulation of acetylcholine at nicotinic and muscarinic acetylcholine receptors in the peripheral nervous system. The resultant effect is exaggerated cholinergic response such as muscle fasciculations, cramps, weakness, muscle twitching, respiratory difficulty, tremor, GI tract disturbances, and paralysis (Abou-Donia et al., 1996). Finally, death occurs from asphyxia. It should be clearly noted that a therapeutic oral dose of PB for myasthenia gravis is 200–1400 mg/day but that much lower dose was taken in the Persian Gulf.

Permethrin, a third-generation synthetic pyrethroid, has been approved for use as an insecticide by the U.S. Environmental Protection Agency (EPA). This compound has also been used to impregnate army battle-dress uniforms in the field. Formulations for application include a 0.5% aerosol and a 40% solution applied either with a 2-gallon compressed air sprayer or via a passive absorption method in a plastic bag (for uniform impregnation). The impregnation method available to soldiers prior to and during the Gulf War was the aerosol spray can method. The aerosol spray can supply and distribution were limited within the war theater (less than 5% of deployed units had distributional access) (McCain et al.,

1997). Permethrin modifies sodium channels to open longer during a depolarizing pulse, evoking repetitive after-discharges by a single stimulus. This repetitive nerve action is associated with hyperactivity, tremors, ataxia, convulsions, and eventually paralysis.

DEET is an aromatic amide used as a personal insect repellent against mosquitoes, biting flies, and ticks, among other insects. It has been used since 1946 by the U.S. Army and since 1957 by the general population. Approximately 30% of the U.S. population uses DEET as a lotion, stick, or spray at concentrations between 10% and 100% active ingredient. DEET is an EPA-approved insect repellant that is widely used commercially. Several formulations using various concentrations of DEET are available. It is the active ingredient in products such as Deep Woods Off and Cutter Insect Repellent. Formulations prepared for the U.S. Army include 75% DEET in ethanol, 33% extended duration formulation, and 19% in stick. Entomologists assigned in the Persian Gulf during the conflict indicated a very low usage of personal repellents, including DEET, even at times and in areas where mosquitoes were present and biting. The cool seasonal climatic conditions that prevailed at the time of the war (January and February 1991) resulted in the near absence of biting insects. Extensive and repeated topical applications of DEET resulted in human poisoning including two deaths (de Garbino and Laborde, 1983; Roland et al., 1985). Symptoms of poisoning are characterized by tremors, restlessness, slurred speech, seizures, impaired cognitive functions, and coma (Institute of Medicine, 1995). The exact mechanism underlying DEET toxicity is unknown. Pathological findings, following DEET administration, indicate that this compound is a demyelinating agent that produces spongiform myelinopathy, primarily of the cerebellar roof nuclei.

In light of the established safety of PB, it was surprising that approximately half of all military personnel seen in health-care facilities during the Gulf War complained of PB side effects consistent with muscarinic stimulation (Institute of Medicine, 1995). One of the conclusions reached by the Committee to Review the Health Consequences of Service during the Persian Gulf War was that "studies are needed to resolve uncertainties about whether PB, DEET, and permethrin exert additive effects" (Institute of Medicine, 1995). The Committee also recommended for immediate action: that "appropriate laboratory animal studies of interactions between DEET, PB, and permethrin should be conducted." Regardless of the need for further studies, it is clear that contaminant mixture exposure produced a Gulf War syndrome in humans.

REFERENCES

Abou-Donia MB, Wilmarth KR, Jensen KF, et al. (1996). Neurotoxicity resulting from coexposure to pyridostigmine bromide, DEET, and permethrin: implications of gulf war chemical exposures. J Toxicol Environ Health 48, 35–56.

Bayen S, Koroleva E, Lee HK, et al. (2005). Persistent organic pollutants and heavy metals in typical seafoods consumed in Singapore. J Toxicol Environ Health A 68, 151–66.

Berry C, La Vecchia C, Nicotera P (2010). Paraquat and Parkinson's disease. Cell Death Differ 17, 1115–25.

Brown M (2006). Toxicological assessments of gulf war veterans. Philos Trans R Soc Lond B Biol Sci 361, 649–79.

Choi SM, Yoo SD, Lee BM (2004). Toxicological characteristics of endocrine-disrupting chemicals: developmental toxicity, carcinogenicity, and mutagenicity. J Toxicol Environ Health B Crit Rev 7, 1–24.

Clegg DJ, van Gemert M (1999). Expert panel report of human studies on chlorpyrifos and/ or other organophosphate exposures. J Toxicol Environ Health B 2, 257–79.

Coulston F (1985). Reconsideration of the dilemma of DDT for the establishment of an acceptable daily intake. Reg Toxicol Pharmacol 5, 332–83.

de Garbino JP, Laborde A (1983). Toxicity of an insect repellent: N,N-diethyltoluamide. Vet Hum Toxicol 25, 422–3.

Doherty JD (1979). Insecticides affecting ion transport. Pharmacol Ther 7, 123–51.

Ecobichon DJ (1998). Toxic effects of pesticides. In: Klaassen CD, ed. Casarett and Doull'sToxicology. New York, NY: McGraw-Hill, Inc.

FAO (1990). Pesticide Residues in Food—1990. Report of the FAO and WHO Groups of Experts on Pesticide Residues. FAO Plant Production and Protection Paper No. 102. Rome: Food and Agricultural Organization of the United States.

FDA (1987). Residues in Foods. Washington, DC.: Food and Drug Administration.

Frawley JP, Fuyat HN, Hagen EC, et al. (1957). Marked potentiation in mammalian toxicity from simultaneous administration of two anticholinesterase compounds. J Pharmacol Exp Ther 121, 96–106.

Hayes WJ Jr (1982). Pesticides Studied in Man. Baltimore, MD: Williams & Wilkins.

IARC (1977). Monographs on the Evaluation of Carcinogenic Risk of Chemicals to Man, vol. 15. Some Fumigants, the Herbicides 2,4-D and 2,4,5-T, Chlorinated Dibenzodioxins and Miscellaneous Industrial Chemicals. Lyon, France: International Agency for Research in Cancer.

IARC (1983). Monographs on the Evaluation of Carcinogenic Risk of Chemicals to Man, vol. 30. Miscellaneous Pesticides. Lyon, France: International Agency for Research in Cancer.

Infante-Rivard C, Weichenthal S (2007). Pesticides and childhood cancer: an update of zahm and ward's 1998 review. J Toxicol Environ Health B 10, 81–99.

Institute of Medicine (1995). Health Consequences of Service During the Persian Gulf War: Initial Findings and Recommendations for Immediate Action. Washington, DC.: National Academy Press.

Juhász E, Szabó R, Keserü M, et al. (2006). Teratogenicity testing of a 2,4-D containing herbicide formulation and three heavy metals in chicken embryos. Commun Agric Appl Biol Sci. 71, 111–14.

Koller LD (1979). Effects of environmental contaminants on the immune system. Adv Vet Sci Com Med 23, 267–95.

Lu FC (1995). A review of the acceptable daily intakes of pesticides assessed by WHO. Reg Toxicol Pharmacol 21, 352–64.

Lu FC, Jessup DC, Lavallée A (1965). Toxicity of pesticides to young versus adult rats. Food Cosmet Toxicol 5, 591–6.

McCain WC, Lee R, Johnson MS, et al. (1997). Acute oral toxicity study of pyridostigmine bromide, permethrin, and DEET in the laboratory rat. J Toxicol Environ Health 50, 113–24.

Murphy SD (1969). Mechanisms of pesticide interactions in vertebrates. Residue Rev 25, 201–21.

Narahashi T (1980). Nerve membrane as a target of environmental toxicants. In: Spencer P, Schaumberg HH, eds. Neurotoxicology. Baltimore, MD: Williams & Wilkins.

Peakall DB (1970). Pesticides and the reproduction of birds. Sci Am 222, 72–8.

Pope CN (1999). Organophosphorus pesticides: do they all have the same mechanism of toxicity? J Toxicol Environ Health B 2, 161–81.

Roland EH, Jan JE, Rigg JM (1985). Toxic encephalopathy in a child after brief exposure to insect repellents. Can Med Assoc J 132, 155–6.

Roy D, Palangat M, Chen C-W, et al. (1997). Biochemical and molecular changes at the cellular level in response to exposure to environmental estrogen-like chemicals. J Toxicol Environ Health 50, 1–29.

Smith P, Heath D (1976). Paraquat. CRC Crit Rev Toxicol 4, 411–45.

Steinhoff D, Weber H, Mohr U, et al. (1983). Evaluation of amitrole (aminotriazole) for potential carcinogenicity in orally dosed rats, mice and golden hamster. Toxicol Appl Pharmacol 69, 161–9.

Street JC (1981). Pesticides and the immune system. In: Sharma RP, ed. Immunologic Considerations in Toxicology. Boca Raton, FL: CRC Press.

Vial T, Nicolas B, Descotes J (1996). Clinical immunotoxicity of pesticides. J Toxicol Environ Health 48, 215–29.

Wang XQ, Gas PY, Lin YZ, et al. (1988). Studies on hexachlorocyclohexane and DDT contents in human cerumen and their relationship to cancer mortality. Biomed Environ Sci 1, 138–51.

Weil CS, Woodside MD, Carpenter CP, et al. (1972). Current status of tests of carbaryl for reproductive and teratogenic effects. Toxicol Appl Pharmacol 21, 390–404.

Weselak M, Arbuckle TE, Foster W (2007). Pesticide exposures and developmental outcomes: the epidemiological evidence. J Toxicol Environ Health B 10, 41–80.

Wigle DT, Arbuckle TE, Turner MC, et al. (2008). Epidemiologic evidence of relationships between reproductive and child health outcomes and environmental chemical contaminants. J Toxicol Environ Health B 11, 373–517.

Wills JH, Jameson E, Coulston F (1968). Effects of oral doses of carbaryl on man. Clin Toxicol 1, 265–71.

Woodwell GM (1967). Toxic substances and ecological cycles. Sci Am 216, 24.

World Health Organization (1970). Pesticide Residues in Food. WHO Tech Rep Ser 458. Geneva, Switzerland: WHO.

World Health Organization (1974). Pesticide Residues in Food. Report of the 1973 Joint FAO/WHO Meeting. Tech Rep Ser 545. Geneva, Switzerland: WHO.

Appendix 1   Toxicological Findings and Evaluation on Certain Insecticides

Pesticides	LD_{50} (mg/kg)	NOAEL (mg/kg)			ADI (mg/kg)
		Rat	Dog	Human	
Azinphosmethyl	13	0.45	0.74	0.3	0.005
Chlorfenvinphos	15	0.05	0.05		0.002
Diazinon	108	0.02	0.02	0.025	0.002
Dichlorvos	80		0.05 (NOEL)	0.04	0.004
Dimethoate	215	0.4		0.2	0.02
Disulfoton	6.8	0.06	0.03	0.01	0.0003
Malathion	1375	5.0		0.2	0.02
Mevinphos	6.1	0.02	0.025	0.014	0.0015
Parathion	13			0.05	0.005
Parathion-methyl	14	0.1	0.375	0.3	0.02
Trichlorfon	630	2.5	1.25		0.01
Aldicarb	0.8	0.125	0.25	0.025	0.003
Carbaryl	500~850	10		0.06	0.01
Propoxur	83	12.5	50		0.02
DDT	113	0.05			0.01
Aldrin/dieldrin	40	0.025	0.025		0.0001
Chlordane	335	0.25	0.05		0.0005
Endrin	18	0.05	0.025		0.002
Heptacholor	100	0.25	0.025		0.0001
Lindane	88	1.25	1.75		0.008
Methoxychlor	6000	10			0.1

Abbreviations: ADI, acceptable daily intake; DDT, dichlorodiphenyltrichloroethane; NOAEL, no-observed-adverse-effect level; NOEL, no-observed-effect level. *Source*: LD50s from Gaines, other data from various WHO reports, summarized in Lu (1995).

22

Nanotoxicity

INTRODUCTION

Advances in nanoscience and nanoengineering technology have provided benefits and presented risks to human safety. Nanoparticles (NPs) are now being used in many consumer products, such as, foods, cosmetics, biosensors, electronic devices, and drug delivery systems and their applications continue to increase rapidly (Zhao and Castranova, 2011). In general, a NP is defined as a particle with a diameter between 1 nm and 100 nm (SCENIHR, 2010; ISO, 2008), and NPs enter cells either via energy-dependent endocytosis, transmembrane channels, or membrane penetration and may produce adverse effects.

TYPES OF NANOMATERIALS: CLASSIFICATION

One nanometer (nm) is one billionth of a meter and the term "nanomaterials" refers to any engineered materials of 100 nm or less in at least one direction. Nanomaterials (NMs) are classified as NPs, nanofibers, and nanoplates (ISO, 2008) (Fig. 22.1). NMs can be classified as carbon-based NMs, metal-based NMs, dendrimers, and nanocomposites (as summarized below) (Choi and Frangioni, 2010).

1. **Carbon-Based Nanomaterials**: Carbon nanomaterials (CNMs) exist in several forms, such as, hollow spheres, ellipsoids, rings, or tubes. Spherical and ellipsoidal CNMs are called fullerenes, whereas, cylindrical CNMs are termed nanotubes. Carbon fullerenes (also termed buckminster fullerenes in full or bulky balls) are similar to graphite in structure, insoluble, and nonreactive. The most common and smallest fullerene is C_{60}. Carbon nanotubes (CNTs) can be further divided into single-walled carbon nanotubes (SWCNTs) and multiwalled nanotubes (MWCNTs). CNMs are used in the electronics industry and for material engineering.

2. **Metal-Based Nanomaterials**: These include metals (silver, gold), metal oxides (iron oxide, aluminum oxide, cerium oxide, copper oxide, ZnO, and TiO_2), and quantum dots (also called nanocrystals, made from ZnSe, ZnS, CdSe, CdTe,

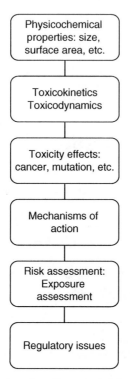

Figure 22.1 ISO TS 27687 categories of nanomaterials: nanoparticles, nanofibers, and nanoplates (ISO, 2008).

PbSe, and PbS compounds). These metal-based NMs are used in consumer products, cosmetics, semiconductors, and in the automobile industry. Of the metal-based NMs, the oxides of zinc and copper are known to be particularly toxic.

3. **Dendrimers**: Dendrimers are hyperbranched materials and nanosized polymers. Dendrimers are used in nanomedicine, for drug delivery and catalysis, and as chemical sensors and reaction vessels.

4. **Nanocomposites**: Nanocomposites are combinations of NPs with other materials or NPs, and are used in auto parts, for drug delivery, in electronics, and in packaging materials, to enhance mechanical, thermal, and flame-retardant properties (Hu and Gao, 2010).

Auffan et al. (2009) proposed that for specific "nano-effects," the particles must be below 30 nm, but particles larger than 30 nm also exhibit NP-like properties.

EXPOSURE SOURCES

Exposure sources are numerous and vary from natural to anthropogenic sources. Humans are exposed to smoke or ash produced by cigarettes, automobile exhausts, combustion, power plants, fires, and volcanoes. Meteorological changes can also generate NPs. Aerosols generated by human activities (automobiles and industrial exhausts) are estimated to constitute 10% of the total, and the remaining 90% of the air-borne aerosols of dust and particulate matter (PM) are generated naturally by volcanic eruptions, forest fires, vegetation, and by sea spray (Taylor, 2002). Humans are exposed to NPs from foods, cosmetics, electronics, medical devices, drugs, and consumer products (e.g., detergents and paper).

PHYSICOCHEMICAL PROPERTIES OF NANOMATERIALS

NPs have various physicochemical properties that depend on size and chemical composition. As the physicochemical properties of NPs can affect both the pharmacological and toxicological effects of NPs in biological systems, information on the physicochemical properties (e.g., size, shape, surface area, surface charge, surface chemistry, solubility, structure, stability, surface porosity, electric properties, conductivity, agglomeration, magnetic properties) is considered important (Johnston et al., 2010).

Physicochemical properties govern the toxicokinetics (e.g., absorption, distribution, metabolism, excretion, and storage) of NPs, toxicodynamics (interactions with biomolecules), and toxicological outcomes. The intratracheal instillation of ultrafine TiO_2 particles (20 nm) was found to produce pulmonary inflammation in rats and mice, and its toxicity was found to be correlated with a greater surface area per unit mass (Oberdörster et al., 2000). Furthermore, as the degree of sidewall functionalization of SWCNTs increases, SWCNTs become less cytotoxic to cultured human dermal fibroblasts (HDF) (Sayes et al., 2006). Smaller NPs have substantially greater specific surface areas. NPs can produce unique optical effects, because their sizes produce quantum effects. For example, the colors of gold NPs change size-dependently from red to black in solution, whereas gold slabs are usually yellow. Furthermore, the melting point of gold NPs of 2.5 nm is ~300°C, whereas that of gold slabs is 1064°C (Buffat and Borel, 1976).

The physicochemical properties of NP can be characterized by using various analytical techniques such as AFM (atomic force microscopy), DLS (dynamic light scattering), DMA (dynamic mechanical analysis), FFF (field flow fractionation), ICP-MS (inductively coupled plasma–mass spectrometry), MALDI-TOF (matrix-assisted laser desorption/ionization time-of-flight mass spectrometry), NMR (nuclear magnetic resonance), SEM (scanning electron microscopy), TEM (transmission electron microscopy), UV/Vis absorption spectroscopy, XPS (x-ray photoelectron spectroscopy), and XRD (x-ray diffraction).

Examples of the Size Range of Different Materials

- DNA molecules have a diameter of 2–12 nm
- Viruses typically have a maximum dimension of 10–100 nm
- A single red blood cell (RBC) has a diameter of 2500–5000 nm
- A human hair has a thickness of 10,000–50,000 nm

USAGES AND EFFECTS OF NANOMATERIALS

NMs are being used in more than 500 consumer products and this number is expected to grow. Although it is estimated that consumer products involving nanotechnology applications will value $1 trillion in the world market by 2012 (Service, 2004; Burnett and Tyshenko, 2010), this is expected to reach approximately $3 trillion by 2015. NPs can be made of many materials, but the specific types of NPs mentioned above are being widely used. NPs are used in the medical and food industries, in cosmetics, electronics, textiles, and in other consumer products such as deodorants, detergents, shampoos, soaps, and toothpastes (Table 22.1; Zhao and Castranova, 2011). According to a report from the Wilson Center (2008), 20 countries use 803 types of nanoproducts and the numbers continue to increase rapidly.

Nanomedicine is an emerging area for the development of new drugs, diagnostics, treatments, medical devices, and drug delivery systems (Armstead and Li, 2011). Different types of NPs have also been applied in biomedicine as imaging agents. Liposomes are commonly used NPs for the delivery of drugs or biomolecules such as siRNAs. Silver NPs have effective antibacterial properties against pathogenic bacteria (Gram-negative and Gram-positive), and smaller silver NPs enhance these effects, due to their larger surface area to volume ratios (Panacek et al., 2006).

TOXICITIES OF NANOMATERIALS

The development and application of NMs introduced safety issues, and thus, nanotoxicology has emerged as an important part of toxicology and nanoscience. The major concerns relate to the introduction of NMs and nanoproducts without safety evaluations. However, lessons were learned regarding the importance of the toxicologies of NPs from the data reported on asbestos, metal fumes, and smokes, before the era of nanotechnology (Pacurari et al., 2010). The applications of asbestos in building construction produced various lung diseases (e.g., asbestosis and mesothelioma) in the exposed workers. In addition, smokes produce various types of diseases such as cancer, respiratory disorders, GI tract diseases, skin diseases, and reproductive diseases. Some key factors such as the physicochemical properties and toxicokinetics/toxicodynamics need to be considered for nanotoxicity (Fig. 22.2).

Similar safety concerns have been raised about CNTs because they have asbestos-like shapes (Helland et al., 2007). In a 14-week inhalation toxicity study, MWCNTs were found in the lungs, and there was scarring and fibrosis of the lungs, but none of these symptoms were seen in mice exposed to carbon black, which was composed of graphene, the same substance from which nanotubes were made, but in the form of a compact particle (Donaldson and Poland, 2009). Recent epidemiological studies of fine particles showed that small NMs induced damage in the pulmonary, cardiovascular, and nervous systems (Krug and Wick, 2011). Routes of exposure to NPs were via the skin, ingestion, and/or inhalation, and toxic responses could be local or systemic, depending on the physicochemical properties of the NPs concerned.

Table 22.1 List of Commercial Products Containing Nanoparticles

Categories	Subcategories	Products	Exposure route
Food			
Food conservation	Storage	Food containers, baby (milk) bottles, mugs	Dermal/oral
	Cleaning	Sterilizing spray	Inhalation/dermal
Food equipment	Cooking utensils	Cutting/chopping boards	Dermal
Food consumption	Supplements	AgNPs in water	Oral
Consumer Products			
Personal care/cosmetics	Skin care	(Body) cream, beauty soap, etc.	Dermal
	Oral hygiene	Tooth brush	Oral
	Hair care	Hair brush, hair masks	Dermal
	Cleaning	Elimination spray	Dermal
	Baby care	Pacifier, teether	Dermal
	Other	Deodorant	Dermal
Textile	Clothing	Fabrics/fibers, socks, underwear	Dermal
	Other textiles	Sheet, towels, sleeves	Dermal
	Toys	Plush toys	Dermal/oral
Electronics	Personal care	Hair dryers, shavers	Dermal
	Household appliance	Refrigerators, washing machines	Dermal
		Humidifier	-
	Computer hardware	Notebooks, (laser) mouse, keyboards	Dermal
	Mobile devices	Mobile phone	Dermal
Household products/ home improvement	Cleaning	Laundry soap Detergents, fabric softener	Dermal
	Coating	Spray	Dermal
	Others	Pet products, algaecide	Dermal
Filtration, purification, neutralization, sanitization	Filtration	Air filters	Inhalation
	Cleaning	Disinfectant/aerosol spray	Inhalation/dermal
Medical Products			
Medical instruments	Breathing masks, endotracheal tube	Inhalation	
	Gastrointestinal tube	Oral	
	Orthopedic implants	Intramedullary	
	Contact lens	Ophthalmic	
	Incontinence material	Dermal	
	Catheters	Intravascular/urethral/ Intrathecal/intravesical	
Others	Sling for reconstructive pelvic surgery	Intraperitoneal	
	Surgical mask/textile	Inhalation/dermal	
	Wound dressings	Dermal	
	Pharmaceuticals	Oral/dermal	

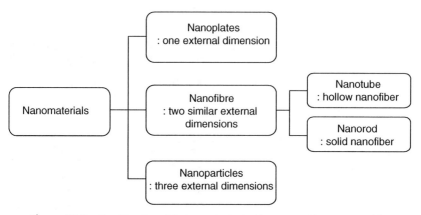

Figure 22.2   Consideration of the key toxicological issues posed by nanomaterials.

Skin Toxicity

NPs are applied in over 200 commercial skin products, such as, sunscreens, cosmetics, and personal care products. Nano TiO_2 (titanium dioxide, a potent photocatalyst) and nano zinc oxide (ZnO) are utilized as additives in sunscreens to protect the skin from UV radiation. Currently NP usages are being examined, as treatments for dermatological conditions (Wiesenthal et al., 2011). Wu et al., (2009) reported that TiO_2 NPs (4 nm, 60 nm) can penetrate the skin of pig ears after treatment for 30 days, and that TiO_2 NPs (21 nm) reached the brain in hairless mice after treatment for 60 days. In this investigation, severe pathological changes of the mouse skin and liver were observed, and the SOD activity and malondialdehyde (MDA) levels were significantly changed. Furthermore, it was also reported that typical exposure to SWCNTs produced dermal toxicity, reactive oxygen species (ROS) generation, and inflammation (Shvedova et al., 2003 and Murray et al., 2009). Although there are three types of TiO_2 (rutile, anatase, and brookite), the anatase form has raised concerns over its toxicity.

Pulmonary Diseases

Nano particles can produce pulmonary diseases, such as, asthma, cystic fibrosis (CF), and chronic obstructive pulmonary disease (COPD) by altering the mucus rheology in the respiratory tract (Chen et al., 2010). Occupational exposure to NPs (e.g., carbon black, dust, aerosols, fire, and welding fumes) may produce fibrosis, emphysema, bronchitis, pulmonary inflammation, and pulmonary edema. Furthermore, pneumoconiosis might also be associated directly or indirectly with uncharacterized NPs. The underlying mechanisms of NP-induced pulmonary toxicity include generation of oxidative stress, DNA damage, and inflammation leading to fibrosis and pneumoconiosis (Li et al., 2010).

Mutation

Shinohara et al. (2009) reported negative results for the micronucleus (MN) test, after treating ICR mice with fullerene C_{60}. SWCNTs were not found to induce MN formation in Chinese hamster lung (CHL) cells, but Totsuka et al. (2009) showed that fullerene C_{60} NPs, depending on the concentration, increased MN frequency in A549 cells. Asakura et al. (2010) reported that MWCNTs significantly increased the rate of polyploidy in CHL/IU cells, as determined by a chromosomal aberration test. In the Ames test, some NPs such as CNTs, fullerenes C_{60}, and ZnO were found to be negative. On the other hand, carbon black NPs were reported to induce genotoxicity in the lungs and livers of C57BL/6 mice (Bourdon et al., 2012) and silver NPs were reported to produce DNA damage, chromosomal aberrations, and MN formation (Ahamed et al., 2008; Asharani et al., 2009a; 2009b; Kawata et al., 2009).

Cancer

Various types of NPs have been investigated for tumorigenicity in animals, but the results are contradictory. CNTs may induce granulomas (microscopic nodules) in lungs and skin, and mesothelioma, the type of cancer produced by exposure to asbestos (Poland et al., 2008). MWCNTs (3500 ppm iron content; diameter 100 nm; approximate length 1–5 μm, 25 weeks) induced mesothelioma in the peritoneal cavity of male p53 (+/−) mice (C57BL/6 background), by intraperitoneal injection (Takagi et al., 2008), but another study reported a negative result in male CD1 mice treated intranasally, intratracheally, orally, or intraperitoneally with MWCNTs (approximately 30–50 nm in diameter and 100–300 mm in length) (Carrero-Sanchez et al., 2006). On the other hand, SWCNT was found to be negative for tumor formation in rats and mice (Warheit et al., 2004).

Carbon black was classified as a possible human carcinogen (Group 2B) in 2010, by the International Agency for Research on Cancer (IARC, 2012). Furthermore, the inhalation of TiO_2 NPs (28 nm) produced lung tumors in female rats (Heinrich et al., 1995), and hydrophilic anatase TiO_2 NPs (200 nm) induced a significant incidence of lung tumors (29.5–63.6%) by intratracheal instillation in female rats (Pott and Roller, 2005). In addition, the tumor incidence of chronically inhaled TiO_2 NPs was found to correlate better with a specific surface area than with a particle mass.

Immunotoxicity

Interactions between NPs and the immune system can produce undesirable immune responses, such as, immunostimulation or immunosuppression, which may promote inflammation, autoimmune disorders, and increase susceptibility to infections and cancer (Zolnik et al., 2010). *In vitro* and in vivo studies have demonstrated that NPs and ultrafine particles activate proinflammatory cytokines, chemokines, and adhesion molecules, which lead to the recruitment of inflammatory cells and disrupt immune defense (Chang, 2010). NPs can be taken up and processed by dendritic cells in the regional lymph nodes; they interact with self-proteins, modify their antigenicities, alter immune responses, and induce autoimmunity (Di Gioacchino et al., 2011). Furthermore, CoCr NPs can elevate cytotoxicity, induce DNA damage and chromosomal aberrations, and possibly stimulate metal hypersensitivity (Gill et al., 2012).

Neurotoxicity

NPs (combustion-derived, manufactured, or engineered) can reach the brain by inhalation and may be associated with neurodegeneration via neuroinflammation, oxidative stress, and alterations of gene expression (Win-Shwe and Fujimaki, 2011). Some NPs cross the blood–brain barrier either by passive diffusion or by carrier-mediated endocytosis (Hoet et al., 2004). Another potential route of entry for NPs may be via the ionic channels (i.e., Na^+, K^+, Ca^{2+}) present in the neuron cell membranes. The inhalation of NPs present in PM or ultrafine PM increases cardiopulmonary morbidity and mortality (Pope et al., 2004) and may increase the inflammatory processes in the brain via MAP kinase signaling pathways and via the translocations of NPs to the central nervous system (Kleinman et al., 2008). In primary rat brain microvessel endothelial cells, silver NPs may interact with the cerebral microvasculature, and induce proinflammatory cascades, inflammation, and neurotoxicity (Trickler et al., 2010).

Endocrine Disruption and Reproductive Toxicity

Several reports demonstrated that NPs disrupt the endocrine system. Prenatal exposure of pregnant F344 rats to NP-rich diesel exhaust (NP-DE) suppressed testicular function in male rats after birth (Li et al., 2009). Furthermore, the relative weights of the seminal vesicles and prostate, to the body weight, were decreased, as were the serum hormones (testosterone, progesterone, corticosterone, and FSH), steroidogenic acute regulatory protein (StAR), and 17beta-hydroxysteroid dehydrogenase mRNA in the testes. NP-DE increased testosterone biosynthesis, StAR, and cytochrome P450 side-chain cleavage (P450scc)-mRNA expressions via growth hormone signaling, which might be the mechanism underlying reproductive toxicity in male rats (Ramdhan et al., 2009). Furthermore, TiO_2 produced reproductive toxicity in zebra fish by reducing the number of zebra fish eggs by 29.5% after 13 weeks of TiO(2) exposure (0.1 mg/L) (Wang et al., 2011).

MECHANISMS OF NANOTOXICITY

NMs exert adverse effects such as mutagenicity and carcinogenicity, and these effects are organ specific (e.g., skin, kidney, brain, lung, endocrine system, and immune system) in vitro and in vivo. Two specific characteristics of NMs are involved: (*i*) Transportation of NMs and the processes of phagocytosis and endocytosis (Beyersmann and Hartwig, 2008; Park et al., 2010) and (*ii*) surface area per unit mass or volume (Oberdörster et al., 2000).

Free Radical Generation

Although the toxic mechanisms of NPs are not clearly understood, it has been proposed that the formation of ROS or free radicals may be associated with nanotoxicity types, including mutagenicity and carcinogenicity (Pacurari et al., 2010). NMs like C_{60} fullerenes, CNTs, TiO_2, and silver NPs have been reported to produce ROS in vitro and in vivo (Shvedova et al., 2003; Oberdörster et al., 2005). Free radicals, such as hydroxyl radicals or superoxide anions generated by NPs can attack biomolecules (e.g., lipids, proteins, DNA), produce oxidative damage products (e.g., MDA, carbonyl contents, 8-OHdG), and deplete antioxidant proteins.

ROS generation by NPs has several possible sources: (*i*) Directly from the surfaces of NPs, (*ii*) the Fenton reaction catalysis associated with metals like Fe and Cu, (*iii*) homeostasis disruption due to effects on respiratory cellular organelles, and mitochondria, and (*iv*) the activations of ROS generating cells, macrophages, and neutrophils (Krug and Wick, 2011).

INFLAMMATION

NPs with a positive charge may induce inflammation, which is one of the critical responses to NP exposure, leading to the induction of cytokines, interleukins (IL-8, IL-6, IL-2), and TNF-α (Nel et al., 2006). ROS generation may also disturb the immune systems in the cells, and the oxidative stress or damage produced by the free radicals can lead to inflammation, mutation, and cancer.

Mitochondrial Perturbation and Cell Cycle Arrest

In Ag-NP-induced cytotoxicity and genotoxicity, perturbation of the mitochondrial respiratory chain led to the production of ROS, interruption of ATP synthesis, and production of DNA damage as suggested by Asharani et al.(2009b). Mitochondrial damage in turn produced cellular membrane damage, opened permeability transition pores, interfered with energy transfer, and led to apoptosis and cytotoxicity.

Furthermore, interactions between Ag-NPs and DNA may result in cell cycle arrest in the G(2)/M phase by PKCζ downregulation (Lee et al., 2011). In another in vitro study, Ag-NP induced apoptosis was found to be possibly mediated by the mitochondria-dependent jun-N terminal kinase pathway and ROS (Hsin et al., 2008).

REFERENCES

Ahamed M, Karns M, Goodson M, et al. (2008). DNA damage response to different surface chemistry of silver nanoparticles in mammalian cells. Toxicol Appl Pharmacol 233, 404–10.

Armstead AL, Li B (2011). Nanomedicine as an emerging approach against intracellular pathogens. Int J Nanomedicine 6, 3281–93.

Asakura, M, Sasaki, T, Sugiyama, T, et al (2010). Genotoxicity and cytotoxicity of multi-wall carbon nanotubes in cultured Chinese hamster lung cells in comparison with chrysotile A fibers. J. Occup. Health 52(3):155–66.

Asharani PV, Hande MP, Valiyaveettil S (2009a). Anti-proliferative activity of silver nanoparticles. BMC Cell Biol 10, 65.

Asharani PV, Low Kah Mun G., Hande MP, et al. (2009b). Cytotoxicity and genotoxicity of silver nanoparticles in human cells. ACS Nano 3, 279–90.

Auffan M, Rose J, Bottero JY, et al. (2009). Towards a definition of inorganic nanoparticles from an environmental, health and safety perspective. Nat Nanotechnol 4, 634–41.

Beyersmann D, Hartwig A (2008). Carcinogenic metal compounds: recent insight into molecular and cellular mechanisms. Arch Toxicol 82, 493–512.

Bourdon JA, Saber AT, Jacobsen NR, et al. (2012). Carbon black nanoparticle instillation induces sustained inflammation and genotoxicity in mouse lung and liver. Part Fibre Toxicol 9:5.

Buffat P, Borel JP (1976). Size effect on the melting temperature of gold particles. Physical Rev A 13, 2287.

Burnett K, Tyshenko MG (2010). A comparison of human capital levels and the future prospect of the nanotechnology industry in early sector investors and recent emerging markets. Intl J Nanotechnol 7, 187–208.

Carrero-Sanchez JC, Elias AL, Mancilla R, et al. (2006). Biocompatibility and toxicological studies of carbon nanotubes doped with nitrogen. Nano Lett 6, 1609–16.

Chang C (2010). The immune effects of naturally occurring and synthetic nanoparticles. J Autoimmun 34, J234–46.

Chen EY, Wang YC, Chen CS, et al. (2010). Functionalized positive nanoparticles reduce mucin swelling and dispersion. PLoS One 5, e15434.

Choi HS, Frangioni JV (2010). Nanoparticles for biomedical imaging: fundamentals of clinical translation. Mol Imaging 9, 291–310.

Di Gioacchino M, Petrarca C, Lazzarin F, et al. (2011). Immunotoxicity of nanoparticles. Int J Immunopathol Pharmacol 24(1 Suppl), 65S–71S.

Donaldson K, Poland CA (2009). Nanotoxicology: new insights into nanotubes. Nature Nanotechnol 4, 708–10.

Gill HS, Grammatopoulos G, Adshead S, et al. (2012). Molecular and immune toxicity of CoCr nanoparticles in MoM hip arthroplasty. Trends Mol Med 18, 145–55.

Heinrich U, Fuhst R, Rittinghausen S, et al. (1995). Chronic inhalation exposure of Wistar rats and two different strains of mice to diesel engine exhaust, carbon black, and titanium dioxide. Inhal Toxicol 7, 533–56.

Helland A, Wick P, Koehler A, et al. (2007). Reviewing the environmental and human health knowledge base of carbon nanotubes. Environ Health Perspect 115, 1125–31.

Hoet PH, Bruske-Hohlfeld I, Salata OV (2004). Nanoparticles—known and unknown health risks. J Nanobiotechnol 2, 12. (doi:10.1186/1477-3155-2-12).

Hsin YH, Chen CF, Huang S, et al. (2008). The apoptotic effect of nanosilver is mediated by a ROS- and JNK-dependent mechanism involving the mitochondrial pathway in NIH3T3 cells. Toxicol Lett 179, 130–9.

Hu SH, Gao X (2010). Nanocomposites with spatially separated functionalities for combined imaging and magnetolytic therapy. J Am Chem Soc 132, 7234–7.

IARC (International Agency for Research on Cancer) (2012). IARC Monographs on the Evaluation of Carcinogenic Risks to Humans. Available from: http://monographs.iarc.fr/.

ISO (International Organization for Standardization) (2008). Nanotechnologies-Terminology and definitions for nanoobjects-Nanoparticle, nanofiber and nanoplate. ISO/TS 27687:2008.

Johnston HJ, Hutchison GR, Christensen FM, et al. (2010). The biological mechanisms and physicochemical characteristics responsible for driving fullerene toxicity. Toxicol Sci 114, 162–82.

Kawata K, Osawa M, Okabe S (2009). In vitro toxicity of silver nanoparticles at noncytotoxic doses to HepG2 human hepatoma cells. Environ Sci Technol 43, 6046–51.

Kleinman MT, Araujo JA, Nel A, et al. (2008). Inhaled ultrafine particulate matter affects CNS inflammatory processes and may act via MAP kinase signaling pathways. Toxicol Lett 178, 127–30.

Krug HF, Wick P (2011). Nanotoxicology: an interdisciplinary challenge. Angew Chem Int Ed Engl 50, 1260–78.

Lee YS, Kim DW, Lee YH, et al. (2011). Silver nanoparticles induce apoptosis and G2/M arrest via PKCζ-dependent signaling in A549 lung cells. Arch Toxicol 85, 1529–40.

Li JJ, Muralikrishnan S, Ng CT, et al. (2010). Nanoparticle-induced pulmonary toxicity. Exp Biol Med (Maywood) 235, 1025–33.

Li C, Taneda S, Taya K, et al. (2009). Effects of in utero exposure to nanoparticle-rich diesel exhaust on testicular function in immature male rats. Toxicol Lett 185, 1–8.

Murray AR, Kisin E, Leonard SS, et al. (2009). Oxidative stress and inflammatory response in dermal toxicity of single-walled carbon nanotubes. Toxicology 257, 161–71.

Nel A, Xia T, Madler L, etal. (2006). Toxic potential of materials at the nanolevel. Science 311, 622–7.

Oberdörster G, Finkelstein JN, Johnston C, et al. (2000). Acute pulmonary effects of ultrafine particles in rats and mice. Res Rep Health Eff Inst 96, 5–74. disc. 75–86.

Oberdörster, G., Oberdörster, E., Oberdörster, J. (2005). Nanotoxicology: an emerging discipline evolving from studies of ultrafine particles. Environ Health Perspect 113, 823–39.

Pacurari, M., Castranova, V., Vallyathan, V. 2010. Single-and multiwalled carbon nanotubes versus asbestos: are the carbon nanotubes a new risk to humans? J. Toxicol. Environ health A 73: 378–95.

Panacek A, Kvítek L, Prucek R, et al. (2006). Silver colloid nanoparticles: synthesis, characterization, and their antibacterial activity. J Phys Chem B 110, 16248–53.

Park EJ, Yi J, Kim Y, et al. (2010). Silver nanoparticles induce cytotoxicity by a trojan-horse type mechanism. Toxicol In Vitro 24, 872–8.

Poland CA, Duffin R, Kinloch I, et al. 2008 Carbon nano-tubes introduced into the abdominal cavity of mice show asbestos-like pathogenicity in a pilot study. Nat Nanotechnol 3, 423–8.

Pope CA, Burnett RT, Thurston GD, et al. (2004). Cardiovascular mortality and long-term exposure to particulate air pollution: epidemiological evidence of general pathophysiological pathways of disease. Circulation 109, 71–7.

Pott F, Roller M (2005). Carcinogenicity study with nineteen granular dusts in rats. Eur J Oncol 10, 249.

Ramdhan DH, Ito Y, Yanagiba Y, et al. (2009). Nanoparticle-rich diesel exhaust may disrupt testosterone biosynthesis and metabolism via growth hormone. Toxicol Lett 191, 103–8.

Sayes CM, Liang F, Hudson JL, et al. (2006). Functionalization density dependence of single-walled carbon nanotubes cytotoxicity in vitro. Toxicol Lett 161, 135–42.

Scenihr (2010). Scientific committee on emerging and newly identified health risks. scientific basis for the definition of the term "nanomaterial". Available from: http://ec.europa.eu/health/scientific_committees/emerging/docs/scenihr_o_032.pdf.

Service RF (2004). Nanotechnology grows up. Science 304, 1732–4.

Shinohara N, Matsumoto K, Endoh S, et al. 2009. In vitro and in vivo genotoxicity tests on fullerene C60 nanoparticles. Toxicol Lett 191, 289–96.

Shvedova, A.A., Castranova, V, Kisin, E.R., et al 2003. Exposure to carbon nanotubes material: assessment of nanotube cytotoxicity using human keratinocyte cells. J. Toxicol. Environ. Health A 66: 1909–26.

Takagi A, Hirose A, Nishimura T, et al (2008). Induction of mesothelioma in p53+/- mouse by intraperitoneal application of multi-wall carbon nanotube. J Toxicol Sci 33, 105–16.

Taylor D A (2002) Dust in the wind Environ Health Perspect 110, A80–7.

Totsuka Y, Higuchi T, Imai T, et al. (2009). Genotoxicity of nano/microparticles in in vitro micronuclei, in vivo comet and mutation assay systems. Part Fibre Toxicol 6, 23.

Trickler WJ, Lantz SM, Murdock RC, et al. (2010). Silver nanoparticle induced blood-brain barrier inflammation and increased permeability in primary rat brain microvessel endothelial cells. Toxicol Sci 118,160–70.

Wang J, Zhu X, Zhang X, et al. (2011). Disruption of zebrafish (Danio rerio) reproduction upon chronic exposure to TiO_2 nanoparticles. Chemosphere 83, 461–7.

Warheit DB, Laurence BR, Reed KL, et al (2004). Comparative pulmonary toxicity assessment of single-wall carbon nanotubes in rats. Toxicol Sci 77, 117–25.

Wiesenthal A, Hunter L, Wang S, et al. (2011). Nanoparticles: small and mighty. Int J Dermatol 50, 247–54.

Win-Shwe TT, Fujimaki H (2011). Nanoparticles and neurotoxicity. Int J Mol Sci 12, 6267–80

Wilson Centre (Woodrow Wilson International Centre for Scholars) (2008). Project on emerging nanotechnologies. consumer products inventory of nanotechnology products. Available from: http://www.nanotechproject.org/inventories/consumer/

Wu J, Liu W, Xue C, et al. 2009. Toxicity and penetration of TiO_2 nanoparticles in hairless mice and porcine skin after subchronic dermal exposure. Toxicol Lett 191, 1–8.

Zhao, J., Castranova, V. 2011. Toxicology of nanomaterials used in medicine. J. Toxicol. Environ. Health B 14: 593–632.

Zolnik BS, González-Fernández A, Sadrieh N, et al. (2010). Nanoparticles and the immune system. Endocrinology 151, 458–65.

23

Toxicity of metals

INTRODUCTION

Metals are a unique class of toxicants. They occur and persist in nature, but their chemical forms may be changed because of physicochemical, biological, or anthropogenic activities. Their toxicity may be drastically altered as they assume different chemical forms. Most of them have some value to humans because of their varied use in industry, agriculture, or medicine. Some are essential elements, required in various biochemical/physiological functions. On the other hand, they may pose health hazards to the public because of their presence in food, water, or air, and to workers engaged in mining, smelting, and a variety of industrial activities.

Occurrence

Most of the metals and "metalloids" occur in nature, dispersed in rocks, ores, soil, water, and air. However, their distribution is grossly uneven. In general, levels of metal sources are relatively low in soil, water, and air. These levels may be increased by geological activities such as degassing, which releases, for example, 25,000 to 125,000 tons of mercury a year. Anthropogenic activities such as mining of mercury contribute about 10,000 tons a year. It must be noted that anthropogenic activities may be more significant in relation to human exposure because they increase the levels of the metals at the site of the human activities.

Uses and Human Exposure

In ancient times, certain metals such as copper, iron, and tin were used to make utensils, machinery, and weapons. Mining and smelting were undertaken to supply such demands. These activities increased their environmental levels. In addition, as the ores often contain other metals, such as lead and arsenic, the levels of these "contaminants" were also increased.

In later years, a greater variety of metals have found uses in industry, agriculture, and medicine. For example, mercury is used extensively in the chloralkali industry as the cathode in the electrolysis of salt in water to produce chlorine and sodium hydroxide, both of which are important raw materials in the chemical industry. Lead is used in storage batteries and the cable industry. However, the use of various lead compounds as insecticides, fuel additives, and pigments in paints has gradually been discontinued.

More recently, the aerospace industry and medicodental profession require materials that have strength, resistance to corrosion, and nonirritant properties. Alloys of titanium and other metals are becoming even more important.

These human activities have increased the extent of exposure not only to occupational workers but also to the consumers of these products. In addition, the toxicity of a metal may be significantly altered by changes in its chemical form. For example, inorganic mercury compounds are toxic primarily to the kidney, whereas methyl mercury is a CNS toxicant.

CERTAIN COMMON FEATURES

Metals have a wide range of toxicity. Some, for example lead and mercury, are very toxic; others are almost nontoxic, such as titanium. They also possess a variety of toxic properties. Nevertheless, there are a number of toxicological features that are shared to some extent by many metals.

Site of Action

Enzyme

A major action of toxic metals is the inhibition of enzymes. This action usually occurs as a result of the interaction between the metal and the SH group of the enzyme. An enzyme may also be inhibited by a toxic metal through displacement of an essential metal cofactor of the enzyme. For example, lead may displace zinc in the zinc-dependent enzyme, δ-aminolevulinic acid dehydratase (ALAD).

Another mechanism by which metals interfere with the functions of enzymes is by inhibiting their synthesis. For example, nickel and platinum inhibit the δ-aminolevulinic acid synthetase (ALAS), thereby interfere with the synthesis of heme, which is an important component of hemoglobin and cytochrome (Maines and Kappas, 1977). The enzymes can be protected from toxic metals by the administration of "chelating agents," such as dimercaprol British anti-lewisite (BAL), that form stable bonds with the metals.

Enzymes differ in their susceptibility to metals. Figure 23.1 depicts the synthesis of heme and the various enzymes involved, most of which may be inhibited by lead. However, they differ in susceptibility. Inhibition of ALAD occurs at a blood lead level (Bl–Pb) of 10 μg/dL or lower. As a result, δ-aminolevulinic acid will not be processed to become porphobilinogen and thus will be spilled over

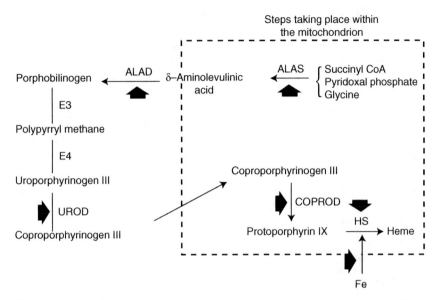

Figure 23.1   A schematic diagram representing the reactions involved in heme synthesis. Large arrows indicate steps that are inhibited by lead. For further explanation, see section on lead. *Abbreviations*: ALAD, δ-aminolevulinic acid dehydratase; ALAS, δ-aminolevulinic acid synthetase; COPROD, coproporphyrinogen oxidase; and HS, heme synthetase; UROD, uroporphyrinogen decarboxylase. *Source*: From Jaworski (1978).

into urine at a Bl–Pb of 40 µg/dL, and anemia will only occur at a Bl–Pb of about 50 µ/dL (WHO, 1977).

Subcellular Organelles

In general, the adverse effects of metals result from reactions between them and intracellular components. For a metal to exert its toxic effect on a cell, it must enter the cell. The entry across the membrane is facilitated if it is lipophilic such as methyl mercury. When it is bound to a protein, it is absorbed by endocytosis. Passive diffusion is another form of entry of metals such as lead.

After their entry into the cell, metals may affect different organelles. For example, the endoplasmic reticulum contains a variety of enzymes. These microsomal enzymes are inhibited by many metals, such as cadmium, cobalt, methyl mercury, and tin. Toxic metals also disrupt the structure of the endoplasmic reticulum. The lysosomes are another site of action of metals such as cadmium (as conjugate of metallothionein). Cadmium is accumulated in the lysosomes of renal proximal tubular cells. In the lysosomes, the cadmium complex degrades and releases cadmium. The cadmium ion inhibits the proteolytic enzymes in the lysosomes and produces cell injury. The mitochondria, because of their high metabolic activity and rapid membrane transport, are also a common target of metals. The respiratory enzymes in these organelles are readily inhibited by metals. A number of metals enter the nucleus and may form inclusion bodies. For example, chronic exposure to lead induces inclusion bodies in the nuclei of renal proximal tubular cells. Lead also stimulates DNA, RNA, and protein synthesis. The lead-induced renal adenocarcinoma has been attributed to this mechanism (Goering et al., 1987).

It is therefore evident that the subcellular organelles either enhance or impede the movement of metals across these biological membranes, thereby affecting their toxicity. In addition, certain proteins in cytosol, lysosomes, and nuclei may bind with toxic metals such as cadmium, lead, and mercury, thereby reducing their availability for adverse effects on sensitive organelles and metabolic sites (Fowler et al., 1984).

Factors Affecting Toxicity

Levels and Duration of Exposure

As with other toxicants, the toxic effects of metals are related to the level and duration of exposure. In general, the higher the levels and the longer the duration, the greater are the toxic effects. However, apart from these quantitative differences, changes in the level and duration of exposure may alter the nature of the toxic effects. For example, ingestion of a single, large dose of cadmium induces gastrointestinal tract (GIT) disturbances. Repeated intakes of smaller amounts of cadmium result in renal dysfunction.

Chemical Form

A notable example is mercury. Its inorganic compounds are essentially renal toxicants, while methyl mercury and ethyl mercury compounds are more toxic to the nervous system. The latter type of mercury compounds is lipophilic and thus they readily cross the blood–brain barrier. Similarly, tetraethyl lead readily enters the myelin sheath and affects the nervous system. Organic compounds of metals are generally excreted in the bile, while their inorganic compounds are excreted in the urine. Furthermore, the former are biodegradable and the latter are not (Furst, 1987).

Metal–Protein Complexes

Perhaps as protective mechanisms, various metal–protein complexes are formed in the body. For example, the complexes formed with lead, bismuth, and mercury–selenium are microscopically visible as "inclusion bodies" in the affected cells. Iron may combine with protein to form ferritin, which is water soluble, or hemosiderin, which is not. Cadmium and several other metals (e.g., zinc) combine with metallo-thionein, a low-molecular-weight protein. The cadmium complex is less toxic than Cd^{2+}. However, in the renal tubule cells, the cadmium–metallothionein is degraded by the cysteine protease in lysosomes to release Cd^{2+} and produces toxic effects (Squibb and Fowler, 1984; Min et al., 1992).

Host Factor

As with most other toxicants, young and old animals are in general more suscep-tible to metals than that of young adults (Luebke et al., 2006a, 2006b). Young children appear to be especially susceptible to lead because of the generally greater sensitivity and the greater extent of GIT absorption. Furthermore, they have, on a unit body weight basis, a greater intake of food, which is the main source of lead.

Dietary factors such as deficiencies of protein and vitamins C and D enhance the toxicity of lead and cadmium. Certain metals such as lead and mercury cross the placenta, thus affecting the fetus. There is evidence that prena-tally exposed children are affected more severely than their mothers: it was found in a study that the median dose that produced ataxia in the mothers was 2.7 ± 0.18 mg/kg, whereas that in the prenatally exposed children was 1.23 ± 0.87 (Clarkson, 1981). It is worth noting that metals such as lead, cadmium, and mer-cury bind to albumin and casein, which are subsequently transported to the breast milk and then transferred to the lactating infant. The consequences of milk metal exposure remains unknown but accounts for higher levels seen in these infants (Berlin et al., 2002; Wang and Needham, 2007). As age is a factor in metal-induced toxicity, the lactational component can be significant especially for mercury and neuronal effects.

Biological Indicators/Biomarkers

Exposure to metals can usually be quantitatively assessed. Some of the indicators reveal the extent and the approximate time of exposure. Others are early signs of biological effects.

The presence and level of the metal in blood and urine are often used as indicators of recent exposure. As the metal compounds are distributed, stored, or excreted, the levels in blood and urine generally diminish.

Many metals are accumulated in hair and nails. Their levels generally bear a relationship with those in blood at the time when the hair and nails are formed. Therefore hair, which grows at a relatively constant rate, has been used to deter-mine the level of exposure at various times in the past. In the case of black-foot disease, the ingestion of arsenic was correlated with the levels of metal in hair and fingernails and thus reflected a useful biomarker of exposure (Lin et al., 1998). For example, this procedure has been used extensively to ascertain the intake of methyl mercury among the inhabitants in the areas where methyl mercury poisoning was reported. Using different approaches, a fairly reliable conversion factor has been established. Thus the level of methyl mercury in hair is about 250-fold higher than that in blood, and their relation to the daily intake, after a steady state is reached, is as follows: $0.2\,\mu g/g$ in blood = $50\,\mu g/g$ in hair = $3\,\mu g/kg$ body weight per day (WHO, 1976).

Such biological indicators are also useful in assessing the average blood level of selenium of inhabitants. In areas where there was selenosis it was $3.2\,mg/L$; where there was selenium deficiency syndrome, it was $0.021\,mg/L$; and in an area where there was neither overexposure nor deficiency, it was $0.095\,mg/L$ (WHO, 1987).

Minimal inhibition of ALAD by lead represents a special type of "indicator of exposure" in that this biological effect does not seem to indicate an adverse effect.

COMMON TOXIC EFFECTS

Carcinogenicity

A number of metals were shown to be carcinogenic in humans or animals or both. As listed in Appendix 1 of chapter 7, arsenic and its compounds, beryllium, cadmium, certain chromium compounds, and nickel and its compounds were categorized as human carcinogens (Group 1) (IARC, 2012). Cisplatin, cobalt metal with tungsten carbide, and lead compounds (inorganic) are probable human carcinogens (Group 2A). Cobalt and cobalt compounds; cobalt metal without tungsten carbide, cobalt sulfate, and other soluble cobalt(II) salts; iron-dextran complex; lead; and nickel (metallic and alloys) are possible human carcinogens (Group 2B). Certain other metals may be carcinogenic, but the available information is insufficient to confirm this suggestion.

The aforementioned metals as well as several others might be carcinogenic through multiple mechanisms of action such as the substitution of Ni^{2+}, Co^{2+}, or Cd^{2+} for Zn^{2+} in finger loops of transforming proteins (Sunderman and Barber, 1988) and injury to cytoskeleton by certain metals (Chou, 1989) that affects the fidelity of the polymerase involved in DNA biosynthesis. The carcinogenicity of arsenic involves oxidative stress and induction of the cascade of heat shock proteins (Bernstam and Nriagu, 2000).

Immune Function

Exposure to certain metals may result in the inhibition of immune functions (Sweet and Zelikoff, 2001). Other metals such as beryllium, chromium, nickel, gold, platinum, lead, tributyltin oxide, and zirconium may induce immunotoxicity including hypersensitivity reactions (Lubeke et al., 2006a). The clinical manifestations and mechanism of action of several metals are listed in Table 23.1.

Table 23.1 Hypersensitivity Reactions to Metals

Metal	Type of Reaction[a]	Clinical Features	Mechanism of Reactions
Platinum, beryllium	I	Asthma, conjunctivitis, urticaria, anaphylaxis	IgE reacts with antigen on mast cell/basophil to release vasoreactive amines
Gold, salts of mercury	II	Thrombocytopenia	IgG binds to complement and antigen on cells, resulting in their destruction
Mercury vapor, gold	III	Glomerular nephritis, proteinuria	Antigen, antibody, and complement deposit on epithelial surface of glomerular basement
Chromium, nickel Beryllium, zirconium	IV	Contact dermatitis Granuloma formation	Sensitized T cells react with antigen to cause delayed hypersensitivity reaction

[a]For descriptions see the section on "Hypersensitivity and Allergy," chapter 11.

Nervous System

Because of its susceptibility, the nervous system is a common target for heavy metals. However, even with the same metal, its physicochemical form often determines the nature of the toxicity. As noted above, metallic mercury vapor and methyl mercury readily enter the nervous system and induce toxic effects. Inorganic mercury compounds are unlikely to enter the nervous system in significant amounts and thus usually are not neurotoxic. Similarly, the organic compounds of lead are mainly neurotoxic, whereas inorganic lead compounds affect the synthesis of heme first. However, at much higher levels of exposure, they may induce encephalopathy. In young children, a moderate level of exposure to these compounds may result in a deficit of mental functions. Other neurotoxic metals include copper, triethyltin, gold, lithium, iron, and manganese. For additional information, see Bondy and Prasad (1988).

Kidney

The kidney, as the main excretory organ in the body, is also a common target organ. Cadmium affects the renal proximal tubular cells, producing urinary excretion of small molecule proteins, amino acids, and glucose. In addition, inorganic mercury compounds, lead, chromium, and platinum also induce kidney damage, mainly in the proximal tubules (see chap. 14).

Respiratory System

The respiratory system is the primary target organ of most metals following occupational exposure. There are several types of responses. Many induce irritation and inflammation of the respiratory tract; the anatomical structures affected depend on the metal and the duration of exposure. With acute exposures, chromium affects the nasal passage, arsenic the bronchi, and beryllium the lungs. Prolonged exposure may produce fibrosis (aluminum and iron), carcinoma (arsenic, chromium, and nickel), or granuloma (beryllium). These effects are included in Appendix 1 of chapter 12 and Table 26.2 of chapter 26. The welding fumes or metalloid aerosol may produce various lung diseases including cancer.

METALS OF MAJOR TOXICOLOGICAL CONCERN

Lead, mercury, arsenic, and cadmium are metals of major health concern because of their impact on large numbers of populations resulting from environmental pollution as well as the serious nature of their adverse effects. Several other metals also pose serious toxicological problems.

Mercury

General Considerations

The elemental form of mercury exists in liquid form. It is released from the earth's crust through degassing. It is also present in the environment as inorganic and organic compounds. Elemental mercury may be converted to inorganic compounds by oxidation and revert to elemental mercury by reduction. Inorganic mercury may become organic mercury through the action of certain anaerobic bacteria, and degrade to inorganic mercury slowly.

A variety of anthropogenic activities may raise its levels in the environment. Some of these activities are mining, smelting (to produce metals from their sulfide ores), burning of fossil fuel, and production of steel, cement, and phosphate. Its principal users include the chlor-alkali plants, paper-pulp industry, and electrical equipment manufacturers. These uses fortunately have decreased in recent years.

The mercury level in the ambient air is extremely low. The level in water in unpolluted areas is about 0.1 μg/L, but it may be as high as 80 μg/L near mercury ore deposits. Its level in food, except fish, is very low, generally in the range of 5 to 20 μg/kg. Most fish contain higher levels; the levels in tuna and swordfish usually range from 200 to 1000 μg/kg.

Toxicity

Because of the massive outbreaks of poisoning from consuming grain treated with mercury fungicide or fish contaminated with methyl mercury (Appendix 2 of chap. 1), extensive investigations were conducted. The populations studied ranged

Table 23.2 Daily Intake of Methyl Mercury by Certain Populations

Population	Daily Intake (g)	
	Average	Range
"Normal"	–	1–20
Fisherman	300	Up to 1000
Niigata	1500	250–5000
Iraq	4500	Up to 12,000

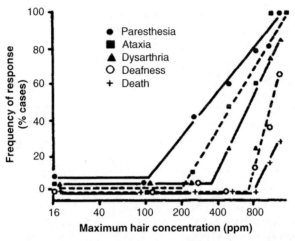

Figure 23.2 The frequency of signs and symptoms of methyl mercury poisoning in adult victims in Iraq plotted according to the estimated maximum hair concentration. Hair samples are not available for all patients and are estimated based on the patient's history of exposure, observed blood levels, blood half-times, and a hair-to-blood concentration ratio of 250 to 1. *Source*: From Clarkson (1987).

from "normal" subjects to those fatally poisoned. Table 23.2 lists some of these population groups. The "fishermen" were exposed to higher-than-normal levels but showed no signs of poisoning. Those involved in the Niigata episode were exposed to smaller intakes than those in the Iraq episode, and hence the latency in Niigata was generally two to three years, whereas in Iraq the latency was two to three months.

These studies revealed that the adverse effects are related to the nervous system, which is extremely sensitive to this toxicant and readily invaded by it. Paresthesia is usually the earliest symptom. Constricted visual field is pathogno-monic. At higher levels of exposure ataxia, dysarthria, deafness, and eventually death occur. Figure 23.2 shows graphically the dose–response and dose–effect relationships. Pathologically, the major damage is atrophy in the occipital lobe, the cerebellar folia, and calcarine cortex. There are also degenerative changes in the axons and myelin sheaths of peripheral nerves.

From these studies it was concluded that methyl mercury poisoning would be unlikely if the daily intake corresponded to a blood level of 20 μg/dL and a hair level of 50 μg/g (WHO, 1976). Other studies have indicated that fetal brain is much more susceptible to methyl mercury than that of adults. This difference is due to the ease of transport across the placenta, the preferential uptake by the fetal brain, and the inhibitory action on cell division and cell migration, both of which are essential for the proper development of fetal brain (Clarkson, 1991).

Elemental mercury *vapor* constitutes a hazard virtually only in occupational settings. Its target organ is also the CNS. The usual symptoms are tremors and mental disturbances. Among workers exposed to mercury vapor the triad of excitability, tremors, and gingivitis have long been observed (Goldwater, 1972). After a continual exposure to a time-weighted air concentration of 0.05 mgHg/m³, sensitive workers may exhibit nonspecific (neurasthenic) symptoms, and at a concentration of 0.1–0.2 mg/m³, they may have tremors (WHO, 1976).

Inorganic mercury *salts* are either monovalent or divalent. The divalent mercuric chloride ($HgCl_2$), the "corrosive sublimate," is corrosive on contact. After ingestion, it causes abdominal cramps and bloody diarrhea, with corrosive ulceration, bleeding, and necrosis of the GIT. These effects are followed by *renal* damage, mainly necrosis and sloughing off of the proximal tubular cells, thereby blocking the tubules and producing oliguria, anuria, and uremia. It may also damage the glomerulus, possibly as a result of disturbed immune function. The monovalent salt calomel, the mercurous chloride (Hg_2Cl_2), is less corrosive and less toxic. However, Hg_2Cl_2 may produce the "pink disease," characterized by *dermal* vasodilation, hyperkeratosis, and hypersecretion of the sweat glands. This effect is probably a hypersensitivity reaction, since it is not dose related. Exposure to mercury results in increased susceptibility to infections as evidenced by immunosuppression, and enhanced allergic responses and autoimmune disease as evidenced by immunostimulation (Sweet and Zelikoff, 2001). Mercury exposure was associated with infertility as evidenced by luteal insufficiency and menstrual irregularities (Gerhard et al., 1998).

Lead

General Considerations

Lead is more ubiquitous than most other toxic metals. The environmental levels have been increasing because of lead mining, smelting, refining, and various industrial uses.

Generally, the lead levels in soil range from 5 to 25 mg/kg, in ground water from 1 to 60 μg/L and somewhat lower in natural surface water, and in air under 1 μg/m³, but may be much higher in certain workplaces and areas with heavy motor traffic.

The major industrial uses, such as fuel additives, and lead pigments in paints, which contributed greatly to the lead levels in the environment, have been gradually phased out. However, its uses in storage batteries and cables have not been significantly reduced. Drinking water may be appreciably contaminated by lead from the use of lead and PVC pipes. Glazed ceramic food-ware is another source of lead, as noted in chapter 20. For most people, the major source of their lead intake is food, which contributes generally 100–300 μg/day.

Infants and young children are likely exposed to a greater extent than adults, because of their habit of licking, chewing, or eating foreign objects, such as soil and flakes of old paints from the wall. As the immune system is immature in children, lead produces greater immunotoxic effects in children (Luebke et al., 2006a, 2006b), which can manifest as higher incidence of infections and asthma. In addition, prenatal exposure to lead could be a risk factor to increase blood pressure in female (Zhang et al., 2011).

Toxicity

The *hematopoietic system* is extremely sensitive to the effect of lead. The main component of hemoglobin is heme, which is synthesized from glycine and succinyl coenzyme A, with pyridoxal phosphate as cofactor. After a number of steps, it finally combines with iron to form heme. The initial and final steps take place in the mitochondria, with the intermediate steps in the cytoplasm, as shown in Figure 23.1. Among the seven enzymes involved in these steps, five are susceptible to the inhibitory effect of lead. ALAD and heme synthetase are the most susceptible, whereas ALAS, uroporphyrinogen decarboxylase, and copro-porphyrinogen oxidase are less sensitive to inhibition by lead. Only two of them are not affected, namely, porphobilinogen deaminase and uroporphyrinogen cosynthetase.

While clinical anemia is evident only when there is moderate exposure to lead, with its level in blood around 50 μg/dL, a number of other effects may be observed at much lower levels of exposure. For example, ALAD inhibition becomes perceptible at a Bl–Pb level just over 10 μg/dL and free erythrocyte porphyrins (FEPs) at 20–25 μg/dL. ALAD inhibition, and possibly FEP, may be considered as an indicator of exposure rather than an indicator of toxicity. The impaired heme synthesis may result in anemia that is hypochromatic and microcytic. The anemia may be due partly to the greater fragility of the erythrocyte membrane (WHO, 1977).

The *nervous system* is also one of the main targets of lead. After high levels of exposure, with a Bl–Pb level over 80 μg/dL, encephalopathy may occur. There are damages to the arterioles and capillaries, resulting in cerebral edema, increased cerebrospinal fluid pressure, neuronal degeneration, and glial proliferation. Clinically this condition is associated with ataxia, stupor, coma, and convulsions. In children, this clinical syndrome may occur with a Bl–Pb level of

70 µg/dL. At further lower levels (40–50 µg/dL), children may exhibit hyperactivity, decreased attention span, and a lowering of IQ scores (Ernhardt et al., 1981; Schnaas et al., 2006). These subtle manifestations may be a result of impairment of the function of neurotransmitters and calcium ion. Peripheral neuropathy is characterized by wrist drop and foot drop, signs of damage to the motor nerves. Lead produces degeneration of Schwann cells followed by demyelination and possibly axonal degeneration. This syndrome occurs mainly among occupational workers.

Lead generally affects the kidney insidiously, resulting in chronic renal failure after long-term exposure. The proximal tubule is the main target. An early sign of lead toxicity on the kidney is the excretion of the lysosomal enzyme N-acetyl-β-d-glucosaminidase (Verschoor et al., 1987). One characteristic of lead poisoning is the presence of lead "inclusion bodies" in the nucleus of tubular cells. These bodies consist of fibrillary lead–protein complexes. In the skeletal system, lead produces osteoporosis and osteomalacia because bone is not only a target organ but a storage depot for lead.

Other Effects

Carcinogenicity of lead has been demonstrated in kidneys of rodents, but there is little human data in this respect (IARC, 1980). Lead also adversely affects *reproductive functions*, mainly through its gametotoxicity in both male and female animals, resulting in low sperm counts, decreased sperm motility, sterility, abortion, and neonatal deaths.

Young children are likely to be exposed to higher levels of lead, as noted above, and their immune system is still immature resulting in higher susceptibility to infections. Furthermore, infants and unborn fetuses are also more sensitive to the toxicity of this metal.

Organic lead compounds such as tetraethyl lead and tetramethyl lead are readily absorbed after inhalation and dermal exposures, and rapidly enter the CNS with ensuing encephalopathy. This hazard concerns essentially occupational workers, but not the general public, because the small amounts emitted from automobile exhaust readily degrade.

Cadmium

General Considerations

Cadmium occurs in nature mainly in lead and zinc ores, and is thus released near the mines and smelters of these metals. Cadmium is used as a pigment (such as in ceramics), in electroplating, and in making alloys and alkali storage batteries. Its level in the air is usually in the range of ng/m^3, but may amount to several mg/m^3 in certain workplaces. The level in water is very low (around 1 µg/L) except in contaminated areas. Most foods contain trace amounts of cadmium. Grains and cereal products usually constitute the main source of cadmium.

Although meat, poultry, and fish have relatively low levels of cadmium, liver, kidneys, and shellfish have much higher levels. The environmental levels are raised by smelting and industrial uses. An additional source is the use of sludge as a food crop fertilizer.

Apart from these environmental sources, humans may be exposed to cadmium through cigarette smoking: a pack a day may double the cadmium intake. Extensively decorated and improperly fired ceramic foodware is another source of cadmium (see chap. 20). Occupational exposure occurs mainly in smelters.

Toxicity

The *acute* effects of cadmium exposure result mainly from local irritation. After ingestion, the clinical manifestations are nausea, vomiting, and abdominal pain; after inhalation, the lesions include pulmonary edema and chemical pneumonitis.

Cadmium is excreted slowly with a half-life of about 15–30 years. After chronic exposure, *kidney* lesions predominate. The primary site of action is the proximal tubules. Damage to these tubules generally occurs when the cadmium level in the kidney reaches $200 \mu g/g$, the "critical concentration." This tubular damage results in their inability to reabsorb small-molecular proteins, the major one of which is β_2-microglobulin. Other proteins include retinol-binding protein, lysozyme, ribonuclease, and immunoglobulin light chains (Lauwerys et al., 1979). Similarly, aminoaciduria is another result of damage to tubular cells that normally reabsorb the amino acids filtered through the glomeruli. Other related effects are glycosuria and decreased tubular reabsorption of phosphate.

At later stages, there may be hypercalcinuria, which, probably in conjunction with altered bone metabolism, may lead to *osteomalacia*. However, the connection between cadmium and *itai-itai* disease, characterized by chronic renal disease and bone deformity, reported in Toyama, Japan where the cadmium level in rice was high (see Appendix 2 of chap. 1), has not been firmly established (Nomiyama, 1980).

Effects on the *respiratory system* result from inhalation exposure. Chronic bronchitis, progressive fibrosis of the lower airway, and rupture of septae between alveoli lead to emphysema.

Other effects include *hypertension*, which may be the result of sodium retention, vasoconstriction, and hyperreninemia. *Carcinoma* of the prostate has been reported among occupational workers (Kipling and Waterhause, 1967). Cadmium inhibits *N*-acetyltransferase 1 and 2 (NAT1, NAT2), phase II-metabolizing enzymes that play an important role in the metabolism of carcinogenic aromatic amines (Joseph, 2009; Ragunathan et al., 2010). Cadmium also binds to a cysteine-rich metalloprotein, metallothionein (MT)-1 or MT-2, which protects cadmium-induced toxicities including nephrotoxicity, immunotoxicity, and osteotoxicity (Klaassen et al., 2009).

Other Metals

Arsenic

Although arsenic is a ubiquitous metalloid, its levels in water and ambient air are generally low. The major source of human exposure is food, which contains somewhat less than l mg/kg. However, its level in seafood may reach 5 mg/kg.

In certain parts of Taiwan, South America, and Bangladesh, the water perhaps contains hundreds of milligrams of arsenic per liter. In these areas, the inhabitants may suffer from dermal hyperkeratosis and hyperpigmentation. A more serious condition is gangrene of lower extremities, the *black foot disease*, resulting from peripheral endarteritis (Lin et al., 1998; Chowdhury et al., 2000).

Cancer of the skin and liver is also observed in those areas, as well as among patients who had been taking Fowler's solution ($KAsO_2$) as a therapy for leukemia (Bernstam and Nriagu, 2000). Cancer of the lung may occur among workers exposed to arsenic in copper smelters and plants that manufacture arsenic-containing pesticide (Pinto et al., 1978; Enterline et al., 1987; Viren and Silvers, 1994). Unlike other human carcinogens, arsenic has not been shown to be carcinogenic to laboratory animals, but was found to produce developmental toxicity as evidenced by malformations, growth retardation, and death (Golub et al., 1998). Furthermore, mutagenesis tests have been essentially negative. The mechanism of arsenic carcinogenesis might be associated with epigenetic changes such as modifications of DNA and histone methylation (Zhou et al., 2008; Marsit et al., 2006).

Other effects include toxicity to *liver* parenchyma, resulting clinically in jaundice in early stages and in cirrhosis and ascites, and carcinoma later. *Acutely*, very large doses of arsenic compounds induce GIT damage with vomiting and bloody diarrhea, muscular cramps, and cardiac abnormality (WHO, 1981). Exposure to excessive amounts of arsenic may interfere with heme formation as evidenced by the increased urinary excretion of porphyrins (Xie et al., 2001).

Beryllium

Beryllium is released into the environment mainly through combustion of fossil fuel and is used in ceramic plants and in making alloys. Beryllium and its alloys have a number of applications in nuclear, space, and other industries.

The major toxic effect is *berylliosis*, resulting from long-term inhalation exposures. This disease of the lungs is characterized by granulomas, which in time become fibrotic tissues. These lesions reduce the number of alveoli and consequently pulmonary functions.

After dermal contact, beryllium produces *hypersensitivity reactions* of the skin. The reaction is cell mediated, and therefore delayed (type IV allergy). The soluble compounds of Be induce papulovesicular lesions, whereas the insoluble compounds induce granulomatous lesions.

Beryllium was shown to be carcinogenic to several species of animals (Kuschner, 1981). Epidemiological data suggest that Be is a human carcinogen (IARC, 1994).

Chromium

Chromium occurs in ores. Mining, smelting, and industrial uses tend to increase its environmental levels. It is used in making stainless steel, various alloys, and pigments. Fossil fuel–powered plants and cement-producing plants are also sources of environmental pollution. However, its levels in air, water, and food are generally very low. The major human exposure is occupational.

Chromium is a human carcinogen, inducing lung cancers among workers exposed to it. The carcinogenicity is generally attributed to the hexavalent Cr^{6+}, which is corrosive and water insoluble. It has been suggested that Cr^{6+}, which is more readily taken up by cells, converts to Cr^{3+} intracellularly. The trivalent chromium ion, which is more active biologically, binds to nucleic acid and initiates the carcinogenesis process. The mechanisms of Cr^{6+} carcinogenicity are associated with both genotoxic (e.g., Cr-DNA-adducts, crosslinks, strand breaks via oxidative stress) (Zhitkovich, 2005)(Jomova and Valko, 2011) and epigenetic events (e.g., histone modification) (Sun et al., 2009). It should be noted that there is no clear evidence to correlate occupational chromium exposure with increased incidence of cancer in the United Kingdom (Rowbotham et al., 2000). It is worth noting that chromium is present in cigarettes and it was postulated that the rise in cancer incidence in chromium workers was due to the smoking component. The Cr^{6+} is corrosive and produces *ulceration* of the nasal passages and skin. It also induces *hypersensitivity reactions* of the skin. Acutely, it induces *renal* tubular necrosis.

Nickel

Nickel occurs in ores. Smelting and industrial uses tend to increase its levels in the environment. Its many industrial uses include in the manufacture of storage batteries, electrical contacts and similar devices; electroplating, and as catalysts. It is also emitted from coal gasification.

Nickel is a human carcinogen among occupational workers. Nasal cancer appears to be the predominant type of neoplasm. Nickel also induces cancer of the lungs, larynx, stomach, and possibly also the kidney.

It is one of the most common causative agents of dermal hypersensitivity reactions among the general public. The reactions usually follow contact with nickel-containing metal objects such as coins and jewelry.

RISK/BENEFIT CONSIDERATIONS

The metals discussed in the previous section offer certain benefits because of their industrial and minor medical uses. However, they pose serious toxicological risks either to the population at large or specific occupational workers. On the other hand, there are two groups of metals that are more valuable. One group, the essential metals, is required in certain physiological functions and the other is used for a variety of medical purposes. These three groups of metals are different in their risk/benefit considerations.

Toxic Metals

The general population is at risk to these metals mainly through *food*. Tolerances, or equivalents, are established for various food stuffs to ensure that the total intake will not exceed the amount that is considered acceptable from a toxicological point of view.

However, more targeted action is taken in certain cases. For example, the main source of methyl mercury is fish. The levels in swordfish range from about 0.5 to 1.2 ppm, and in tuna from 0.2 to 0.5 ppm, whereas those in most other kinds of fish are 0.1 ppm or lower. The permissible levels for methyl mercury set by most nations range from 0.4 to 1 ppm. Assuming a daily consumption of fish being 200 g, the intake of methyl mercury would not exceed 0.2 mg. An intake at this level is considered unlikely to induce methyl mercury toxicity (WHO, 1976). The safety is provided by the fact that most of the fish samples contain much less methyl mercury than the 1 ppm permitted. The Joint FAO/WHO Expert Committee on Food Additives and Contaminants established a "tolerable intake" of 0.2 mg/week, thus allowing a safety factor of 7, which the Committee considered adequate in this case (WHO, 1972). The rationale was the availability of the exceptionally extensive data obtained from populations exposed to the full gamut of intake levels, ranging from "normal" to questionably poisoned, minimally poisoned, seriously poisoned, and fatally poisoned (Table 23.2), as well as the fact that most of the investigations were thoroughly conducted and properly reported. Second, fish is considered as an important source of nutrients, which should not be discarded for minimal or nonexistent risks. The intake was set on a weekly basis because fish is consumed, in many parts of the world, once a week.

Similarly, targeted action has been taken with respect to cadmium in rice in Japan, where rice is the main source of this contaminant. Permissible levels of release of lead and cadmium from ceramic foodware have been established internationally (WHO, 1979) and in many nations. See also chapter 20.

There are also tolerances for toxic metals such as arsenic, cadmium, and lead in water and foods for the protection of the health of consumers.

Occupational workers are likely exposed to higher levels of toxic metals in mining, smelting, manufacturing, and similar occupations. The main routes of entry into the body are the skin and respiratory tract. For their protection, threshold limit values of toxicants in air are established. For additional information, see chapter 25.

Essential Metals

Selenium is a typical element that is toxic at high levels of intake and induces a deficiency syndrome when the intake is too low.

Human *overexposure* to selenium has been observed in China as well as in few isolated regions in the Americas. The clinical manifestations include hair loss, nail pathology, and tooth decay. In animals overexposure induces more severe ill effects including retarded growth, liver necrosis, enlargement of spleen and pancreas, anemia, and various disorders of reproductive function.

Deficiency of selenium results in muscular dystrophy in sheep and cattle, exudative diathesis in chicken, and liver necrosis in swine and rats. In rats it may also produce reproductive failures, vascular changes, and cataracts. Selenium is a component of glutathione peroxidase, which is responsible for the destruction of H_2O_2 and lipid peroxides. Its function is, therefore, closely related to that of vitamin E, the biological antioxidant. This close relation is reflected in the fact that the minimal intake of selenium in rats is 0.01 mg/kg, but if there is also a vitamin E deficiency, an intake of 0.05 mg/kg will be needed.

It was only in the late 1970s that selenium was recognized as an essential element in humans. In certain regions in China, where the selenium levels were low in soil and food, a special type of *cardiomyopathy* was noted. It was known as Keshan disease because it was first observed there. The selenium levels in the blood, urine, and hair of the inhabitants were low. As expected, the blood glutathione peroxidase activity was also low. When they were given a sodium selenite supplement, the incidence of this endemic cardiopathy dropped sharply. There is also an endemic *osteoarthropathy* observed in China. It is known as Kashin–Beck disease, and is believed to be due to selenium deficiency; however, the evidence of its etiology is not as strong as that of Keshan disease. Selenium deficiency associated with muscular pain has been reported from New Zealand.

For the general population, selenium exposure is essentially from food, especially cereals. The average daily intake of selenium of inhabitants in areas where there were cases of Keshan disease was about 0.011 mg, whereas in areas where there were cases of selenosis, it was about 5 mg (Yang et al., 1983). It has been estimated that there is about a 100-fold margin between the highest no-toxic-effect level and the lowest level at which deficiency syndrome is avoided. However, this margin is subject to the influence of various modifying factors. For example, vitamin E deficiency increases the toxicity as well as the physiological requirements of selenium, thus effectively reducing the margin. Methyl mercury increases the effect of selenium deficiency, whereas inorganic mercury increases the toxicity of methylated selenium compounds. A hypothetical dose–response (all effects) relationship of selenium is depicted in Figure 4.1 of chapter 4, which shows that ill effects are induced when the dose is too low (curve A), whereas other ill effects are induced when the dose is too high (curve B). Furthermore, because of the great individual variations in susceptibility resulting from host and environmental factors, it is not clear whether there is a dose that can be considered as devoid of deficiency as well as toxic effect on a population basis. Additional details on various aspects of the selenium problem and reference citations may be found in a WHO document (WHO, 1987).

Cobalt, copper, and *iron* are all essential metal elements required in the proper development of erythrocytes. Iron is a component of hemoglobin, and copper facilitates the utilization of iron in the synthesis of hemoglobin. Thus deficiency of either metal results in hypochromatic, microcytic anemia. Cobalt is a component of vitamin B_{12}, which is required in the development of erythrocyte. Its deficiency results in pernicious anemia.

Excessive intake of cobalt results in polycythemia, an overproduction of erythrocytes, and cardiomyopathy. The heart lesion was observed under special conditions, as discussed in chapter 27. Excess copper storage in the body is not a result of overexposure to copper but rather a genetic disorder (Wilson's disease). Copper is accumulated in brain, liver, kidney, and cornea. Clinical manifestations are thus related to disorders of these organs. Overexposure to iron may result from excessive intake of iron or frequent blood transfusion. The excess iron is deposited as hemosiderin mainly in liver, causing liver dysfunction. Iron binds to ambient air particles and is postulated to be responsible for cardiovascular disturbances and increased morbidity associated with air pollutant exposure. In addition, iron binds to asbestos bodies and is believed to be associated with the observed asbestosis in humans.

Occupational exposure to cobalt induces respiratory irritation and dermal hypersensitivity reactions. Certain iron industry workers have been reported as having pneumoconiosis and increased lung cancer incidence associated with iron binding to particles and subsequent release. Acute oral poisonings have been reported after consuming improperly canned vegetable juices containing excessive amounts of copper and after taking large doses of iron supplement medications. The clinical manifestations relate mainly to GIT irritation.

Other essential metals include manganese and molybdenum, which are cofactors in a number of enzyme systems such as phosphorylase, xanthine oxidase, and aldehyde oxidase. However, these metals are so plentiful in the human diet that no cases of deficiency syndrome have been reported. These metals have a variety of industrial uses, notably in making high-temperature-resistant steel alloys. Occupational exposure to manganese results in pneumonitis acutely, and encephalopathy chronically. Overexposure to manganese in animals orally induces GIT disturbances followed by fatty degeneration of liver and kidney.

Zinc is the cofactor in scores of metalloenzymes and is therefore an essential element. Deficiency of zinc thus induces a great variety of effects on the nervous system, hematopoietic system, skin, liver, eye, testis, etc. Zinc is readily excreted, and excessive intake by the oral route is thus unlikely to induce toxic effects. Occupational exposure to Zn_2O_3 fume leads to "metal fume fever" (Goyer, 1996).

Metals Used in Medicine

Therapeutic Agents

A number of metal compounds have been used in medicine. For example, compounds of mercury have been used as diuretics and vaccines. Because of their toxicity, their uses have been discontinued. Those that are less toxic include compounds of aluminum as antacid, bismuth as astringent, gold for rheumatoid arthritis, lithium for mental depression, platinum complexes as antitumor agents, and thallium as depilatory. They may produce toxic effects on the nervous system (e.g., aluminum, bismuth, lithium, and thallium), kidneys (e.g., bismuth, gold, and lithium), skin (e.g., gold and platinum), and cardiovascular, and GI systems (e.g., lithium and thallium). Although used as antitumor agents, platinum complexes may induce tumors.

Other Uses

Aluminum in hemodialysis for chronic renal failure has resulted in fatal neurological syndrome. The use of barium and gallium, in conjunction with X-ray, as a radiopaque agent and radioactive tracer has proved to be relatively safe. However, accidental ingestion of soluble Ba salts has resulted in serious GIT, muscular, and cardiovascular disturbances. Therapeutic use of radiogallium has resulted in disease conditions related to radioactivity. Of special interest is titanium. It is inert and resistant to corrosion and thus has been used widely in surgical and dental implants. It is present in trace amounts in a variety of foods of plant origin, and titanium dioxide has been used as a color additive because of its low toxicity.

REFERENCES

Berlin CM, Kacew S, Lawrence R, et al. (2002). Criteria for chemical selection for programs on human milk surveillance and research for environmental chemicals. J Toxicol Environ Health A 65, 1839–51.

Bernstam L, Nriagu J (2000). Molecular aspects of arsenic stress. J Toxicol Environ Health B 3, 293–322.

Bondy SC, Prasad KN (1988). Metal Neurotoxicity. Boca Raton, FL: CRC Press.

Chou IN (1989). Distinct cytoskeletal injuries induced by As, Cd, Co, Cr, and Ni compounds. Biomed Environ Sci 2, 358–65.

Chowdhury UK, Biswas BK, Chowdhury RT (2000). Groundwater arsenic contamination in Bangladesh and West Bengal. Environ Health Perspect 108, 393–7.

Clarkson TW (1981). Dose–response relationships for adult and prenatal exposures to methyl mercury. In: Bery GG, Maillie HD, eds. Measurements of Risk. New York, NY: Plenum Press, 111–30.

Clarkson TW (1987). Metal toxicity in the central nervous system. Environ Health Perspect 75, 59–64.

Clarkson TW (1991). Methyl mercury. Fundam Appl Toxicol 16, 20–1.

Enterline PE, Henderson VL, Marsh GM (1987). Exposure to arsenic and respiratory cancer: a reanalysis. Am J Epidemiol 125, 929–38.

Ernhardt CB, Landa B, Schnell NB (1981). Subclinical levels of lead and developmental deficits: a multivariate follow-up reassessment. Pediatrics 67, 911–19.

Fowler BA, Abel J, Elinder CG (1984). Structure, mechanism and toxicity. In: Nriagu J, ed. Changing Metal Cycles and Human Health. New York, NY: Springer-Verlag.

Furst A (1987). Relationships of toxicological effects to chemical forms of inorganic compounds. In: Brown SS, Kodama Y, eds. Toxicology of Metals. Chichester, UK: Halstead Press.

Gerhard I, Monga B, Waldbrenner A, et al. (1998). Heavy metals and infertility. J Toxicol Environ Health A 54, 593–611.

Goering PL, Mistry P, Fowler BA (1987). Mechanism of metal toxicity. In: Haley TJ, Berndt WO, eds. Handbook of Toxicology. New York, NY: Hemisphere.

Goldwater LJ (1972). Mercury: A History of Quicksilver. Baltimore, MD: York Press.

Golub MS, Macintosh MS, Baumrind N (1998). Developmental and reproductive toxicity of inorganic arsenic: animal studies and human concerns. J Toxicol Environ Health B 1, 199–241.

Goyer RA (1996). Toxic effects of metals. In: Klaassen CD, ed. Casarett and Doull's Toxicology. New York, NY: McGraw-Hill, 691–736.

IARC (1980). Monograph on the Evaluation of the Carcinogenic Risks of Chemicals to Humans. Some Metals and Metallic Compounds, vol. 23. Lyon, France: International Agency for Research on Cancer.

IARC (1994). Monograph on the Evaluation of Risks to Humans. Cadmium, Mercury, Benyllium and the Glass Industry, vol. 58. Lyons, France: International Agency for Research on Cancer.

IARC (2012). Monograph on the Evaluation of the Carcinogenic Risks of Chemicals to Humans. Agents Classified by the IARC Monographs, Volumes 1–102. Lyon, France: International Agency for Research on Cancer.

Jaworski JK (1978). The Effects of Lead in the Canadian Environment. Ottawa, Canada: National Research Council Canada.

Jomova K, Valko M (2011). Advances in metal-induced oxidative stress and human disease. Toxicology 283, 65–87.

Joseph P (2009.) Mechanisms of cadmium carcinogenesis. Toxicol Appl Pharmacol 238, 272–9.

Kipling M, Waterhause J (1967). Cadmium and prostatic carcinoma. Lancet 1, 730–1.

Klaassen CD, Jie L, Bhalchandra DA (2009). Metallothionein protection of cadmium toxicity. Toxicol Appl Pharmacol 238, 215–20.

Kuschner M (1981). The carcinogenicity of beryllium. Environ Health Perspect 40, 101–6.

Lauwerys RR, Roels HA, Poncket JP, et al. (1979). Investigations on the lung and kidney function in workers exposed to cadmium. Environ Health Perspect 28, 137–46.

Lin T-H, Huang Y-L, Wang M-Y (1998). Arsenic species in drinking water, hair fingernails and urine of patients with blackfoot disease. J Toxicol Environ Health A 53, 85–93.

Luebke RW, Chen DH, Dietert R, et al. (2006a). The comparative immunotoxicity of five selected compounds following developmental or adult exposure. J Toxicol Environ Health B 9, 1–26.

Luebke RW, Chen DH, Dietert R, et al. (2006b). Immune system maturity and sensitivity to chemical exposure. J Toxicol Environ Health A 69, 811–25.

Maines MD, Kappas A (1977). Metals as regulators of heme metabolism. Science 198, 1215–21.

Marsit C, Karagas M, Danaee H, et al. (2006). Carcinogen exposure and gene promoter hypermethylation in bladder cancer. Carcinogenesis 27, 112–16.

Min KS, Nakatsubo T, Fujita Y, et al. (1992). Degradation of cadmium metallothionein in vitro by lysosomal proteases. Toxicol Appl Pharmacol 113, 299–305.

Nomiyama K (1980). Recent progress and perspectives in cadmium health effects studies. Sci Total Environ 14, 199–232.

Pinto SS, Henderson V, Enterline PE (1978). Mortality experience of arsenic exposed workers. Arch Environ Health 33, 325–31.

Ragunathan N, Dairou J, Sanfins E, et al. (2010). Cadmium alters the biotransformation of carcinogenic aromatic amines by arylamine N-acetyltransferase xenobiotic-metabolizing enzymes: molecular, cellular, and in vivo studies. Environ Health Perspect. 118, 1685–91

Rowbotham AL, Levy LS, Shuker LK (2000). Chromium in the environment: an evaluation of exposure of the UK general population and possible adverse health effects. J Toxicol Environ Health B 3, 145–78.

Schnaas L, Rothenberg SJ, Flores MF, et al. (2006). Reduced intellectual development in children with prenatal lead exposure. Environ Health Perspect. 114, 791–7.

Squibb KS, Fowler BA (1984). Intracellular metabolism of circulating cadmium–metallothionein in the kidney. Environ Health Perspect 54, 31–5.

Sun H, Zhou X, Chen H, et al. (2009). Modulation of histone methylation and MLH1 gene silencing by hexavalent chromium. Toxicol Appl Pharmacol 237, 258–66.

Sunderman FW Jr, Barber AM (1988). Fingerloops, oncogenes and metals. Ann Clin Lab Sci 18, 267–88.

Sweet LI, Zelikoff JT (2001). Toxicology and immunotoxicology of mercury: a comparative review in fish and humans. J Toxicol Environ Health B 4, 161–205.

Verschoor M, Wibowo A, Herber R, et al. (1987). Influence of occupational low-level lead exposure on renal parameters. Am J Ind Med 12, 341–51.

Viren JR, Silvers A (1994). Unit risk estimates for airborne arsenic exposure: an updated view based on recent data from two copper smelter cohorts. Reg Toxicol Pharmacol 20, 125–38.

Wang RY, Needham LL (2007). Environmental chemicals: from the environment to food, to breast to the infant. J Toxicol Environ Health B 10, 597–609.

WHO (1972). Evaluation of Certain Food Additives and the Contaminants Mercury, Lead and Cadmium. Tech Rep Ser 505. Geneva, Switzerland: World Health Organization.

WHO (1976). Mercury. Environmental Health Criteria 1. Geneva, Swirzerland: World Health Organization.

WHO (1977). Lead. Environmental Health Criteria 3. Geneva, Switzerland: World Health Organization.

WHO (1979). Ceramic Foodware Safety. Document HCS/79.7. Geneva, Switzerland: World Health Organization.

WHO (1981). Arsenic. Environmental Health Criteria 18. Geneva, Switzerland: World Health Organization.

WHO (1987). Selenium. Environmental Health Criteria 58. Geneva, Switzerland: World Health Organization.

Xie Y, Kondo M, Koga H, et al. (2001). Urinary porphyrins in patients with endemic chronic arsenic poisoning caused by burning coal in China. Environ Health Prevent Med 5, 180–5.

Yang G, Wang S, Zhou R, et al. (1983). Endemic selenium intoxication of humans in China. Am J Clin Nutr 37, 872–81.

Zhang A, Hu H, Sánchez BN, et al. (2011). Association between prenatal lead exposure and blood pressure in female offspring. Environ Health Perspect 120, 445–50.

Zhitkovich A. (2005). Importance of chromium-DNA adducts in mutagenicity and toxicity of chromium (VI). Chem Res Toxicol 18, 3–11.

Zhou X, Sun H, Ellen T, et al. (2008). Arsenite alters global histone H3 methylation. Carcinogenesis 29, 1831–6.

24

Over-the-counter preparations

GENERAL REMARKS

Pharmaceutical agents required by law to be prescribed to patients are called prescription drugs. However, over the years there have been an escalating number of products available to treat various ailments for which a written prescription is not necessary. This latter group of compounds is termed over-the-counter (OTC) drugs. The OTC drugs are believed to be relatively safe and effective in the view of the general public simply because the regulatory agencies allow these drugs to be sold without medical advice. It is the popular belief that if a drug needs to be prescribed then it must be regulated, as there are inherent adverse effects. However, the public does not know that many of these OTC products have not undergone extensive clinical testing and may not be safe. Although it may be laudable to treat serious illnesses and make available the compounds that are prescribed and required for these purposes, one must question the trend toward easy access of an uneducated public to more OTC drugs that are self-administered and have not undergone proper testing.

It is safe to assume with respect to OTC drugs that the public

(i) is generally overwhelmed and confused by the wide array of products available;
(ii) will probably use those that are most heavily advertised;
(iii) will use these drugs inadvertently and inappropriately in some cases; and
(iv) may be subjected to adverse effects (Kacew, 1999).

A paradox exists with respect to public awareness and drug use. De Jongvan den Berg et al. (1992, 1993) found that increased awareness of adverse drug effects led to a decrease in the use of prescription drugs during pregnancy. However, because of the perception that OTC drugs are safe, there was a disproportionate rise in the quantity of OTC medications such as laxatives and vitamins, which were self-administered. From an epidemiological point of view, the population most at risk for adverse effects from OTC drugs is children, resulting from the absence of safety caps, attractive packages, administration of overdoses by parents, etc. It is worthwhile to note that Kacew (1992, 1997) clearly demonstrated that pharmacokinetics and pharmacodynamics are different between children and adults, which consequently this difference was associated with differences in responsiveness to drugs. Thus, prediction of therapeutic effectiveness based on adult data can lead to grave consequences in children (Kogan et al., 1994; Smith and Kogan, 1997).

PREVALENCE IN SOCIETY

In 1989, the American public spent approximately $10 billion on an estimated 300,000 OTC products to medicate themselves for self-diagnosed ailments ranging from acne to warts, colds, headaches, upset stomach, constipation, etc. (Koda-Kimble, 1992). These 300,000 products represent about 700 active ingredients in various forms and combinations. It is thus apparent that many are no more than "me too" products advertised to the public in ways that suggest that there are significant differences between them. Almost $2 billion per year is spent by the American public on cough and cold remedies (Rosendahl, 1998). There are more than 800 OTC preparations for the common cold (Lowenstein and Parrino, 1987), over 100 for treatment of diarrhea (Dukes, 1990), over 200 different systemic analgesic products, almost all of which contain aspirin (acetylsalicylic acid, ASA), paracetamol (acetaminophen, APAP), salicylamide, phenacetin, ibuprofen, or a combination of these agents as primary ingredients (Leist and Banwell, 1974). OTC drugs can be made different from one another in the following ways:

(i)   addition of questionable ingredients such as caffeine or antihistamines;
(ii) creation of an identity by brand names chosen to suggest a specific use of strength ("feminine pain," "arthritis," "maximum," "extra"); or
(iii) indication of their special dosage form (enteric-coated tablets, liquids, sustained-release products, powder, seltzers etc.).

Hence, the consumer could utilize a product without the realization that an analgesic agent was being ingested (Kacew, 1994).

OTC preparations also contain excipients and/or inactive ingredients such as dyes, sweeteners, flavorings, or preservatives. The so-called "hidden ingredients" in OTC products may on their own initiate adverse effects or potentiate the actions of the active components (Golightly et al., 1998; Kumar et al., 1993).The findings that excipients cause adverse effects, including skin disorders, gastrointestinal upset, and cardiovascular abnormalities, clearly indicate that OTC drugs should not be used merely due to the improper perception of safety from adverse effects.

The enormity and severity of OTC drug usage in our society have received little, if any, attention. In addition to the economics, it has been estimated that 70% of illnesses, predominantly in the adult population, are treated with OTC agents (Knapp and Knapp, 1972; Conn, 1991; Chrischelles et al., 1992). However, of greater concern is the fact that 48–63% of children, a population known to be far more susceptible to drug-induced adverse effects (Lock and Kacew, 1988; Kacew, 1997) received OTC drugs during a two-week period (Dunnell and Cartwright, 1972; Kovar, 1994) and that approximately 40% of these children received at least two preparations (Kogan et al., 1994; Smith and Kogan, 1997). Due to serious adverse events and infant deaths associated with OTC cough and cold remedies, there are suggestions that the OTC drugs should not be given to infants and very young children (Vassilev et al., 2010; Rimsza and Newberry, 2008).

It is worthwhile noting that during pregnancy, both mother and fetus are equally exposed to a chemical, but the risk of fetal toxicity far exceeds that of the mother or neonate (Kacew, 1997, 1999). Hence, the presumption of safety for the mother cannot be applied with certainty to the fetus. The hair cream Le Kair contains estrogens (Koda-Kimble, 1992) and presumably, if used appropriately does not produce toxicity. However, there have been reports that the use of estrogenic cosmetics resulted in gynecomastia in the child (Kacew, 1999). Although a correlation between estrogenic OTC products and fetal toxicity has not been examined, it is known that estrogens are teratogenic (Lock and Kacew, 1988; Safe, 1998). It should be noted that various foods are estrogenic (Safe, 1998) and thus the combination of certain foods and OTC products may potentially affect fetal development. This latter scenario is further compounded, as there are numerous environmental estrogenic contaminants to which a pregnant mother is inadvertently exposed on a daily basis (Shore et al., 1993). Since estrogens are lipophilic and accumulate in tissue fat, the potential for fetal exposure to excess estrogens is dependent on diet and environment. These compounds can certainly convert a relatively safe OTC into a toxic agent.

ADVERSE CONSEQUENCES

As a general rule, all drugs, including OTC preparations, should be avoided whenever possible. High-risk subpopulations have been identified, including children and geriatrics. Of even greater risk is the use of OTC in pregnancy where the fetus is the target (Hays and Pagliaro, 1987; Karboski, 1992). Although it is falsely perceived that OTC preparations are virtually without any adverse fetal consequences, the reverse may be the case. Palatnick and Tenenbein (1998) recently reported a case of fetal death in a 17-year-old, 37-week-pregnant girl who had ingested aspirin daily for one month. Autopsy of the fetus revealed petechiae of lungs, heart, thymus, and kidneys. Clearly, the amount of aspirin taken was excessive but the drug was also readily available. Aspirin is not contraindicated for the treatment of headaches during pregnancy (Underhill, 1994), but it is stressed that aspirin and other nonsteroidal anti-inflammatory products should be avoided during the third trimester (Bonati et al., 1990; Koren et al., 1998). It is of interest that ingestion of aspirin during the first 20 weeks of gestation does not significantly affect IQ at four years of age (Klebanoff and Berendes, 1988). These confusing messages are relayed to the public with the recommendation that even though aspirin can be taken safely during pregnancy, paracetamol has been recommended as the drug of choice. However, due to the increased use of paracetamol (APAP), poisoning cases with APAP exceeded those of other nonsteroidal anti-inflammatory drugs and APAP toxicity was recorded as the single most common cause of liver failure in the United States and United Kingdom, and associated with nearly 500 results in fatality per year (Davern et al., 2006).

Under pressure from the pharmaceutical industry, a number of prescribed drugs have been switched to OTC status (Fletcher et al., 1995). Although the effects of the antidiarrheal agent loperamide on fetal outcome have not been established, administration of this drug to infants produced paralytic ileus and persistent drowsiness in 20% of the cases (Motala et al., 1990). The recent inclusion of the antiulcerogenic histamine blocker, cimetidine, in the OTC list is a further example of a drug with potential effects on the fetus and easy public accessibility. The finding that cimetidine concentrations in neonatal plasma exceeded those in the mother's suggested that there was a substantial uptake by the fetus (Somogi and Gugler, 1983). The fact that cimetidine is known to inhibit hepatic microsomal enzymes and was reported to produce fetal liver toxicity when used in late pregnancy (Glode et al., 1980) indicates that self-administration of this drug for reflux esophagitis during pregnancy could have adverse consequences. This could be of particular concern if a pregnant epileptic mother with impaired liver function were to ingest cimetidine; plasma concentrations of anticonvulsants would be increased, with adverse consequences for the fetus. In patients who are taking tricyclic antidepressants for depression, cimetidine potentiates the actions of the antidepressant resulting in cardiovascular abnormalities, hallucinations, vomiting, and hypotension. In the elderly, cimetidine causes confusion, which could have dire consequences, as this population tends to be more forgetful.

A number of current OTC products are associated with adverse consequences. Industry has applied pressure to make certain drugs more accessible and, because of a presumed history of safety and the public perception that self-administered therapies will hasten recovery, even more compounds will be transferred from prescription to nonprescription status (Splinter et al., 1997). Consequently, a larger assortment of OTC drugs will be available to the pregnant mother and geriatric populations. Indeed, Rubin et al. (1993) reported that OTC preparations were used 1.5-fold more often than prescription drugs during pregnancy; this figure is presumably underestimated because they failed to include vitamins in their study. It is disturbing to note that approximately 50% of products taken during pregnancy are OTC medications (Rayburn et al., 1982). With aging, there is also an increased use of drugs.

Clearly, some pregnant women are self-medicating themselves during a period of fetal vulnerability. Although it is stressed that pregnant women should not drink or smoke, these activities still occur during pregnancy. Indeed, the maternal characteristics associated with increased OTC medication use were Caucasians, smoking more than 20 cigarettes per day, and drinking alcohol (Buitendijk and Bracken, 1991). Hence, it is likely that despite warnings, pregnant women will use OTC medications, the choice of which is expanding. An example of this problem arises with the use of imidazolines as topical vasoconstrictors for nasal decongestion. These compounds are used for sinusitis, colds, and allergic rhinitis, and are known to produce CNS depression, bradycardia, hypotension, and miosis (Liebelt and Shannon, 1993). There is a lack of clinical data regarding the use of these compounds in high-risk subpopulations, yet the potential for adverse effects is quite serious as these drugs produce vasoconstriction.

The misconception that frequent bowel movements are essential has resulted in the misuse of cathartics amongst some women, especially the geriatric populations. Saline cathartic magnesium sulfate induces hypotonia, CNS, and respiratory depression. Bulk-forming laxatives can produce cramping and nausea, and result in fluid loss and electrolyte imbalance. In patients with congestive heart failure, this type of OTC product is contraindicated.

Ingestion of a proper diet is sufficient to provide the necessary requirement for vitamins and iron. However, the erroneous belief that vitamin supplements provide extra energy and create a feeling of "well-being" has resulted in the ingestion of quantities of vitamins vastly in excess of the recommended dietary allowance. This widespread nutritional self-medication promoted through effective massive advertising can have dire consequences in susceptible populations. Vitamin A in the fetus is associated with spontaneous abortion, hydrocephalus, and cardiac anomalies, while in the adult there are menstrual irregularities, exophthalmos, and skin hyperpigmentation. With vitamin D, hypercalcemia occurs in the adult and is manifested as anorexia, fatigue, kidney dysfunction, and aortic stenosis. In the fetus, hypervitaminosis D results in elfin facies, mental retardation, and aortic stenosis. Liver dysfunction, jaundice, and hemorrhage occur as a result of excessive vitamin K intake. Excessive iron intake results in vomiting, cyanosis, and circulatory collapse. In the fetus, there are congenital anomalies and GIT upset. This reiterates the fact that essential nutritional OTC in excess is not safe. The use of OTC mixtures of vitamins and minerals is not effective in abolishing iron deficiency anemia and this practice should be discouraged. Although there is an increased demand for iron in pregnancy, the prophylactic use of iron to correct any deficiency should be carried out with caution.

An issue that still remains to be considered is the interaction between two OTC preparations or between a prescribed medication and an OTC preparation. In a situation where a mother is being treated for a peptic ulcer with cimetidine, it is conceivable that there is simultaneous consumption of large quantities of tea (theophylline). Cimetidine, by preventing the metabolism of theophylline, results in increased theophylline concentrations and potentially a higher risk of toxicity. Aspirin displaces oral hypoglycemic agents from protein-binding sites, which can lead to severe manifestations in diabetes. Another example is the ingestion of iron to correct iron-deficiency anemia. If the mother is ingesting iron plus a multivitamin

Table 24.1   Select Over-the-Counter Preparations: Their Adverse Effects and Susceptible Populations

Susceptible Populations	OTC Preparation	Adverse Effects
Pregnant women	Aspirin	Fetal death with internal hemorrhage
	Cimetidine	Liver toxicity
	Imidazolines	Mental depression, hypertension, miosis
	Vitamin A	Spontaneous abortion, hydrocephalus, cardiac anomalies
	Vitamin D	Mental retardation, hemorrhage
	Vitamin K	Liver dysfunction
Infants	Loperamide	Paralytic ileus, persistent drowsiness
Geriatric patients	Saline laxatives	Hypotonia, CNS, and respiratory depression
	Bulk laxatives	Cramping, nausea, fluid loss, electrolyte imbalance
General	Hyperglycemic drugs and aspirin	Aggravation of diabetes
	Multivitamin preparation + iron	Interference of iron absorption
	Cimetidine + tea	Cimetidine interferes with metabolism of theophylline

preparation, the latter preparation interferes with iron absorption. Consequently, less iron is available and the hematological response is impaired.

The omnipresence of OTC preparations and concerted advertising may be a fact of life; however, increased awareness of the dangers associated with the use of self-medication must be stressed. Table 24.1 lists examples of OTC preparations that have been reported to produce adverse effects.

REFERENCES

Bonati M, Bortolus R, Machetti F, et al. (1990). Drug use in pregnancy: an overview of epidemiological (drug utilization) studies. Eur J Clin Pharmacol 38, 325–8.

Buitendijk S, Bracken MB (1991). Medication in early pregnancy: prevalence of use and relationship to maternal characteristics. Am J Obstet Gynecol 165, 33–40.

Chrischelles EA, Foley DJ, Wallace RB, et al. (1992). Use of medications by persons 65 and over; data from the established populations for epidemiologic studies of the elderly. J Gerontol 47, M137–44.

Conn VS (1991). Older adults: factors that predict the use of over-the-counter medication. J Adv Nurs 16, 1190–6.

Davern TJ 2nd, James LP, Hinson JA, et al. (2006). Measurement of serum acetaminophen-protein adducts in patients with acute liver failure; acute liver failure study group. Gastroenterology 130, 687–94.

De Jong-van den Berg LTW, Van Den Berg PB, Haaijer-Ruskamp FM, et al. (1992). Handling of risk-bearing drugs during pregnancy: do we choose less risky alternatives? Pharm Weekbl Sci 14, 38–45.

De Jong-van den Berg LTW, Waardenburg CM, Haaijer-Ruskamp FM, et al. (1993). Drug use in pregnancy: a comparative appraisal of data collecting methods. Eur J Clin Pharmacol 45, 9–14.

Dukes GE (1990). Over-the-counter antidiarrheal medications used for the self-treatment of acute non-specific diarrhea. Am J Med 88, 24S–6S.

Dunnell K, Cartwright A, eds. (1972). Medicine Takers, Prescribers and Hoarders. New York, NY: Routledge and Kegan Paul.

Fletcher P, Stephen R, Du Pont H (1995). Benefit/risk considerations with respect to OTC-descheduling of loperamide. Arzeimittelforschung 45, 608–13.

Glode G, Saccar CL, Pereira GR (1980). Cimetidine in pregnancy and apparent transient liver impairment in the newborn. Am J Dis Child 134, 87–8.

Golightly LK, Smolinske SS, Bennett ML, et al. (1998). Pharmaceutical excipients: adverse effects associated with "inactive" ingredients in drug products (Part II). Concepts Toxicol Rev 3, 209–40.

Hays DP, Pagliaro LA (1987). Human teratogens. In: Pagliaro LA, Pagliaro AM, eds. Problems in Pediatric Drug Therapy. Hamilton, IL: Drug Intelligence Publications, 51–191.

Kacew S (1992). General principles in pharmacology and toxicology applicable to children. In: Guzelian PS, Henry CJ, Olin SS, eds. Similarities and Differences Between Children and Adults. Washington, DC.: ILSI Press.

Kacew S (1994). Fetal consequences and risks attributed to the use of over-the-counter (OTC) preparations during pregnancy. Int J Clin Pharmacol Ther 32, 335–43.

Kacew S (1997). General principles in pediatric pharmacology and toxicology. In: Kacew S, Lambert GH, eds. Environmental Toxicology and Pharmacology of Human Development. Washington, DC.: Taylor & Francis.

Kacew S (1999). Effect of over-the-counter drugs on the unborn child. Pediatr Drugs 1, 75–80.

Karboski JA (1992). Medication selection for pregnant women. Drug Ther 22, 53–61.

Klebanoff MA, Berendes HW (1988). Aspirin exposure during the first 20 weeks of gestation and IQ at four years of age. Teratology 37, 249–55.

Knapp DA, Knapp DE(1972). Decision-making and self-medication between medication and preliminary findings. Am J Hosp Pharm 29, 1004–12.

Koda-Kimble MA (1992). Therapeutic and toxic potential of over-the-counter agents. In: Katzung BG, ed. Basic and Clinical Pharmacology. Norwalk, CT: Appleton and Lange.

Kogan MD, Pappas G, Yu SM, et al. (1994). Over-the-counter medication use among pre-school aged children in the United States. J Am Med Assoc 272, 1025–30.

Koren G, Pastuszak A, Ito S (1998). Drugs in pregnancy. N Engl J Med 338, 1128–37.

Kovar MG (1994). Use of medications and vitamin-mineral supplements by children and youths. Public Health Rep 100, 470–3.

Kumar A, Rawlings RD, Bearman DC (1993). The mystery ingredients: sweeteners, flavorings, dyes, and preservatives in analgesic/antipyretic, antihistamine/decongestant, liquid theophylline preparations. Pediatrics 91: 927–33.

Leist ER, Banwell JG (1974). Products containing aspirin. N Engl J Med 291, 710–12.

Liebelt EL, Shannon M (1993). Small doses, big problems: a selected review of highly toxic common medications. Pediatr Emerg Care 9, 292–7.

Lock S, Kacew S (1988). General principles, in pediatric pharmacology and toxicology. In: Kacew S, Lock S, eds. Toxicologic and Pharmacologic Principles in Pediatrics. Washington, DC.: Hemisphere Publishing, 1–15.

Lowenstein SR, Parrino TA (1987). Management of common cold. Adv Intern Med 32,207–34.

Motala C, Hill ID, Mann MD, et al. (1990). Effect of loperamide on stool output and duration of acute infectious diarrhea in infants. J Pediatr 117, 467–71.

Palatnick W, Tenenbein M (1998). Aspirin poisoning during pregnancy: increased fetal sensitivity. Am J Perinatol 15, 39–41.

Rayburn W, Wible-Kaut J, Bledsoe P (1982). Changing trends in drug use during pregnancy. J Reprod Med 27, 569–75.

Rosendahl I (1998). Expense of physician care spurs OTC, self-care market. Drug Top 132, 62–3.

Rubin JP, Ferencz C, Loffredo C (1993). Use of prescription and nonprescription drugs in pregnancy. J Clin Epidemiol 46, 581–9.

Rimsza ME, Newberry S (2008). Unexpected infant deaths associated with use of cough and cold medications. Pediatr. 122, 318–22.

Safe S (1998). Dietary estrogens: an overview (abstract). J Toxicol Sci 42, 352.

Shore LS, Gurevitz M, Shemesh M (1993). Estrogen, an environmental pollutant. Bull Environ Contam Toxicol 51, 361–6.

Smith MBH, Kogan MD (1997). Over-the-counter medication use and toxicity in children. In: Kacew S, Lambert GH, eds. Environmental Toxicology and Pharmacology of Human Development. Washington, DC.: Taylor & Francis.

Somogi A, Gugler R (1983). Clinical pharmacokinetics of cimetidine. Clin Pharmacokinet 8, 463–95.

Splinter M, Sagraves R, Nightengale B, et al. (1997). Prenatal use of medications by women giving birth at a university hospital. South Med J 90, 498–502.

Underhill R (1994). OTC products (correspondence). Pharm J 253, 112.

Vassilev ZP, Kabadi S, Villa R (2010). Safety and efficacy of over-the-counter cough and cold medicines for use in children. Expert Opin Drug Saf 9, 233–42.

25

Environmental pollutants

GENERAL REMARKS

The environment consists of air, water, and soil; biota is sometimes included as one of the environmental media. Toxic substances may originate from any one medium; however, they are generally transported to other media. Humans are exposed to environmental pollutants from a variety of pathways. Figure 25.1 illustrates the transportation of lead to humans, via air, water, food, dusts, etc. The lead that enters humans is returned to the environment via excreta, refuse, dumps, incinerators, etc. Many other pollutants also have complex routes of environmental transport and affect humans. A number of more important pollutants are briefly described in this chapter.

AIR POLLUTANTS

Introduction

Past Disasters

Several episodes of severe air pollution affecting the health and lives of large numbers of people have been reported. The notable ones occurred in Meusee Valley, Belgium (December 1930); Donora, Pennsylvania (October 1948); London, England (December 1952); Los Angeles, California (August or September 1942, 1952, 1955); and Piscataway, New Jersey (September 1971). These episodes fell into two categories. One type occurred in winters, especially during the night, when domestic burning of coal was an important source of pollution, and the other occurred in summers, during daytime, when photo oxidation of automobile exhaust was the major source of pollutants. In either case, the meteorological conditions, low wind, and high barometric pressure kept the pollutants at ground level. The major effects were related to distress of respiratory and, to a lesser extent, cardiovascular systems. A number of deaths were reported from the air

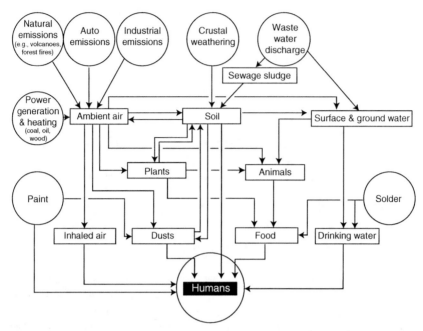

Figure 25.1   Environmental pathways of human exposure to lead. *Source*: From OECD (1993).

pollution episodes, either directly from the exposure to air pollutants or from strains on pre-existing diseases or deficiencies in these systems (Waldbott, 1978). In the case of the London smog in 1952, there was an outbreak of a severe influenza epidemic, which could be attributed to the fraction of elevated mortality for this period (Bell et al., 2004).

Current Condition

As a result of these tragic events, measures have been taken to reduce the extent of air pollution. Nevertheless, the health problem remains, although somewhat abated. For example, Mar et al. (2000) reported that elevated levels of CO and NO_2 in Phoenix were associated with increased total non-accidental mortality, and increased frequency of mortality due to cardiovascular involvement was associated with higher levels of CO, NO_2, SO_2, and particulate matter. Similar observations in other cities are cited in a review (Dominic et al., 2005; Krewski et al., 2003).

The most important anthropogenic source of ambient air pollutants in many developed nations is automobiles (Krewski and Rainham, 2007). Other sources include combustion (coal, natural gas, fuel oil, incineration of refuse, and wood stoves), metallurgical industry (see chap. 23), and chemical industry (solvents, chemical intermediates, etc.).

Outdoor Pollutants

Reducing Type of Pollutants

Composition and Sources

The major pollutants are sulfur oxides and suspended particulate matter. The former includes sulfur dioxide, sulfuric acid, and sulfates; the latter includes finely divided solids and liquids. Particles of $0.1-10\,\mu m$ in diameter settle very slowly, with a velocity of $8 \times 10^{-7}\,m/sec$ to $3 \times 10^{-3}\,m/sec$, while larger particles ($1000\,\mu m$ in diameter) settle at a velocity of $3.9\,m/sec$ (Fuchs, 1964). Thus, particles smaller than $10\,\mu m$ are suspended in air and are inhalable, as noted in chapter 2.

The main sources of these pollutants are domestic burning of coal and other fuels for heating and cooking and industrial combustion of these fuels to generate energy. Smelting of ores also generates these and other pollutants.

Diverse Effects

SO_2 is easily and highly soluble; hence it is readily absorbed in the nose and upper respiratory tract, where it induces irritation. This is followed with thickening of the mucus layer in trachea and hypertrophy of goblet cells.

The irritation produces cough, expectoration, dyspnea, and bronchoconstriction. Respiratory functions are impaired, manifesting as decreased tidal volume, increased pulmonary resistance, and higher respiratory rate. Among exposed individuals, there is a rise in the incidence of respiratory tract infections, which may be attributable in part to an interference of the respiratory tract clearance mechanisms. Under normal conditions, this mechanism is responsible for removing bacteria and other particles from the tract. Aerosols of sulfuric acid, formed from SO_3, are even more irritating than sulfur dioxide, which forms sulfurous acid (Costa and Amdur, 1996).

The effects of these sulfur pollutants are enhanced by the presence of suspended sulfur dioxide and smoke (suspended particulate matter) and produce deaths, especially among the elderly and those with pre-existing diseases of the respiratory tract and heart, as those in Belgium (1930), Pennsylvania (1948), and London (1952).

Even at lower concentrations (e.g., $SO_2 \geq 500\,\mu g/m^3$ and smoke $\geq 500\,\mu g/m^3$), there is likely to be excess incidence of mortality among the elderly and the chronically sick. When exposure to these pollutants takes place at half of these concentrations, there is likely to be a worsening of existing respiratory disease (WHO, 1979). Willis et al. (2003) reported that an increased risk of mortality attributed to cardiopulmonary complications was correlated with atmospheric sulfur dioxide concentrations.

Photochemical Oxidants

Composition and Sources

This group of air pollutants consists of nitrogen dioxide (NO_2), ozone (O_3), and a number of other oxides of nitrogen (N_2O, NO, NO_2, N_2O_3, N_2O_4, and N_2O_5). N_2O

is the most abundant among these chemicals, but it is generated by anaerobic processes in the soil and in the surface layer of the oceans, and hence is not an important air pollutant, as far as human health is concerned. The last three oxides of nitrogen can be formed from NO and/or NO_2. However, their levels are very low and are not known to produce any harmful effects.

NO is the main oxide formed from man-made sources. However, after its discharge from the sources to the atmosphere, it reacts with O_2 to form NO_2. This reaction is facilitated in the presence of ozone.

Ozone is the most ubiquitous photochemical oxidant. At times, it constitutes as much as 90% of the oxidants in smog. Ozone is also a natural constituent of the upper atmosphere, formed by the photolysis of oxygen. Atmospheric circulation carries some to the lower levels.

The main sources of photochemical oxidants are automobiles and industrial combustion. Domestic heating and power stations also generate significant amounts. Ozone is also produced by a variety of high-voltage electrical equipment. Formaldehyde, which is one of the photochemical oxidants, will be discussed under section, "Indoor Air Pollutants/Sick Building Syndrome."

Adverse Effects

In contrast to CO_2, NO_2 is hardly soluble in water. It, therefore, passes through the upper respiratory tract to the terminal bronchioles and alveoli, where it forms nitric and nitrous acids. These acids are irritant and corrosive. Acute exposure produces pulmonary edema and congestion and damage ciliated epithelium and type I cells (see chap. 12), which are then replaced by the less-sensitive nonciliated epithelial cells and cuboidal type II cells. Chronic exposure produces emphysema. Resistance to bacterial and viral infections is decreased (WHO, 1977).

After inhalation exposure, ozone reacts with organic matter in the respiratory tract. Similar to NO_2, its main effects are on the epithelial cells of the nasal cavity, terminal bronchioles, and alveoli, affecting the more susceptible ciliated epithelial cells and type I cells. The endothelia surrounding these structures are also damaged, resulting in pulmonary edema. Chronic exposure results in emphysema, atelectasis, focal necrosis, and sometimes bronchopneumonia. In the nasal mucosa, there is destruction of the epithelial lining and release of cytokines, and consequent inflammatory processes develop (Nikasinovic et al., 2003). Resistance to bacterial and viral infection is decreased. Because of the oxidative activity of ozone, vitamin C decreases its toxicity, whereas vitamin E deficiency has the opposite effect (WHO, 1978).

Apart from their toxic effects on the respiratory tract, these air pollutants also produce eye irritation in adults (see chap. 16). Recently, focus of air pollutants has concentrated on neonates, infants, and children (Foos et al., 2008). It is well established that the lung is not mature and full development of architecture and functionality do not occur until age 18. Children have a larger lung surface area per kilogram and under normal circumstances, breathe a greater amount of air. Further, the immune system is still immature. Thus maternal exposure to air pollutants during pregnancy results in fetal loss, while infant exposure is correlated with a higher frequency of mortality. The effect of air pollutants on children is an increased incidence of cough, bronchitis, and asthma.

Indoor Air Pollutants/"Sick Building Syndrome"

In recent years, the importance of indoor pollutants has become increasingly appreciated. The more efficient insulation of modern buildings, resulting in inadequate ventilation and in the use of certain insulation materials, has intensified the problem. Some of the more important pollutants and reactions are described in the chapter. Additional details are provided in articles by Karol (1991) and Samet (1993).

Formaldehyde

This organic chemical is a product of photo oxidation of natural and man-made hydrocarbons. Formaldehyde is more important as a component of urea formaldehyde foam insulation material, which has been widely used in mobile homes and, to a lesser extent, in conventional houses. Because of its volatility and toxicity, it has been a significant indoor air pollutant.

Formaldehyde is water soluble and irritates the eyes, nose, and upper respiratory tract. At higher concentrations, it also affects the bronchioles and alveoli, and induces pulmonary edema and pneumonia. The dose–effect relationship of formaldehyde is listed in Table 25.1. In addition, it has been reported to induce nasal cancers in rodents, while in humans there is an increased incidence of micronucleated buccal and mucosal cells (Liteplo and Meek, 2003). Some studies reported evidence of genetic defects in humans. In 2004, formaldehyde was upgraded from Group 2A (a probable human carcinogen) to Group 1 (a human carcinogen) by International Agency for Research on Cancer (IARC). Formaldehyde can produce not only nasal cancer, but also common cancer including leukemia (Golden, 2011). Furthermore, formaldehyde was also associated with the increased incidence of asthma in children (McGwin et al., 2010). The modes of action of formaldehyde are related to both genotoxic and epigenetic mechanisms (Rager et al., 2010).

Asbestos

Asbestos is a naturally occurring silicate fiber. Because of its heat and electrical insulation properties, it has been widely used in houses, ships, automobiles, etc. Workers in certain occupations are the main population at risk. However, the general public may also be exposed to it through the air and, to a lesser extent, the drinking water because it is used as a water filter (Paustenbach et al., 2004).

After inhalation, asbestos enters the alveoli and produces parenchymal asbestosis consisting of fibrosis and asbestos bodies (Vallyathan et al., 1998). Iron bound to asbestos fibers is also believed to be involved in the toxic manifestations

Table 25.1 Acute Human Health Effects of Formaldehyde at Various Concentrations

Reported Effects	Formaldehyde Concentration (ppm)
None reported	0.0–0.05
Neurophysiologic effects	0.05–1.5
Odor threshold	0.05–1.0
Eye irritation[a]	0.1–2.0
Upper airway irritation	0.10–25
Lower airway and pulmonary effects	5–30
Pulmonary edema, inflammation, pneumonia	50–100
Death	>100

[a]As measured by the determination of optical chronaxy, electroencephalography, and sensitivity of dark-adapted eyes to light. The low concentration (0.01 ppm) was observed in the presence of other pollutants that may have been acting synergistically.
Source: From NRC, Committee on Aldehydes (1981).

observed. It may pierce the alveoli and produce pleural asbestosis. It also produces lung carcinoma, the incidence of which is significantly higher among cigarette smokers (Vallyathan et al., 1998). Mesothelioma is a rare type of malignant tumor, which may originate from the pleural and peritoneal surfaces after inhalation and ingestion, respectively.

Asbestos fibrosis appears to result from its entering the cells (macrophages and lymphocytes), breaking the lysosomal membrane, and releasing hydroxylases. It produces tumors either by carrying carcinogenic hydrocarbons into the body or by acting as co-carcinogen (Vallyathan et al., 1998).

CO, NO_2, SO_2, and Suspended Particulate Matter

These substances exist indoors as well as outdoors. In fact, this type of indoor air pollution may be more important than that which exists outdoors. This is because people in general spend more time indoors and because domestic heating may involve burning coal or other fuel without adequate ventilation. However, the predominant source of air pollutants arises from vehicular generation (Krewski and Rainham, 2007).

Others

Various volatile organic compounds (benzene, toluene, xylene, ethyl benzene, etc.) are present in offices and homes, arising from paints, adhesives, cleaners, cosmetics, furnishings, and printed materials. In addition, there are many types of biological material such as bacteria, viruses, fungi, fungal spores, and dandruff. These substances may induce allergic reactions. The mixture of pollutants produces a garnet of reactions, which has been named "Sick Building Syndrome." The common symptoms of this syndrome include irritation of eyes, nose, and throat, headaches, fatigue, and nasal congestion (Samet et al., 1988).

The presence of nanoparticles in electronics, various household items, and televisions is ubiquitous. In animals exposed to high concentrations of nanoparticles via the respiratory route it is established that these compounds exert adverse effects on lung functions. Although humans are clearly exposed to nanoparticles, a direct correlation to adverse effects has not been established. However, considering the fact that nanoparticles are ubiquitous, further investigations are needed to establish the safety of these compounds.

WATER AND SOIL POLLUTANTS

General Considerations

Various pollutants are discharged into environmental media. Those that predominate in the air are described in the preceding section. Others are discharged in wastewater as effluent, or stored in dump sites. Generally these will contaminate both the water and soil.

Water and soil contaminants include pesticides and metals, which have been discussed in chapters 23 and 24. Asbestos is also an important environmental pollutant. Its major health hazard is related to inhalation exposure as outlined in the preceding section. It is also present in water because of various mining, milling, and industrial applications as well as its use in filter pads for wine, beer and so on (Paustenbach et al., 2004).

A great variety of organic chemicals, including some solvents and pesticides, have been detected in water, and most of these are present at extremely low levels. However, some of them are more persistent. In addition, a number of inorganic ions may also present health hazards. Both of these groups are described below. Drugs are released into water from human urine. Hormonal steroids are released into water from livestock and produce endocrine disruption.

Synthetic Persistent Chemicals

Polychlorinated Biphenyls

Polychlorinated biphenyls (PCBs) are manufactured by the progressive chlorination of biphenyl. Commercial products are mixtures of biphenyl with a different degree of chlorine substitution. These products have a variety of uses in electric insulators, and rubber and paper industries, as plasticizers. PCBs are stable and hence are persistent in the environment with levels in water ranging from 0.5 to 500 ppb, depending on the extent of contamination. PCBs are lipophilic, and are thus bioaccumulated in aquatic organisms; fish caught from certain lakes contain 520 ppm PCBs. Because of extreme persistence and toxicity, many nations have suspended or restricted their use. However, they will remain in the environment for a long time.

PCBs, being lipophilic, are stored in adipose tissue and secreted in milk. PCBs are a potent inducer of microsomal enzymes (Hu and Bunce, 1999). As a result, they enhance the metabolism of steroids such as estradiol and androsterone, a fact that may account for some of their effects on reproductive function. Because of this effect on enzymes, they can modify the toxicity of other chemicals and act as a promoter of carcinogenesis.

PCBs exert a variety of toxic effects in animals. For example, they induce hepatic adenoma and carcinoma. Among the *reproductive functions* affected are lengthened estrus cycles and decreased frequency of implanted ova in mice, lowered fertility in mink and Rhesus monkey, and reduced hatchability of eggs in birds. With respect to the *immune system*, they produce atrophy of lymphoid tissue in chickens and rabbits, and suppress a variety of humoral and cell-mediated immunity functions. The illnesses reported in Japan due to exposure to PCBs were referred to as Yusho disease and in Taiwan as Yu-Cheng disease.

An outbreak of poisoning occurred in Japan in 1968, resulting from a consumption of rice oil contaminated with PCBs, which affected more than 1000 people. The major clinical manifestations were chloracne, hyperkeratosis, and darkening of skin. Immunosuppression was also noted. Various subjective symptoms were reported, such as numbness of the limbs, coughing, expectoration, general fatigue, and eye discharge. There may also be an increase of liver and lung cancer among the male patients.

Polybrominated Biphenyls

Polybrominated biphenyls (PBBs) are used as fire retardants. They gained notoriety because of a large-scale contamination of cattle feed in Michigan in 1973. The beef was contaminated with PBBs (Weber and Greim, 1997). They are similar to PCBs in many aspects, such as biotransformation, storage, and effects on reproduction, carcinogenesis, immune system, and skin (chloracne). The actions of PBBs on thyroid function and central nervous system disturbances in animals resulted in the banning of some of these chemicals by the European Union and the United States environmental protection agency (USEPA).

2,3,7,8-Tetrachlorodibenzo-p-dioxin

2,3,7,8-tetrachlorodibenzo-*p*-dioxin (TCDD) attracted wide attention after its accidental release from a factory in Seveso, Italy, in 1976. While its level in water is low, it is important toxicologically because of its extreme potency. Furthermore, TCDD is a contaminant of other chemicals, notably the herbicide 2,4,5-T, which was extensively used as a defoliant in the Vietnam War. TCDD is extremely toxic, with LD_{50}s ranging from 0.0006 to 0.115 mg/kg in different species of animals (NRC, 1977).

TCDD is a potent inducer of microsomal enzymes, by binding to a specific receptor (Hu and Bunce, 1999). TCDD is a potent carcinogen (2 ppb in rats), inducing cancer in a variety of organs such as liver, respiratory tract, and oral cavity (Kociba et al., 1977). At somewhat higher doses, it is hepatotoxic, immunosuppressive, teratogenic, and fetotoxic. In humans, the predominant effect of TCDD is chloracne. In the past, it was not reported to be carcinogenic in humans despite its extremely potent carcinogenicity in rats (Zack and Suskind,

1980). However, epidemiological studies have shown that TCDD can produce cancer in humans and was finally classified as a human carcinogen, Group 1 by IARC in 1997 (IARC, 1997; Baan et al., 2009; Warner et al., 2011).

Other Organic Chemicals

Phthalate esters are extensively used in plastics and are widely distributed in the environment, especially water. Their acute toxicity is low, but di(2-ethylhexyl) phthalate was shown to be carcinogenic and adversely affect reproductive functions in animals (Conference on Phthalates, 1982). *Trihalomethanes* are formed through the chlorination of water. These chemicals comprise chloroform, bromodichloromethane, dibromochloromethane, and bromoform. They are found in drinking water from less than 0.1–311 ppb. Among them, chloroform had the highest concentration. At high doses, these chemicals are hepatotoxic, produce reproductive and developmental effects, and may be carcinogenic (Teuschler et al., 2004).

Inorganic Ions

Nitrates

The increase of nitrates in soil and water results mainly from intensive application of fertilizers, but also from wastes (excreta) of humans and farm animals. They are converted to nitrites in soil, water, and the gastrointestinal tract through microbial action. Nitrites induce methemoglobinemia, thus reducing the oxygen-carrying capacity of hemoglobin as noted in chapter 4. Furthermore, they may react with certain amines to form nitrosamines, most of which are carcinogenic (chaps. 7 and 20).

Phosphates

These substances arise mainly from fertilizers and detergents. They have very low toxicity, but their presence in a body of stagnant water results in excessive growth of algae. The algae reduce the oxygenation of the water, resulting in fish kill. Certain "algae," the cyanobacteria, contain hepatotoxins and neurotoxins (see the respective sections on these toxins).

Fluoride

The natural level of fluoride in water varies greatly, depending on the location. Industrial activities may also raise its level. While fluoride has been added to water to about 1 ppm to reduce dental cavity formation, excessive levels in water (10 ppm) are likely to produce fluorosis. The enamel on the teeth is weakened, resulting in surface pitting. Changes in the bones, including osteosclerosis and exostoses, usually affect the spine and produce knee deformity known as genu valgum. At lower levels of fluoride intake, chalky-white patches appear on the surface of the dental enamel. These patches are then stained yellow or brown and give rise to the characteristic "mottled" appearance (Dean, 1942).

Arsenic

In certain areas of Taiwan, South America, and Bangladesh, high levels of arsenic have been reported to be associated with black foot disease, a peripheral vascular disorder resulting in gangrene. Arsenic also produces skin lesions and possibly visceral cancers, especially the liver (see chap. 23).

Cyanotoxins/Eutrophication

Eutrophication occurs in lakes and ponds when there are excessive amounts of phosphorus. In general, this results from run-offs contaminated with fertilizers and detergents. Algae tend to thrive in such waters. Some of the algae produce cyanotoxins. Three groups of cyanotoxins are now recognized: one affects the nervous system, the second termed as cylindrospermopsin inhibits protein synthesis and are cytotoxic, while the third termed as microcystins inhibits protein phosphatases in the liver (Chorus et al., 2000; Zurawell et al., 2005).

Neurotoxins

The most important among them is saxitoxin, also known as paralytic shellfish poison. Human exposure to saxitoxin is through consumption of contaminated shellfish. The toxin acts by blocking the conduction of nerve impulse thereby inducing muscle paralysis (see chaps. 17 and 20).

Microcystins

The other type comprises microcystins and nodulins. These toxins are hepatotoxic to wild and domestic animals (Zurawell et al., 2005). In an epidemiological study in several areas in China, Chorus et al. (2000) found a positive correlation between the use of surface water and high rates of primary liver cancer. Subsequently, Wang and Zhu (1996) showed that an extract of *Microcystis aeruginosa* (a major species of cyanobacteria) promoted cell transformation of Syrian hamster embryo cells which had been exposed to a genotoxic carcinogen. It is thus evident that the extract is a carcinogen promoter. Gilroy et al. (2000) showed that a "health food product," made of blue-green algae, was contaminated with microcystins, more than 70% of the samples tested contained ≥1 mg/kg.

In 1996 in Caruaru, Brazil, 100 patients suffered acute liver failure from the use of partially treated municipal water for kidney dialysis. More than half of the patients died. The cause of the outbreak has now been attributed to certain cyanotoxins (Chorus et al., 2000). In addition, a recent report demonstrated that the reproductive toxicity in male rats might be related to reactive oxygen species generation, and inducing oxidative stress in Sertoli cells, and subsequently leading to apoptosis (Li and Han, 2012).

REFERENCES

Baan R, Grosse Y, Straif K, et al. (2009). A review of human carcinogens—Part F: chemical agents and related occupations. Lancet Oncol 10, 1143–4.

Bell ML, Davis DL, Fletcher T (2004). A retrospective assessment of mortality from the London smog episode of 1952: the role of influenza and pollution. Environ Health Perspect. 112, 6–8.

Chorus I, Falconer IR, Salas HJ, et al. (2000). Health risks caused by freshwater cyanobacteria in recreational waters. J Toxicol Environ Health B 3, 323–47.

Conferences on Phthalates (1982). Proceedings of the conference. Environ Health Perspect 45, 11–51.

Costa DL, Amdur MO (1996). Air pollution. In: Klaassen CD, ed. Casarett and Doull's Toxicology. New York, NY: McGraw-Hill, 857–82.

Dean HT (1942). The investigation of physiological effects by the epidemiological method. Am Assoc Adv Sci 19, 23–31.

Dominic F, Mcdermott A, Daniels M, et al. (2005). Revised analyses of the national morbidity mortality and air pollution study: mortality among residents of 90 cities. J Toxicol Environ Health A 68, 1071–92.

Foos B, Marty M, Schwartz J, et al. (2008). Focusing on children's inhalation dosimetry and health effects for risk assessment: an introduction. J Toxicol Environ Health A 71, 149–65.

Fuchs NA (1964). The Mechanisms of Aerosol. Oxford, UK: Pergamon Press, 28.

Gilroy DJ, Kauffman KW, Hall RA, et al. (2000). Assessing potential health risks from microcystin toxins in blue-green algae dietary supplement. Environ Health Perspect 10, 435–49.

Golden R (2011). Identifying an indoor air exposure limit for formaldehyde considering both irritation and cancer hazards. Crit Rev Toxicol 41, 672–721.

Hu K, Bunce NJ (1999). Metabolism of polychlorinated dibenzo-p-dioxins and related dioxin-like compounds. J Toxicol Environ Health B 2, 183–210.

IARC (International Agency for Research on Cancer) (1997). Polychlorinated dibenzo-para-dioxins and polychlorinated dibenzofurans. IARC Monogr Eval Carcinog Risks Hum 33–342.

Li Y, Han X (2012). Microcystin-LR causes cytotoxicity effects in rat testicular sertoli cells. Environ Toxicol Pharmacol. 33, 318–26.

Karol MH (1991). Allergic reactions to indoor air pollutants. Environ Health Perspect 95, 45–51.

Kociba RJ, Keyes DG, Beyer JE (1977). Results of a two-year chronic toxicity and oncogenicity study of 2,3,7,8-tetrachlorodibenzo-p-dioxin in rats. Toxicol Appl Pharmacol 46, 279–303.

Krewski D, Burnett RT, Goldberg MS, et al. (2003). Overview of the reanalysis of the Harvard six cities study and American Cancer society of particulate air pollution and mortality. J Toxicol Environ Health A 66, 1507–51.

Krewski D, Rainham D (2007). Ambient air pollution and population health: overview. J Toxicol Enviorn Health A 70, 275–83.

Liteplo RG, Meek ME (2003). Inhaled formaldehyde: exposure estimation, hazard characterization and exposure response analysis. J Toxicol Environ Health B 6, 85–114.

McGwin G, Lienert J, Kennedy JI (2010). Formaldehyde exposure and asthma in children: a systematic review. Environ Health Perspect 118, 313–17.

Mar TF, Norris GA, Koenig JQ, et al. (2000). Associations between air pollution and mortality in phoenix, 1995–1997. Environ Health Perspect 108, 347–53.

Nikasinovic L, Momas I, Seta N (2003). Nasal, epithelial and inflammatory response to ozone exposure: a review of laboratory-based studies published since 1985. J Toxicol Environ Health B 6, 521–68.

NRC (1977). Drinking Water and Health. Washington, DC.: National Research Council, National Academy of Sciences.

NRC, Committee on Aldehydes (1981). Formaldehyde and Other Aldehydes. Washington, DC.: National Academy Press.

OECD (1993). Risk Reduction Monograph No. 1: Lead Background and National Experience with Reducing Risk. Paris, France: Organization for Economic Cooperation.

Paustenbach DJ, Finley BL, Lu ET, et al. (2004). Environmental and occupational health hazards associated with the presence of asbestos in brake linings and pads (1900 to present): a state of the art review. J Toxicol Environ Health B 7, 25–80.

Rager JE, Smeester L, Jaspers I, et al. (2010). Epigenetic changes induced by air toxics: formaldehyde exposure alters miRNA expression profiles in human lung cells. Environ Health Perspect 119, 494–500.

Samet JM (1993). Indoor air pollution: a public health perspective. Indoor Air 3, 219–26.

Samet JM, Marbury MC, Spengler JD (1988). Health effects and sources of indoor air pollution. part II. Am Rev Respir Dis 137, 221–42.

Teuschler LK, Rice GE, Wilkes CR, et al. (2004). A feasibility study of cumulative risk assessment methods for drinking water disinfection by-product mixtures. J Toxicol Environ Health A 67, 755–77.

Vallyathan V, Green F, Ducatman B, et al. (1998). Roles of epidemiology, pathology, molecular biology and biomarkers in the investigation of occupational lung cancer. J Toxicol Environ Health B 1, 91–116.

Waldbott GK (1978). Health Effects of Environmental Pollutants. St. Louis, MO: C.V. Mosby.

Warner M, Mocarelli P, Samuels S, et al. (2011). Dioxin exposure and cancer risk in the seveso women's health study. Environ Health Perspect. 119, 1700–5.

Wang HB, Zhu HG (1996). Promoting activity of microcystins extracted from waterbloom in SHE cell transformation assay. Biomed Environ Sci 9, 46–51.

Weber LW, Greim H (1997). The toxicity of brominated and mixed-halogenated dibenzo-p-dioxins and dibennzofurans: an overview. J Toxicol Environ Health 50, 195–215.

WHO (1977). Oxides of Nitrogen. Environ Health Criteria 4. Geneva, Switzerland: World Health Organization.

WHO (1978). Photochemical Oxidants. Environ Health Criteria 7. Geneva, Switzerland: World Health Organization.

WHO (1979). Sulfur Oxides and Suspended Particulate Matter. Environ Health Criteria 8.Geneva, Switzerland: World Health Organization.

Willis A, Jerrett M, Burnett RT, et al. (2003). The association between sulfate air pollution and mortality at the county scale: an exploration of the impact of scale on a long-term exposure study. J Toxicol Environ Health A 66, 1605–24.

Zack JA, Suskind RR (1980). The mortality experience of workers exposed to tetrachlorodibenzodioxin in a trichlorophenol process accident. J Occup Med 22, 1–114.

Zurawell RW, Chen H, Burke JM, et al. (2005). Hepatotoxic cyanobacteria: a review of the biological importance of microcystins in freshwater environments. J Toxicol Environ Health B 8, 1–37.

26

Occupational toxicology

GENERAL REMARKS

As noted in previous chapters, humans are exposed to a variety of substances, by ingestion, inhalation, and dermal contact. Unlike the general populations, however, workers are often exposed to much higher levels of specific toxicants. Such exposures may clearly result in adverse effects. In fact, as early as 1775, Pott observed that chimney sweeps having been exposed to soot, developed cancer of the scrotum. Rehn discovered in 1895 that bladder tumors occurred among workers in aniline dye factories.

In the late nineteenth century, certain societal changes prompted the development of a variety of new occupations. One of the changes was the introduction of powerful machinery to facilitate many mining activities. While the machinery increased the output of mining, it also increased the airborne dusts to which miners were exposed.

Another major change was the invention of internal combustion machines, which increased air pollution from motor vehicles. To fuel these vehicles, petroleum was produced in large quantities. In fact, the excess petroleum became an excellent source of new chemicals. These petrochemicals, along with other raw materials, found uses in the production of clothing, furniture, construction material, household, and office commodities, as well as in paints, pesticides, solvents, pharmaceuticals, etc. These and other changes in society increased the number of occupational workers as well as the variety of substances to which the workers are exposed.

Workers engaged in the production, processing, or utilization of these substances are thus exposed to some chemical hazards. The severity of the adverse effects, however, depends not only on the nature of the substance but also on the level and duration of the exposure. Occupational toxicology is thus intended to assess the "permissible" levels of exposure, for a specified duration, to the toxicants encountered in workplaces. For the protection of the workers, the concentrations of the toxicants in the workplaces are to be maintained at or below their corresponding permissible levels. It should be noted that occupational exposure does not happen in a vacuum. A worker can be exposed to more than a single chemical, leading to a mixture of effects. Furthermore, a worker who smokes or drinks, or suffers from a chronic illness such as diabetes or on a chronic medication regime may be more susceptible than the nonsmoking worker to the same chemical. It needs to be clarified that individuals who spray pesticides are also occupational exposure workers exposed to the outdoors where chemical concentration cannot be determined. However, in the context of this chapter occupational refers to jobs done in an indoor setting.

EXPOSURE LIMITS

Food additives and most medications which, if too toxic, can be readily prohibited for use; but occupational toxicants, in general, cannot be eliminated, that is, the workers who are exposed to these toxicants are dependent on the jobs for their income. To protect the health of occupational workers, permissible ("safe") limits of exposure are assessed.

Definitions

Permissible limits of exposure are existent in many countries. In the United States, a yearly booklet listing the threshold limit values (TLVs) is published by the American Conference of Governmental Industrial Hygienists (ACGIH) since 1946 (ACGIH, 2000). The limits refer to airborne concentrations of substances. They represent conditions under which "nearly all workers may be repeatedly exposed day after day without adverse effects." The list includes solvents, metals and their compounds, pesticides, and others. There are three categories of TLV:

1. TLV-TWA (time-weighted average) refers to the TWA concentration for a normal eight-hour workday and a 40-hour work week.
2. TLV-STEL (short-term exposure limit) refers to the STEL to which workers may be exposed. It is defined as a 15-minute TWA exposure. This limit is set mostly to avoid irritation and narcosis, but also to avoid chronic or irreversible tissue damage. The short-term exposure is acceptable provided that the TLV-TWA is not exceeded.
3. TLV-C refers to the ceiling that should not be exceeded during any part of the working exposure.

These limits are expressed in terms of parts per million (ppm) and/or milligrams per cubic meter (mg/m^3). Since 1 mole of an ideal gas at 25°C and 760 mmHg occupies 24.45 L, the following equation can be used to convert the limits: parts of vapor/million parts air (ppm) = C (mg/m^3) × 24.45/(molecular weight of the solvents), where the letter "C" denotes a concentration of chemical For example, 15 mg/m^3 of formaldehyde (MW = 30 g/mol) can be converted to 12.225 ppm [= 15 (mg/m^3) × 24.45/(30 g/mol)]. The Occupational Safety and Health Administration published a list of "permissible exposure limits" which are essentially similar to the TLV of ACGIH. There are other occupational exposure limits such as the maximum allowable concentration. However, the TLV published by ACGIH have been widely accepted, even outside of the United States.

Scientific Basis

The permissible levels of exposure are assessed on the basis of relevant test results in experimental animals as well as in clinical observations and epidemiological studies in humans.

Tests in Animals

These include the various types of tests described in previous chapters. However, with occupational toxicants, the major routes of exposure are the respiratory tract and skin. After inhalation, gases and vapors may exert effects locally, and may also be absorbed. Large particulate matters and liquid droplets ($>10\,\mu m$) do not enter the respiratory tract and affect the nasal mucosa; very small particles ($<0.01\,\mu m$) are likely to be exhaled. Those within the range of $0.01-10\,\mu m$ may be absorbed from the respiratory tract and exert systemic effects and may also induce local effects in the lungs.

Skin is relatively impermeable to most chemicals, but some may be absorbed in sufficient quantities to induce systemic effects. Some toxicants may produce local irritation and hypersensitization.

After absorption, a toxicant is distributed to various parts of the body. Depending on its nature, a small or large portion of it may be stored. In general, it is excreted as it is or after undergoing biotransformation. In general, this process renders the toxicant more water soluble, hence more excretable. However, some chemicals undergo bioactivation, especially in the liver and become more toxic. For additional information on bioactivation, see chapter 3.

Although all organs and systems may be adversely affected by occupational toxicants, the most commonly affected targets, apart from the respiratory tract and skin, are the nervous system, the liver, and the kidneys. In addition, potential adverse effects on the immune system, reproductive function, and fetal development merit special attention.

Human Data

To obtain relevant data from humans, a variety of studies may be used. The *case–control study* is generally used to unravel the etiology of a specific adverse effect. For example, Cole et al. (1972) observed a higher rate of lower urinary tract cancer among workers engaged in the manufacture of dyestuff, rubber, and leather. This observation provided a basis for further confirmatory studies.

Epidemiological studies are more elaborate and usually provide more precise information. Prospective studies are usually carried out to confirm a suspected cause–effect relationship, and/or to provide more precise quantitative data. Retrospective studies involve analysis of clinical data obtained in exposed workers versus a group of unexposed cohort, matched for age, gender, and such lifestyle as smoking and alcohol consumption.

Assessment of Permissibility

With adequate and relevant animal and human data, a "no-observed-adverse-effect level" (NOAEL) can generally be assessed. The permissible exposure level can be obtained by applying an appropriate "safety factor" to the NOAEL. A detailed description of the procedure used in Europe to assess the permissible levels of exposure to pesticides was described by de Raat et al. (1997). Procedures used in the United States, Canada, Germany, and the Czech Republic are outlined in a WHO document (WHO, 2000).

OCCUPATIONAL TOXICANTS

Organic Solvents

Solvents comprise a variety of organic chemicals such as aromatic hydrocarbons [e.g., chloroform and carbon tetrachloride (CCl_4)], alcohols, or glycols, and their ethers. These chemicals are used extensively in paints, inks, thinners, adhesives, pharmaceuticals, cosmetics, etc. Some solvents are used mainly for dry-cleaning clothes and degreasing machinery. Their manufacture and use in industry may pose health hazards to occupational workers. In addition, some of them become components of household products, thereby constituting potential health hazards to the consumer. Their toxic effects are outlined below, and summarized along with their TLV-TWAs in Table 26.1. Chloroform can produce toxic effects in the liver, kidney, central nervous system (CNS), and cardiovascular system (Table 26. 1).

Table 26.1   Toxic Effects and TLV-TWAs of Certain Organic Solvents

Organic Solvents	Toxic Effects	TWA (ppm)
Benzene	Leukemia	0.5
Carbon disulfide	CNS, neuropathy	10
Carbon tetrachloride	Liver	5
Chloroform	CVS, liver, kidney, CNS	10
Dioxane	Skin	20
n-Hexane	Neuropathy, CNS irritation	50
Methanol	Neuropathy, vision CNS	200
Methyl n-butyl ketone	Neuropathy	5
Methylene chloride	CNS, anoxia	50
Toluene	CNS, skin	50
Trichloroethylene	CNS, liver	50

Abbreviations: CNS, central nervous system; CVS, central vascular system; TLV, threshold limit value; TWA, time-weighted average. *Source*: From ACGIH (2000).

General Effects

Most of the solvents exert certain nonspecific effects. These include irritation at the site of contact, and depression of CNS.

Irritation

At room temperature solvents are in the liquid form. When they are in contact with skin, irritation may occur. As they are volatile, inhalation of their vapors may produce irritation of the nasal epithelium and respiratory tract, and they may also produce eye irritation and watering.

CNS Depression

At sufficiently high levels of exposure, a consistent effect of solvents is CNS depression. The clinical manifestation begins with disorientation, giddiness, and euphoria. The last-named effect is responsible for abuse of some of these chemicals. The syndrome may progress to paralysis, unconsciousness, and convulsions. Death may ensue.

The mechanism of action is not clear, but well over half a century ago, Meyer (1937) observed that the narcosis (CNS depression) was related to the solubility of these substances in lipid and was not related to their chemical structure, and hence suggested that narcosis resulted from CNS cell dysfunction following solubilizing of the solvents in the cell membrane.

Interaction

As noted above, most solvents may undergo biotransformation and may elevate the activities of cytochrome P-450 isozymes. Since solvents are often present in mixtures, interaction between them may occur. For example, a solvent, such as benzene, may potentiate the adverse effects of others by enhancing their bioactivation. On the other hand, the toxicity may also be decreased with certain mixtures. For example, toluene may reduce the toxicity of benzene by competitively inhibiting the bioactivation enzyme systems (Andrews et al., 1977). These effects are dependent on normal liver function but become skewed in an alcoholic. The presence of drugs will also affect solvent biotransformation. It is worth noting that there are gender differences and in general men appear to be more susceptible to chemical-induced alterations compared with women.

Specific Effects

Apart from the general effects described earlier, a variety of specific effects may follow exposure to solvents. The diversity of these effects is a result of different reactive metabolites being formed. Some of the specific effects are described next.

Liver

As noted in chapter 13, ethanol is a common cause of fatty liver and liver cirrhosis. These effects likely result from the direct toxicity of ethanol and nutritional deficiency commonly present among alcoholics. Various chlorinated hydrocarbons may produce a variety of liver damages. These include fatty liver as well as liver necrosis, cirrhosis, and cancer. The liver lesions are induced by reactive metabolites of these solvents. For example, the likely metabolite of carbon tetrachloride is trichloromethyl radical, that of chloroform is phosgene, and those of halogenated aromatic hydrocarbons such as bromobenzene are their epoxides (Reid and Krishna, 1973). However, the recurrent cytotoxicity and chronic tissue regeneration may be the cause of carcinogenicity.

Kidneys

As noted in chapter 14, certain chlorinated hydrocarbons such as chloroform and carbon tetrachloride are nephrotoxic in addition to being hepatotoxic. At lower levels of exposure, the renal effects are related to tubular functions, such as glycosuria, amino aciduria, and polyuria. At higher levels, there may be cell death along with elevated BUN and anuria. In humans, CCl_4 affects mainly kidneys when the route of exposure is inhalation, whereas liver is the major target organ when the chemical is ingested. Ethylene glycol is nephrotoxic because of its direct cytotoxicity as well as the blocking of the proximal tubules with the formation of crystals of its metabolite, calcium oxalate. Trichloroethylene, a solvent used as a degreasing agent was shown to produce damage to the proximal tubules as well as nephrocarcinogenicity.

Nervous System

Apart from their effects on CNS, as noted above, aliphatic hydrocarbons and certain ketones such as *n*-hexane and methyl *n*-butyl ketone also affect the peripheral nervous system. The clinical manifestation of this polyneuropathy begins with numbness and paresthesia, as well as motor weakness of both hands and feet. These effects then involve both arms and legs. Pathologically, it is characterized by distal axonopathy (chap. 17). The reactive metabolite of these two solvents is 2,5-hexanedione (Krasavage et al., 1980). Perchloroethylene (tetrachloroethylene) present in dry-cleaning fluids was found to produce central nervous system disturbances.

Hematopoietic System

Benzene is an outstanding example of a solvent affecting this system. It depresses bone marrow in animals and humans, thereby decreasing the circulating erythrocytes, leukocytes, and thrombocytes. In humans exposed to benzene, leukemia has been reported (Snyder, 2000).

Carcinogenesis

As noted above, a number of chlorinated hydrocarbons are known to produce liver tumors. Benzene is carcinogenic in animals and produces leukemia in humans. In addition, dioxane is also a liver carcinogen and produces nasopharyngeal cancers (Andrews and Snyder, 1996).

Diethylene glycol induced bladder tumors in rats fed with large doses of the solvent. In all the tumor-bearing rats, there were bladder stones that were composed of calcium oxalate, a metabolite of this chemical (Fitzhugh and Nelson, 1946). This solvent has thus been considered a secondary carcinogen (chap. 7). Chloroform (Group 2B, a possible human carcinogen) was reported to induce renal tumors only in male rats and mice (Meek et al., 2002) but appears to have a limited evidence for humans. Trichlorethylene (Group 2A, a probable human carcinogen) was found to induce renal tumors that are relevant for humans, whereas perchloroethylene (Group 2A, a probable human carcinogen) was shown to be a weak renal carcinogen.

Other Effects

Testicular degeneration and *cardiovascular abnormalities* have been observed in animals exposed to ethylene glycol monoethyl ether. Methanol may damage the *retina* through its metabolite and affect mainly the part that is responsible for central vision. Methylene chloride produces CNS depression and irritation to the eye and skin. However, it also induces *carboxy hemoglobinemia*, because CO is formed in the biotransformation (WHO, 1984). Chloroform may induce *cardiac arrhythmia*, probably as a result of sensitization of the myocardium to epinephrine. This is one of the reasons why chloroform has been discontinued as a general anesthetic.

It should be noted that certain solvents are practically nontoxic. For example, propylene glycol possesses low toxicities, with LD_{50} values of 32 and 18 mL/kg in rats and rabbits, respectively, and rats fed on this solvent at 1.8 mL/kg for two years showed no adverse effects. This chemical has thus been used as a food additive.

Metals

Metals are mined, smelted, refined, and processed for a great variety of uses. Workers are therefore exposed to metals and their compounds in many ways through their occupations. The target organs and the nature of toxicity, as described in chapter 23, depend on the metal and its chemical form. For example, elemental mercury vapor produces excitability, tremors, and gingivitis. On the other hand, the divalent mercuric chloride is corrosive on contact, whereas the monovalent mercurous chloride causes dermal vasodilatation, hyperkeratosis, and hypersecretion of the sweat gland.

Table 26.2   Toxic Effects and TLV-TWAs of Toxic Metals

Metals	Toxic Effects	TWA (mg/m^3)
Arsenic	Cancer (lung, skin)	0.01
Beryllium	Cancer (lung), berylliosis	0.002
Cadmium	Cancer (lung, prostate), kidney lesions	0.01
Metal Fume Fever		
Cr, metal and Cr III	Skin, irritation	0.5
Cr VI, soluble	Cancer, liver, kidney	0.05
Cr VI, insoluble		0.01
Lead	CNS, GI, blood, kidney, reproduction	0.05
Mercury		
Alkyl	CNS	0.01
Aryl	CNS, neuropathy, eye, kidney	0.1
Inorganic and elemental	CNS, neuropathy, eye	0.025
Nickel, elements	Skin	1.5
Soluble compounds	CNS, skin	0.1
Insoluble compounds	Cancer (lung)	0.2

Abbreviations: CNS, central nervous system; Cr, chromium; TLV, threshold limit value; TWA, time-weighted average. *Source*: From ACGIH (2000).

Table 26.2 lists the main toxic effects and/or target organs as well as the TLV-TWAs of a number of toxic metals. Additional details are provided in chapter 23.

Pesticides

Pesticides are widely used in agriculture and in public health programs to control vector-borne diseases. There are several types of pesticides, that is, insecticides, herbicides, fungicides, rodenticides, and fumigants.

The organochlorine insecticides include aldrin, chlordane, DDT, lindane, and methoxychlor. Their major adverse effects are on the CNS and liver. The organophosphorus insecticides, such as azinphos-methyl (guthion), diazinon, malathion, methyl parathion, and parathion, inhibit acetylcholinesterase (AChE). The inhibition of AChE in the central, peripheral, and autonomic nervous systems produces a variety of adverse effects, as described in chapter 21. Carbaryl, a carbamate insecticide, also inhibits AChE, but its effects are short lived.

The herbicides, 2,4-D and diquat, irritate the skin. Paraquat is stored in the lungs, hence it produces lung edema. The TLV-TWA for this chemical is much lower. The fungicide thiram produces skin irritation and may disturb reproductive function. The fumigant metam sodium produces allergic dermatitis and exacerbates asthma. The irritant effects are attributed to account for the observed neurotoxicity (Pruett et al., 2001).

Table 26.3 lists the main toxic effects and/or target organs as well as the TLV-TWA of the above-mentioned pesticides. Additional details on their toxicity are provided in chapter 21. Their acute toxicity in humans is listed in Appendix 1.

Table 26.3   Toxic Effects and TLV-TWAs of Certain Pesticides

Pesticides	Toxic Effects	TWA (mg/m^3)
Aldrin	Liver	0.25
Azinphos-methyl	AChE inhibition	0.2
Carbaryl	AChE inhibition	0.5
Chlordane	CNS, liver lesion	0.5
2,4-D	Skin irritation	10
DDT	CNS, liver lesion	1
Diazinon	AChE inhibition	0.1
Diquat	Irritation of eye, skin	0.5
Lindane	CNS, liver lesion	0.5
Malathion	AChE inhibition	10
Methoxychlor	CNS, liver lesion	10
Methyl parathion	AChE inhibition	0.2
Paraquat	Lung edema, kidney, liver	0.5
Parathion	AChE inhibition	0.1
Thiram	Skin irritation, reproduction	1

Abbreviations: AChE, acetylcholinesterase; CNS, central nervous system; Cr, chromium; DDT,; TLV, threshold limit value; TWA, time-weighted average.
Source: From ACGIH (2000).

Miscellaneous Toxicants

Particulate Matter

As noted above, particulate matter of sizes in the range of 0.01 to 10 μm ($PM_{0.01}$ to PM_{10}) are readily inhaled and exert adverse effects. A notable example is asbestos. It is widely used to provide thermal and acoustic insulation as well as fire protection, but produces pulmonary fibrosis (asbestosis), and cancers of the bronchus and mesotheliomas of the pleura and peritoneum (Vallyathan et al., 1998). Its TLV-TWA is "1 fiber/cm^3" (ACGIH, 2000).

Other common particulate matters include coal dust, kaolin, silica, and talc. All these substances may induce pulmonary fibrosis (Vallyathan et al., 1998). Coke oven emissions cause tracheobronchial cancers (Vallyathan et al., 1998). Tobacco smoking enhances the toxic effects of particulate matters, such as asbestos (see chap. 5) and cement dust (Table 26.4). Particulate matter is a complex mixture of different sizes, shapes, types, and chemical compositions (Donaldson et al., 2005). Exposure to particulate matter produced from combustion can induce oxidative damage to DNA and lipids (Møller and Loft, 2010) and was associated with cardiovascular and pulmonary diseases (Salvi and Barnes, 2009).

Gases

A number of gases, such as CO, CO_2, NO_2, O_3, and SO_2, are encountered in certain occupational settings. However, these also occur in the general environment, as described in chapter 25.

Table 26.4   Prevalence of Respiratory Symptoms in Cement Workers

Cement Dust Exposure	Smoking History	Prevalence of Respiratory Symptoms (%)	Ratio
−	−	1.6	1
−	+	3.3	2
+	−	9.0	5.6
+	+	11.7	7.3

Source: From Lu and Gu (1989).

Plastics

There are many types of plastics. They are polymerized monomers, with molecular weights generally in the range of 10,000–1,000,000 Da, hence are inert and nontoxic. However, some monomers are toxic. For example, vinyl chloride was reported to induce hepatic malignant tumors (angiosarcomas) among exposed workers (Creech and Johnson, 1974). Vinyl chloride may also produce cancer in the lung, skin, and lymphatic and hematopoietic tissues (WHO, 1999). Acrylamide, unlike other monomers, is readily absorbed through the skin and may induce peripheral neurotoxicity. After absorption it releases cyanide and induces CNS toxicity (Drew, 1993).

Among the additives, the catalyst benzoyl peroxide was found to promote the cancer on mouse skin initiated by genotoxic carcinogen (Slaga et al., 1981). Phthalates, used as plasticizers, produce proliferation of peroxisomes, thereby acting as nongenotoxic carcinogens (Rao and Reddy, 1987).

Toluene diisocyanate is used in the manufacture of flexible polyurethane foams, surface coatings, fibers, sealants, and adhesives. It is a potent irritant to the eyes, skin, and especially respiratory system, producing allergic asthma (Wilder et al., 2011). There is an immunologic component in this syndrome with an increased immunoglobulin E (Karol et al., 1994).

MONITORING

To ensure that the specified permissible exposure limits are complied with, both the workplace and some workers are monitored.

Workplace Monitoring

In general, using appropriate instruments, the air is monitored for concentrations of airborne pollutants. These include gases, vapors, dusts (total, inhalable, and respirable), fibers, liquid droplets, and smokes. For details see, for example, Gray (1993).

Biological Monitoring

Workers exposed to the same workplace environment may not be equally affected by, or even equally exposed to, the toxicants. This is due to differences in age, gender, body build, diet, medication, disease state, etc. In addition, there are differences in work intensity and duration, temperature, humidity, co-exposure to other chemicals, etc. (ACGIH, 2000). ACGIH has, therefore, published a number of biological exposure indices, values used for guidance to assess biological monitoring results. Human samples frequently used for biological monitoring include urine, blood, hair, feces, nail, expired air and human tissues. The commonly used methods involve monitoring of the exposure to the toxicants or their biological effects.

Effects

Inhibition of AChE in whole blood or plasma is a reliable, sensitive indicator of exposure to organophosphorus insecticides such as parathion and methyl parathion and the carbamates such as carbaryl.

Zinc protoporphyrin is a sensitive indicator of a minimal effect of lead. Carboxy hemoglobin is an indicator of the effect of CO.

Exposure

The levels of lead and mercury in blood are good indicators of the extent of exposure to these metals. The level of mercury in urine is also useful. As the volume of urine varies greatly from day to day and between different individuals, the level of mercury in urine is expressed in terms of microns per gram of creatinine, because a fairly constant amount of creatinine is excreted daily. The extent of exposure to benzene and carbon disulfide is also determined in urine and expressed in terms of microns per gram of creatinine.

Another type of monitoring measures the biochemical reaction products, such as mercapturic acids (N-acetyl-l-cysteine S-conjugates) in wine. This procedure has shown to be useful in monitoring benzene, acrolein, acrylamide, acrylonitrile, trichloroethane, etc. (DeRooij et al., 1998).

REFERENCES

ACGIH (2000). Threshold Limit Values for Chemical Substances and Biological Exposure Indices. Cincinnati, OH: Publications Office, American Conference of Governmental Industrial Hygienists.

Andrews LS, Lee EW, Witmer CM, et al. (1977). Effect of toluene on metabolism, disposition, and hematopoietic toxicity of (3H) benzene. Biochem Pharmacol 26, 293–300.

Andrews LS, Snyder R (1996). Toxic effects of solvents and vapors. In: Klaassen CD, ed. Casarett and Doull's Toxicology. New York, NY: McGraw-Hill.

Cole P, Hoover R, Friedell GH (1972). Occupation and cancer of the lower urinary tract. Cancer 29, 1250.

Creech JL, Johnson MN (1974). Angiosarcoma of the liver in the manufacture of PVC. J Occup Med 16, 150–1.

de Raat WK, Stevenson H, Hakkert BC, et al. (1997). Toxicological risk assessment of worker exposure to pesticides. some general principles. Reg Toxicol Pharmacol 25, 204–10.

DeRooij BM, Commandeur JNM, Vermeulen NPE (1998). Mercapturic acids as biomarkers of exposure to electrophilic chemicals: applications to environmental and industrial chemicals. Biomarkers 3, 239–303.

Donaldson K, Tran L, Jimenez LA, et al. (2005). Combustion-derived nanoparticles: a review of their toxicology following inhalation exposure. Part Fibre Toxicol 2, 1–14.

Drew R (1993). Toxicity of plastics. In: Stacey NH, ed. Occupational Toxicology. London, UK and Bristol, PA: Taylor & Francis.

Ecobichon DJ (1999). Occupational Hazards of Pesticide Exposure. Philadelphia, PA: Taylor & Francis.

Fitzhugh OG, Nelson AA (1946). Comparison of the chronic toxicity of triethylene glycol with that of diethylene glycol. J Ind Hyg Toxicol 28, 40–3.

Gray C (1993). Occupational hygiene-interface with toxicology. In: Stacey NT, ed. Occupational Toxicology. London, UK and Bristol, PA: Taylor & Francis, 269–93.

Karol MH, Tollerud DJ, Campbell TP, et al. (1994). Predictive value of airways hyper-responsiveness and circulating IgE for identifying types of responses to tolerance diisocyanate inhalation challenge. Am J Respir Cont Care Med 143, 611–15.

Krasavage WJ, O'Donoghue JL, DiVincenzo GD, et al. (1980). The relative neurotoxicity of methyl n-butyl ketone, n-hexane and their metabolites. Toxicol Appl Pharmacol 52, 433–41.

Lu PL, Gu XQ (1989). New challenges for occupational health services facing economic reform in China. Biomed Environ Sci 2, 17–23.

Meek ME, Beauchamp R, Long G, et al. (2002). Chloroform: exposure estimation, hazard characterization and exposure–response analysis. J Toxicol Environ Health B 5, 283–334.

Meyer KH (1937). Contributions to the theory of narcosis. Faraday Soc Transl 33, 1062–4.

Møller P, Loft S (2010). Oxidative damage to DNA and lipids as biomarkers of exposure to air pollution. Environ Health Perspect. 118, 1126–36.

Pruett SB, Myers LP, Keil DE (2001). Toxicology of metam sodium. J Toxicol Environ Health B 4, 207–22.

Rao MS, Reddy JK (1987). Peroxisome proliferators and cancer: mechanisms and implications. Carcinogenesis 8, 631–6.

Reid WD, Krishna G (1973). Centrolobular hepatic necrosis related to covalent binding of metabolites of halogenated aromatic hydrocarbons. Exp Med Pathol 18, 80–99.

Salvi SS, Barnes PJ (2009). Chronic obstructive pulmonary disease in nonsmokers. Lancet 374, 733–43.

Slaga TW, Klein-Szanto AJP, Triplett LL, et al. (1981). Skin promoting activity of benzoyl peroxide, a widely used free radical generating compound. Science 213, 1023–5.

Snyder R (2000). Overview of the toxicology of benzene. J Toxicol Environ Health A 61, 339–46.

Vallyathan V, Green F, Ducatman B, et al. (1998). Roles of epidemiology, pathology, molecular biology and biomarkers in the investigation of occupational lung cancer. J Toxicol Environ Health B 1, 91–116.

WHO (1984). Methylene chloride. Environ Health Criteria 32. Geneva, Switzerland: World Health Organization.

WHO (1999). Vinyl chloride. Environ Health Criteria 215. Geneva, Switzerland: World Health Organization.

WHO (2000). Human exposure assessment. Environ Health Criteria 214. Geneva, Switzerland: World Health Organization.

Wilder LC, Langley RL, Middleton DC, et al. (2011). Communities near toluene diisocyanate sources: an investigation of exposure and health. J Expo Sci Environ Epidemiol 21, 587–94.

Appendix 1   Acute Pesticide Toxicity, General Signs, and Symptoms in Humans

Pesticide	Symptoms and signs
Insecticides	
Organophosphates, carbamates	*Mild*: headache, dizziness, perspiration, lacrimation, salivation, blurred vision, tightness in chest, twitching of muscles in eyelids, lips, tongue, face
	Moderate: abdominal cramps, nausea, vomiting, diarrhea, bronchial hypersecretions, bradycardia or tachycardia, muscle (skeletal) spasms, tremors, general weakness
	Severe: pinpoint pupils, profuse sweating, urinary and/or fecal incontinence, mental confusion, pulmonary edema, respiratory difficulty, cyanosis, progressive cardiac and respiratory failure, and unconsciousness leading to coma
Organochlorines	*Mild*: systemically, toxic action is confined to the central nervous system with stimulation resulting in dizziness, nausea, vomiting, headache, and disorientation
	Moderate to severe: hyperexcitability, apprehension, weakness of skeletal muscles, incoordination, tremors, seizures, coma, and respiratory failure (progressive clinical findings related to severity of poisoning)
Pyrethroids	Generally of low toxicity but can cause irritation of oral and nasal mucosa. Some agents cause dermal tingling, stinging, or burning sensation followed by numbness (paresthesia). Facial contamination results in lacrimation, pain, photophobia, congestion, and edema of eyelids and conjunctiva
	Ingestion of large amounts may cause salivation, epigastric pain, nausea, vomiting, headache, dizziness, fatigue, coarse muscular twitching in limbs, convulsive seizures, loss of consciousness
Herbicides	
Bipyridyls	Irritation of nose and throat, hemorrhage, eye irritation with conjunctivitis and corneal stripping, skin irritation, and dermatitis
	Ingestion results in initial signs of ulceration of tongue, throat, and esophagus; sternal and abdominal pain; general muscular pain; vomiting; and diarrhea. After 48–72 hr, signs of renal and hepatic damage (oliguria, jaundice), respiratory difficulty (cough, dyspnea, tachypnea, pulmonary edema), and progressive respiratory failure

(continued)

Appendix 1   Acute Pesticide Toxicity, General Signs, and Symptoms in Humans (*continued*)

Pesticide	Symptoms and signs

Phenoxy acids
  Urea
  Triazines
  Chloroaliphatics
  Aryl carbamates
	Generally of low toxicity but, during handling, may cause irritation of eye, nose, throat, and skin. Ingestion may cause gastroenteritis, nausea, vomiting, diarrhea. Respiratory symptoms include burning sensation, cough, and chest pain. Muscle weakness and muscle twitching may be encountered, and central nervous system signs include dizziness, weakness, anorexia, and lethargy

Fungicides
  Dithiocarbamates
  Phenolics
  Chlorobenzenes
  Benzimidazoles
  Thiophanate
	Generally of low toxicity but local contamination of skin may cause itching, rash, and dermatitis. Ingestion of large amounts may cause nausea, vomiting, diarrhea, and muscle weakness. The dithiocarbomates exert a disulfiram-like effect in the presence of alcohol, causing flushing, sweating, dyspnea, hyperpnea, chest pains, and hypotension

Rodenticides
  Fluorinated agents
  Zinc phosphide
  Strychnine
  α-Naphthyl
    thiourea
  Anticoagulants
	Accidental rodenticide poisoning is difficult to achieve because agents are packaged as baits attractive only to the pest. When ingested, these agents may cause nausea, vomiting, intestinal cramps, diarrhea, excitation, abnormal cardiac rhythms, muscle spasms, and seizures. The anticoagulants require laboratory assessment of coagulation status and treatment with vitamin K_1

Source: From Ecobichon (1999).

27

Toxicological evaluation

INTRODUCTION

Importance and Reasonableness

Descriptions in prior chapters make it abundantly clear that chemicals differ greatly in the nature and potency of their toxicity. Because human exposure to chemicals is not always avoidable (it may even be desirable in certain cases), toxicological evaluation of many chemicals must be carried out to determine the level of exposure (or intake in the case of food and water) under which no risk is likely to occur. A comprehensive review by Paustenbach (2000) covers risk assessment. Because of the gaps in our knowledge, it is prudent to be conservative in assessing the safety and risk. But when undue caution is incorporated into the process, the public may be denied chemicals of great value and society may be burdened with unnecessary economic costs, such as pollution prevention measures and environmental cleanup. Therefore, the most important function of toxicology is to establish the scientific basis for regulating the use (and disposal) of chemicals without undue human health hazards or undue cost.

Historical Development

Around the turn of the century, industrialization and urbanization prompted individuals to move from their farms to cities. Away from the farm, they had to consume stored and processed food. Food adulteration became a serious problem. In the United States, the first U.S. Food and Drug Act was enacted in 1906. Similar action was taken in several other countries. At that time, health hazards were based essentially on *qualitative* assessment; the mere presence of a toxic substance in food was considered adulteration and "adulterated" food was banned outright.

To permit judicious use of food additives, Lehman and Fitzhugh of the U.S. Food and Drug Administration initiated in 1954 a *quantitative* assessment by the use of a "100-fold margin of safety" approach. This assessment of food additives stipulated that "the chemical additive should not occur in the total human diet in a quantity greater than 1/100 of the amount that is the maximum safe dosage in long-term animal experiments" (Lehman and Fitzhugh, 1954).

Although this margin of 100 seemed reasonable for food additives, it could not be applied to other chemicals, such as contaminants and pesticide residues, whose levels in food are not readily controllable. Furthermore, it is impracticable on an international level as there will be marked differences among nations, both in dietary pattern and technological usage. In 1961, the Joint Food and Agricultural Organization/World Health Organization (FAO/WHO) Expert Committee on Food Additives (JECFA) therefore coined the term *acceptable daily intake* (ADI). Later that year, this term was adopted by the Joint FAO/WHO Meeting on Pesticide Residues.

In 1977, the U.S. National Research Council extended the concept to the assessment of contaminants in water, and Environmental Protection Agency (EPA) extended it to pollutants in air, with slight variation in the terminology.

In carcinogenic chemicals the Delaney Amendment of 1958 to the Federal Food, Drug, and Cosmetic Act stipulates that "*any chemical that has been shown to be carcinogenic in man or animal shall not be used as a food additive.*" For other chemicals such as veterinary drugs, the concept of "negligible residues" was introduced to regulate carcinogenic chemicals. As will be seen in subsequent sections, these measures were no panacea. Mathematical models were then devised to estimate doses that could be considered as "virtually safe" (Mantel and Bryan, 1961).

NRC (1983) divided the management of risk assessment into the following steps:

Hazard identification: scrutinizing all relevant toxicological and related data to identify the hazard associated with a chemical.
Dose–response assessment: determining the relationship between the magnitude of
the exposure and the probability of adverse health effects.
Exposure assessment: determining the extent of human exposure.
Risk characterization: estimating the nature and magnitude of human risk, and the
uncertainty of the estimate.

MAJOR APPROACHES

At high enough doses, all chemicals produce toxic effects. As the dose is reduced, the severity of the effects as well as the responses diminishes. For a majority of the chemicals, there are threshold doses below which they will not elicit adverse effects. There are a variety of reasons for the thresholds. The chemical in question may not reach the site of action because of its limited absorption and distribution or its prompt elimination. Metabolic detoxication often plays an important role. Furthermore, repair and regeneration of affected cells and excess functional capacity may overcome/compensate any minor, temporary effects.

The "safety" of such chemicals can be estimated by using the "acceptable daily intake" approach, which involves identification of the most sensitive, yet *appropriate*, indicator of adverse effect and the application of a suitable safety factor to the no-observed-adverse-effect level (NOAEL) to compensate for potential differences between animals and humans, and between the relatively small number of test subjects and the large human population which are more heterogeneous.

Genotoxic carcinogens, on the other hand, probably have no threshold doses. The rationale is that a cancer cell can be induced by a single change in the cellular genetic material, and the cancer cell has the capacity of self-replicating. Therefore, theoretically, a single molecule of such a chemical can induce cancer. In the absence of threshold doses, it will be impossible to identify a no-adverse-effect level, thus rendering the ADI approach impracticable. Mathematical models have been designed to estimate, from the dose–response relationship and a variety of assumptions, a "virtually safe dose (VSD)," exposure to which will result in an extremely small risk, say 10^{-6} (one risk in a million).

ACCEPTABLE DAILY INTAKE/REFERENCE DOSES/SAFETY ASSESSMENT

Definition and Usage

As has already been noted, the term ADI was coined by the JECFA in 1961 (WHO, 1962a). It has been adopted by the Joint FAO/WHO Meeting of Experts on Pesticide Residues (WHO, 1962b). This term has been used at all subsequent meetings of these two international expert bodies in their toxicological evaluation, and reevaluation, of large numbers of food additives and pesticides that leave residues in food. The term has also been adopted by a number of other bodies in the toxicological evaluation of chemicals in food, water, and so on as a basis for setting standards, for example, U.S. EPA (Cotruvos, 1988).

ADI is defined as "the daily intake of a chemical which, during an entire lifetime, appears to be without appreciable risk on the basis of all the known facts at the time." It is expressed in milligrams of the chemical per kilogram of body weight (mg/kg). It is worth noting that the ADI is qualified by the expressions "appear to be" and "on the basis of all the known facts at the time." This caution is in keeping with the fact that it is impossible to be absolutely certain about the safety of a chemical and that the ADI may be altered in the light of new toxicological data.

Toxicological evaluations of food additives and pesticides, in terms of ADIs by these international expert bodies, have been used by the regulatory agencies in many countries as an important consideration in the formulation of national regulations. ADIs have also been used collectively by national authorities in the framework of the Codex Alimentarius Commission. The Commission is an intergovernmental body with more than 150 countries as its members. Its principal function is to elaborate international food standards for the protection of the health of the consumer and to facilitate international food trade. These food standards contain provisions for food additives that are accepted by the Commission only when ADIs have been allocated by the Expert Committee on Food Additives. The latter goal is achieved through the removal of "noneconomic" trade barriers based on unjustified claims of health hazards alleged to be associated with certain additives or pesticides. Additional details about the Codex Alimentarius Commission are given in an article by Lu (1988). The close relationship between the Commission, member governments, academia, and industry are shown in Figure 27.3.

There are a number of variations of the terminology. For instance, in dealing with food contaminants, the JECFA in 1972 coined the term "provisional tolerable weekly intake." The procedure used in arriving at such intakes is identical to that for ADIs. The JECFA Committee, however, felt that, unlike food additives, which serves certain useful purposes, contaminants do not. Therefore they are not acceptable but merely "tolerable." Furthermore, the intakes were expressed in terms of "weekly" because the contaminants dealt then (mercury, lead, and cadmium) were cumulative, and vary (especially mercury) in the *daily* intake, but less so on a *weekly* basis.

Another variation is used by U.S. EPA, which assesses "Reference Doses" (RfDs) instead of ADIs, by using essentially the same procedure, except that the safety factor is called "uncertainty factor (UF)." It might be noted that the term ADI is widely used on an international level as well as by regulatory agencies in many nations, including U.S. FDA.

Procedures for Estimating ADIs

The steps involved in estimating ADIs are discussed in detail.

Collection of Adequate Relevant Data

As noted in previous chapters, chemicals produce different toxicities. Consequently, a great variety of toxicity studies must be done (see chap. 20). Furthermore, pharmacokinetic studies facilitate the assessment of the effects on humans from findings obtained in experimental animals. In addition, the data must be obtained from *relevant* studies. For example, findings of epithelial hyperplasia in the forestomach of rats given an irritant fumigant by gavage have little, if any, bearing on the possible adverse effects on humans consuming food that has been fumigated by the fumigant (see Lu and Coulston, 1996).

The assessment of certain chemicals required less data for establishing their ADIs. Examples are food additives obtained from edible animals, plants, and microbes. The extent of testing and the reasons thereof have been described by WHO (1987).

No-Observed-Adverse-Effect Level

This is the maximum dose level that has not induced any sign of toxicity (adverse effect) in the most susceptible but appropriate species of animals tested, and using the most sensitive indicator of toxicity. As a rule, this level is selected from a long-term study. However, certain signs of toxicity such as cataract, delayed neurotoxicity, and effects on reproduction are demonstrable in short-term studies. The NOAEL is not necessarily an absolutely no-effect level; rather it is a "no-observed-adverse-effect-level," because the use of a more sensitive indicator of toxicity or a more susceptible animal species may reveal a lower NOAEL. Hence these chemicals are reassessed whenever significant new toxicological data become available. In addition, an effect might well be demonstrable if a sufficiently large number of animals were used in the tests. However, using experimental data and mathematical extrapolation, Lu (1985) and Lu and Seilken (1991) showed that increasing the number of animals would only reduce the NOAEL slightly. It should also be noted that part of the safety factor is intended to compensate for the limited number used in most tests.

On the other hand, certain effects are generally considered as physiological, adaptive, or otherwise "nontoxic." These effects are therefore excluded in establishing the NOAEL. For example, liver enlargement may result from stimulation in the activity of hepatic mixed-function oxidases and the *de novo* protein synthesis in the smooth endoplasmic reticulum. A decrease of body weight may follow reduced food consumption, which in turn may be a result of unpalatability of the feed due to the chemical. The U.S. EPA has designated that a change in body-weight greater than 10% denotes a relevant adverse manifestation that needs to be considered in the risk assessment. Feeding large amounts of inert substances such as mannitol and cellulose derivatives may produce diarrhea and malnutrition. However, before disregarding these effects in evaluating the toxicity of a chemical, care must be taken to ensure that these are not manifestations of toxicity. Additional studies may have to be done to elucidate the nature of the effect. These various points have been elaborated in several WHO reports and summarized in a review article (Lu, 1988).

NOAEL has been traditionally used for the estimation of ADI, RfD, and tolerable daily intake, but the NOAEL approach cannot provide information about the shape of dose–response curve, and is strictly dependent on the dose selection, dose interval, and sample size. Therefore, a benchmark dose (BMD) model was alternatively introduced and BMD software programs are now available (Davis et al., 2011). In general, the BMD and BMD 95% lower confidence limit were higher than the NOAEL, but lower than the lowest-observed-adverse-effect level (Izadi et al., 2012).

Safety Factors

To extrapolate from the NOAEL in animals to an acceptable intake in humans, a safety factor of at least 100 is generally used (10 for individual variation in humans, 10 for the differences between humans and animals on the basis of a chronic study). This was originally proposed by Lehman and Fitzhugh (1954). This factor is intended to allow for differences in sensitivity of the animal species and humans, to allow for wide variations in susceptibility among the human population, and to allow for the fact that the number of animals tested is small compared to the size of the human population that may be exposed (WHO, 1958, 1974a; Food Safety Council, 1973).

Although the factor 100 is often used, the WHO expert committees have used figures that ranged from 10 to 2000. The size of the safety factor is determined according to the nature of the toxicity, the period of treatment (acute, subacute, chronic), and the quality of data. Therefore, additional modifying factors (MFs) from 3 to 10 can be multiplied by SF 100 to get the final value of safety factor (i.e., the final SF = MF × SF 100). In addition, a larger figure is used to compensate for slight deficiencies in toxicity data, such as relatively small numbers of animals on test. On the other hand, minimal, reversible, and inconsequential effects such as slight inhibition of acetylcholinesterase by an organophosphorus pesticide may justify the use of a smaller safety factor. In addition, available human data may warrant the use of a smaller figure, for example 10, since they obviate the need for interspecies extrapolation.

Biochemical data relating to the absorption, distribution, metabolism (detoxication and bioactivation) and excretion of the toxicant in various species of animals and in humans are often useful in determining the size of the safety factor. These and other bases for altering the safety factor are elaborated in two WHO documents (WHO, 1987, 1990). The reasons for the use of different safety factors, by WHO in the evaluation/re-evaluation of the 230 pesticides in the past three decades, are noted and explained in a review by Lu (1995).

Some toxicologists prefer the use of individual uncertainty (safety) factors in extrapolating from a NOAEL to the corresponding oral RfD. These usually include a factor of 10 for intra-species differences, a 10 for interspecies differences, a 10 for NOAEL derived from short-term toxicity studies, etc. (Dourson and Stara, 1983).

Assessment of Exposure Acceptability

The ADI is used as a yardstick to check the acceptability of the proposed uses. This is done by comparing the ADI with the "potential daily intake" (PDI). PDI is the sum of the products of the amounts of the food (calculated on the basis of the average per capita consumption) and the permitted use levels of the additives in them.

$$1PDI = (F_1 \times L_1) + (F_2 \times L_2) + (F_3 \times L_3) \dots$$ where F_1, F_2, F_3,... are per capita consumption of food commodities and L_1, L_2, L_3,... are use levels of food additives, or maximum residue levels of pesticide residues or other contaminants.

If the PDI exceeds the ADI, the use levels may be lowered or some of the uses may be deleted. The Commission follows the same procedure in accepting the maximum limits for pesticide residues in food. The use of the "PDI" and other estimated intakes by WHO in assessing the acceptability of food additives and pesticides is provided in some detail in a document WHO (1989) and summarized by Lu and Seilken (1991).

Margin of Safety

The ADI approach is not designed to provide quantitative information on the risks involved with intakes higher than the ADI. This is because of the wide "gray area" between the NOAEL and the ADI. However, the margin of safety (MOS) between the estimated intake and the ADI is sometimes used to indicate the degree of confidence in the safety at a specified intake. In general, the MOS should be greater than 100 to ensure human safety on the basis of SF 100 (10 for human variation and 10 for the difference between humans and animals), and lower values are considered unsafe for humans. This MOS approach has been often used for the risk assessment of consumer products including cosmetics.

MATHEMATICAL MODELS/RISK ASSESSMENT

As discussed in chapter 7, there are genotoxic and nongenotoxic carcinogens. It is generally agreed that there are probably no thresholds for genotoxic carcinogens. In view of the theoretical absence of threshold doses and in the absence of a reliable procedure to determine a threshold for a carcinogen for an entire population, estimating the levels of risk has been considered to be more appropriate.

Estimation of Risks

Definition

Risk has been defined as the expected frequency of undesirable effects arising from exposure to a pollutant or the probability that a substance will produce harm in humans under the specified condition. It may be expressed in absolute terms as the risk due to exposure to a specific pollutant. It may also be expressed as a relative risk, which is the ratio of the risk among the exposed population to that among the unexposed (WHO, 1978).

The term was first adopted by the International Commission on Radiological Protection (ICRP, 1966) in evaluating the health hazards related to ionizing radiation. The use of this term stems from the realization that often a clear-cut "safe" or "unsafe" decision cannot be made.

Risks Levels and Virtual Safety

Estimation of risks involves development of suitable dose–response data and extrapolation from the observed dose–response relationship to the expected responses at doses occurring at actual exposure situations. A number of mathematical models have been proposed for this purpose. Such models are also used to estimate the dose that is expected to be associated with a specific level of risk.

Mantel and Bryan (1961) first introduced the concept of virtual safety. The term was defined as a probability of carcinogenicity of less than 1/100 million (10^{-8}) at a statistical assurance level of 99%. The U.S. FDA, however, found that the doses associated with such a low risk level were too small to be enforceable in most actual situations and thus adopted a risk level of 10^{-6} (FDA, 1977). These levels of risk are so low that the doses associated with them are referred to as VSDs.

Commonplace Activities and Their Risks

In order to place the risk levels in perspective, risks associated with certain commonplace activities and natural occurrences are sometimes cited. Table 27.1 includes a number of estimates of such risks. The risks in Table 27.1, apart from lightning, are considerably greater than 10^{-6}. Estimates of risks associated with other common activities and occupations have been compiled by others, for example, Wilson (1980).

The acceptability of a risk depends on, apart from its magnitude, the nature of the activity. In general, risks associated with voluntary, pleasurable, and/or beneficial activities, such as smoking and driving, are more acceptable to the individual. On the other hand, risks associated with activities that are perceived as having no benefit and those that are not controllable by the individual tend to be rejected, such as food colors suspected of being carcinogenic.

Models for Estimating Risk/ Virtually Safe Dose

A number of mathematical models have been developed for the purpose of estimating the risks. In general, they involve extrapolating from the observed dose response to either of the following:

1. The risks at a specific exposure level.
2. The "risk-specific dose" is the dose associated with a specified risk. When the specified risk is low enough, for example, 10^{-5} or 10^{-6}, the dose associated with it is generally known as the VSD.

Table 27.1   Estimated Risks for Certain Activities and Natural Occurrences

Activity	Risk[a]
Smoking (10 cigarettes/day)	1/400
All accidents	1/2000
Driving (16,000 km/yr)	1/5000
All traffic accidents	1/8000
Work in industry	1/30,000
Natural disasters	1/50,000
Being struck by lightning	1/1,000,000

[a]Risk is expressed as probability of death of an individual for a year of exposure and is given in round figures.
Source: Courtesy of the Controller of Her Majesty's Stationery Office, London.

Probability Models

As noted above, Mantel and Bryan (1961) first introduced the concept of virtual safety and developed a model based on the assumption that the responses (tumor formation) will be the same as most other quantal (all-or-none) toxicological responses, namely, normally distributed among the subjects.

This S-shaped dose–response curve can be straightened, as described in chapter 6, by plotting the points on a *probit* basis. Variations of this probit model include *logit* and *Weibull*. These are also known as "tolerance models," as they are based on the probability of individuals in a population whose tolerances to the carcinogen will be exceeded.

Mechanistic Models

Several other models have been designed based on presumed mechanisms of action of carcinogenesis. The *one-hit* model assumes that a critical hit in a cell by a carcinogen may induce a cancer through initiation, promotion, and progression. On the other hand, the *multihit* model assumes that several hits are required for a response to occur. The *multistage* model is built on the assumption that the induction of a carcinogenic response follows random biological events, the time rate of occurrence of each event being in linear proportion to the dose rate.

The conservativeness of these models is achieved through the use of upper confidence limits to responses on the risk estimated, shallow slopes, or the lower confidence limits on the VSD estimated. Figure 27.1 shows the observed responses, the upper confidence limit, and the linear interpolation.

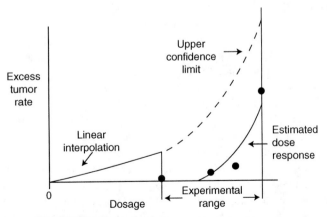

Figure 27.1   Linear extrapolation showing the observed responses, the upper confidence limit of the response at the lowest experimental dose, and the linear interpolation. *Source*: From Gaylor and Kodell (1980).

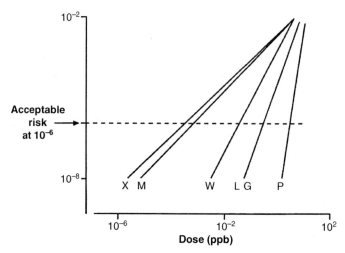

Figure 27.2   The low dose–response relationships based on a set of aflatoxin B$_1$ data, using different models: X, one-hit; M, multistage; W, Weibull; L, logit; G, multihit; and P, probit models. *Source*: From Krewski and Van Ryzin (1981).

Several U.S. regulatory agencies, including EPA (1986), use the linearized multistage model (Anderson, 1986). With this model, it is presumed that no threshold dose exists, a multistage process (i.e., initiation, promotion, and progression) is involved in chemical carcinogenesis, and the time rate of occurrence of each event is linearly proportional to the dose.

Based on a set of aflatoxin B$_1$ carcinogenesis data, low-dose extrapolation was done with various models. The marked difference among them is clearly visible in Figure 27.2. The one-hit and multistage models yielded the most conservative estimates, whereas the probit model yields the least conservative figure. According to the calculations of the Food Safety Council (1980), the VSDs at a risk of 10^{-6} are 3.4 × 10^{-5} ppb (one-hit), 7.9 × 10^{-4} (multistage), 4.0 × 10^{-2} (Weibull), 0.28 (multihit), and 2.5 (probit), respectively.

In addition, *physiologically based pharmacokinetic* modeling has been developed to utilize toxicokinetic differences between the test animals and humans. For example, the target concentration of dichloromethane was about 150-fold higher in mice than in humans; these data provided a much lower, probably more realistic estimate of the risk of this toxicant (Andersen et al., 1987). For additional examples, see Andersen and Krishnan (1994), and Dallas et al. (1995). A modified version, the *biologically based pharmacodynamic* model, also incorporates data on the interaction of the toxicant with tissues and the response of the tissues (Conolly and Andersen, 1991). Although such modeling has certain advantages, it involves complex mathematical equations and the fact that the physiolog-

Table 27.2 Correlation Between Exposure Concentration of Vinyl Chloride (VC), Metabolism, and Induction of Hepatic Angiosarcoma in Rats

Exposure Concentration (ppm of VC)	VC/L of Air (μg)	VC Metabolized (μg)	Percentage Liver Angiosarcoma
50	128	739	2
250	640	2435	7
500	1280	3413	12
2500	6400	5030	22
6000	15,360	5003	22
10,000	25,600	5521	15

Source: From Gehring et al. (1978).

ical parameters regarding various species and strains, disease states, and the like are often ill defined.

Other Variation

The *time-to-response*, instead of the response itself, has also been proposed for the use in the mathematical models (Chand and Hoel, 1974; Sielken, 1981). The importance of this approach has been pointed out by the SOT ED01 Task Force (1981). *Background responses*, that is, those occurring also among the unexposed, are often observed. They can also be incorporated into mathematical models (Hoel, 1980).

The response of an organism to a toxicant is related to the dose and the duration of exposure. It is also affected by *competing risks*. Kalbfleisch et al. (1983) proposed mathematical models that will take these three factors into account.

Since many carcinogens require bioactivation, the importance of incorporating *metabolic data* in evaluating their risks is obvious. For example, vinyl chloride is carcinogenic after bioactivation. Gehring et al. (1978) showed that the tumor incidence in rats exposed to various concentrations of this chemical was proportional to the metabolized amount rather than the exposure concentration (Table 27.2).

Risk Assessment

Risk assessment is done by estimating the risk associated with a toxicant at an ascertained level of exposure, using an appropriate mathematical model described earlier. Where the risk level is low, for example, 10^{-6} or lower, the exposure might be considered acceptable. However, where the risk is higher, various *risk management* decisions may have to be taken. The options consist of lowering the exposure level, shortening the exposure duration, suspending the manufacture/use of chemical, and others.

OTHER PROCEDURES

Noncarcinogenic Chemicals

Not all chemicals require the whole gamut of toxicological testing as described for estimating ADIs. For example, for chemicals to which humans are not likely to be exposed to an appreciable extent, such as indirect food additives and certain pesticides, a *toxicologically insignificant amount* may be estimated on the basis of toxicological data that include at least 90-day feeding studies in two species of mammals and by the use of a larger safety factor (generally 1000) (NAS, 1965). Variations of this principle have been adopted by U.S. FDA and U.S. EPA administratively.

Furthermore, a *decision to reject a chemical* may be made on much more limited data, especially in the course of developing new chemicals. Such data include extreme acute toxicity, positive response in short-term mutagenesis tests, or undesirable features in biochemical studies or short-term feeding studies in animals.

As discussed in the next section, most, if not all, of the nongenotoxic carcinogens are assessed by the ADI approach.

Carcinogenic Chemicals

Chemicals with Questionable Data

The Joint FAO/WHO Expert Committee on Food Additives at its second meeting (WHO, 1958) recommended that "no proved carcinogen should be considered suitable for use as a food additive in any amount." This principle has been followed at subsequent meetings of the Committee and at the Joint FAO/WHO Meetings on Pesticide Residues in not allocating ADIs to proved carcinogens by IARC. *Temporary or conditional ADIs*, however, have been estimated for chemicals with equivocal carcinogenicity data, such as nitrites and amitrole. On the other hand, *discontinuation* of the use of chemicals without essential functions has been recommended. The basis for the decisions on these and other such chemicals has been reviewed and summarized (Lu, 1979). The principle of considering both the soundness of the carcinogenesis data and the usefulness of the chemical is consistent with the policies of many national regulatory agencies (e.g., Somers, 1986).

Secondary and Nongenotoxic Carcinogens

The concept of *secondary carcinogens*, which induce tumors only after certain noncarcinogenic effects, has been accepted by many toxicologists. For example, a WHO scientific group (WHO, 1974b) pointed out that the urinary bladder cancers in rats treated with Myrj 45 (polyoxyethylene monostearate) were induced by the bladder calculi rather than by the chemical directly and that a no-observed-effect level can therefore be established. A variety of other types of nongenotoxic carcinogens have been discussed in chapter 7. Many investigators (e.g., Reitz et al., 1990) have suggested that the predominant mechanism whereby a chemical elicits a carcinogenic response should be considered in extrapolating laboratory data to humans.

INTERNATIONAL ACTIVITIES IN TOXICOLOGICAL EVALUATION

Chemicals in Food

As noted in chapter 20, the World Health Organization and the Food and Agricultural Organization of the United Nations have jointly established the Joint FAO/WHO Expert on Food Additives and Contaminants (JECFA) and the Joint FAO/WHO Meeting on Pesticide Residues (JMPR). JECFA deals with food additives, contaminants, and residues of veterinary drugs, and JMPR deals with residues of pesticides.

The principles of evaluation followed by these two expert bodies, culminating in the assessment of ADIs, are described in detail in two WHO documents (WHO, 1987, 1990). An outline of the principles, along with the historical background of these expert bodies, is provided by Lu (1988). In this article, Lu emphasized two factors contributing to the wide acceptance of the ADIs assessed by JECFA and JMPR. First, there exists a close collaboration between these expert bodies and the research scientists in academia, government, and industry. Second, the ADIs assessed by these expert bodies are used as a basis in the elaboration of international food standards, the Codex Alimentarius. Figure 27.3 depicts the relationship between JMPR and research scientists and that between JMPR and the Codex Alimentarius Commission. Similar relationships exist for JECFA. Copies of the Codex Alimentarius and the Procedural Manual of the Codex Alimentarius Commission are available from FAO, Rome, Italy.

Other Chemicals

WHO, in conjunction with United Nations Environment Program (UNEP), and International Labor Organization (UNEP) have compiled, evaluated, and published more than 200 documents in the "Environmental Health Criteria" series. In general, they deal with subjects such as identity, sources of human exposure, environmental transport, environmental levels, and human exposure, kinetics, and metabolism in animals and humans, effects on laboratory animals and in-vitro systems, effects on humans, and evaluation of human health risks. These topics are critical reviews and summaries of the literature, and citations of references. These documents are thus a good source of toxicological and related topics on environmental and occupational toxicants.

As air, water, and soil are not traded internationally, definitive toxicological assessments are, in general, not included in these documents.

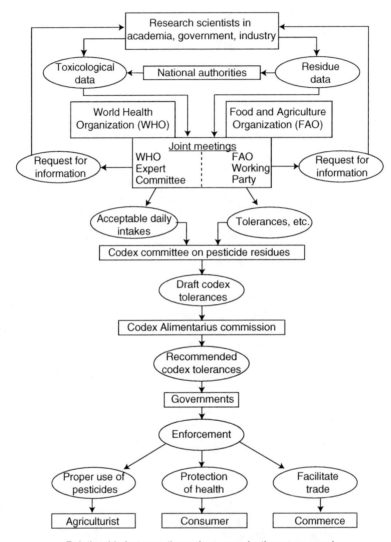

Relationship between the various organizations concerned
with the evaluation and control of pesticide residues

Figure 27.3 The elaborate procedure involved in the allocation of acceptable daily intakes and tolerances (maximum residue levels) of pesticides (or other food chemicals) by the expert committee as well as the inputs from worldwide research scientists are depicted in the upper part of the diagram. The lower part outlines the role of the governments of member states of the intergovernmental organization, the Codex Alimentarius Commission, as well as their impact on the consumer and others. A similar arrangement exists for the handling of food additives and contaminants. *Source*: From Lu (1988).

REFERENCES

Andersen ME, Clewell HJ, Gargas ML, et al. (1987). Physiologically based pharmacokinetics and risk assessment process for methylene chloride. Toxicol Appl Pharmacol 87, 185–205.

Andersen ME, Krishnan K (1994). Physiologically based pharmacokinetics and cancer risk assessment. Environ Health Perspect 102(Suppl. 1), 103–8.

Anderson P (1986). Ninth Symposium on Statistics and the Environment. Washington, DC.: National Academy of Sciences.

Chand N, Hoel W (1974). A comparison of models for determining safe levels of environmental agents. In: Proschan F, Serfling RJ, eds. Reliability and Biometry. Philadelphia, PA: SIAM, 681.

Conolly RB, Andersen ME (1991). Biologically based pharmacodynamic models: tools for toxicological research and risk assessment. Ann Rev Pharmacol Toxicol 31, 503–23.

Cotruvos JA (1988). Drinking water standards and risk assessment. Regul Toxicol Pharmacol 8, 288–99.

Dallas CE, Chen XM, Muraledhara S, et al. (1995). Physiologically based pharmacokinetic model useful in prediction of the influence of species, dose, and exposure route on perchloroethylene pharmacokinetics. J Toxicol Environ Health 44, 301–17.

Davis JA, Gift JS, Zhao QJ (2011). Introduction to benchmark dose methods and U.S. EPA's benchmark dose software (BMDS) version 2.1.1. Toxicol Appl Pharmacol 254, 181–91.

Dourson ML, Stara JF (1983). Regulatory history and experimental support of uncertainty (safety) factors. Regul Toxicol Pharmacol 3, 224–38.

FDA (1977). Chemical compounds in food-producing animals: criteria and procedures for evaluating assays for carcinogenic residues in edible products of animals. Fed Regul 42(35), 10412–37.

EPA (1986). Guides for carcinogenic risk assessment. Fed Regul 51, 33992–4003.

Food Safety Council (1973). Proposed system for food safety assessment. Food Cosmet Toxicol 16, 1–136.

Food Safety Council (1980). Proposed system for food safety assessment. Food Cosmet Toxicol 16(Suppl. 2).

Gaylor DW, Kodell RL (1980). Linear interpolation algorithm for low dose risk assessment of toxic substances. J Environ Pathol Toxicol 4, 305–12.

Gehring PJ, Watanabe PC, Park CN (1978). Resolution of dose–response toxicity for chemicals requiring metabolic activation: example vinyl chloride. Toxicol Appl Pharmacol 44, 581–91.

Hoel DG (1980). Incorporation of background in dose–response models. Fed Proc 39, 73–5.

ICRP (1966). Recommendations of the International Commission on Radiological Protection. ICRP Publication No. 9. Oxford: Pergamon Press.

Izadi H, Grundy JE, Bose R (2012). Evaluation of the benchmark dose for point of departure determination for a variety of chemical classes in applied regulatory settings. Risk Anal 32, 830–5.

Kalbfleisch JD, Krewski D, van Ryzin J (1983). Dose–response models for time to response toxicity data. Can J Stat 11, 25–49.

Krewski D, Van Ryzin J (1981). Dose–response models for quantal response toxicity data. In: Csorgo M, Dawson D, Rao JNK, Shilah E, eds. Statistical and Related Topics. New York, NY: Elsevier/North Holland.

Lehman AJ, Fitzhugh OG (1954). 100-Fold margin of safety. Q Bull Assoc Food Drug Officials US. 33–5.

Lu FC (1979). The safety of food additives. The dynamics of the issue. In: Deichman WB, ed. Toxicology and Occupational Medicine. New York, NY: Elsevier/North-Holland.

Lu FC (1985). Safety assessment of chemicals with thresholded effects. Regul Toxicol Pharmacol 5, 460–4.

Lu FC (1988). Acceptable daily intakes: inception, evolution and application. Regul Toxicol Pharmacol 8, 45–60.

Lu FC (1995). A review of the acceptable daily intakes of pesticides assessed by WHO. Regul Toxicol Pharmacol 21, 352–64.

Lu FC, Coulston F (1996). A safety assessment based on irrelevant data. Ecotoxicol Environ Saf 33, 100–1.

Lu FC, Seilken RL (1991). Assessment of safety/risk of chemicals: inception and evolution of the ADI and dose–response modeling procedures. Toxicol Lett 59, 5–40.

Mantel N, Bryan WR (1961). "Safety" testing of carcinogenic agents. J Natl Cancer Inst 27, 455–70.

National Academy of Sciences (NAS) (1965). Report on "No Residue" and "Zero Tolerance." Washington, DC.: National Academy of Sciences.

National Research Council (1977). Drinking Water and Health, vol. 1. Washington, DC: National Academy of Sciences.

National Research Council (1983). Risk Assessment in the Federal Government: Managing the Process. Washington, DC.: National Academy Press.

Paustenbach DJ (2000). The practice of exposure assessment: a state-of-the-art review. J Toxicol Environ Health Part B 3, 179–291.

Reitz RH, Mendrala AL, Corley R, et al. (1990). Estimating the risk of liver cancer associated with human exposure to chloroform. Toxicol Appl Pharmacol 105, 443–59.

Sielken RL Jr (1981). Re-examination of the ED01 study: risk assessment using time. Fundam Appl Toxicol 1, 88–123.

Somers E (1986). The weight of evidence: regulatory toxicology in Canada. Regul Toxicol Pharmacol 6, 391–8.

SOT ED01 Task Force (1981). Re-examination of the ED01 Study. Fundam Appl Toxicol 1, 26–128.

WHO (1958). Procedures for the Testing of Intentional Food Additives to Establish Their Safety in Use. Second Report. WHO Tech Rep Ser No. 144.

WHO (1962a). Evaluation of the Toxicity of a Number of Antimicrobials and Antioxidants. Sixth Report. WHO Tech Rep Ser No. 228.

WHO (1962b). Principles Governing Consumer Safety in Relation to Pesticide Residues. Report of a Joint FAO/WHO Meeting on Pesticide Residues. WHO Tech Rep Ser No. 240.

WHO (1974a). Toxicological Evaluation of Certain Food Additives with a Review of General Principles and of Specifications. Seventeenth Report. WHO Tech Rep Ser No. 539.

WHO (1974b). Assessment of the Carcinogenicity and Mutagenicity of Chemicals. Report of a WHO Scientific Group. WHO Tech Rep Ser No. 546.

WHO (1978). Principles and Methods for Evaluating the Toxicity of Chemicals. Environ Health Criteria 6. Geneva, Switzerland: World Health Organization.

WHO (1987). Principles for the Safety Assessment of Food Additives and Contaminants in Food. Environ Health Criteria No. 70.

WHO (1989). Guidelines for Predicting Dietary Intakes of Pesticide Residues. Geneva, Switzerland: World Health Organization.

WHO (1990). Principles for the Toxicological Assessment of Pesticide Residues in Food. Environ Health Criteria 104.

Wilson R (1980). Risk-benefit analysis for toxic chemicals. Ecotoxicol Environ Safety 4, 370–83.

FURTHER READING

Crump KS (1984). A new method for determining allowable daily intakes. Fundam Appl Toxicol 4, 854–71.

Dourson ML, Lu FC (1995). Safety/risk assessment of chemicals by different groups. Biomed Environ Sci 8, 1–13.

EPA (1989). Biological Data for Pharmacokinetic Modeling and Risk Assessment. EPA/600/3–90/019, Washington, DC.

FDA (1971). Food and Drug Administration Advisory Committee on Protocols for Safety Evaluation: panel on Carcinogenesis report on cancer testing in the safety evaluation of food additives and pesticides. Toxicol Appl Pharmacol 20, 419–38.

Hart RW, Fishbein L (1985). Interspecies extrapolation of drug and genetic toxicity data. In: Clayson DB, Krewski D, Munro I, eds. Toxicological Risk Assessment, vol. I. Boca Raton, FL: CRC Press.

Munro IC (1988). Risk assessment of carcinogens: present status and future direction. Biomed Environ Sci 1, 51–8.

National Academy of Sciences (NAS) (1984). Toxicity Testing: Strategies to Determine Needs and Priorities. Washington, DC.: National Academy of Sciences.

Ramsey JC, Gehring PJ (1980). Application of pharmacokinetic principles in practice. Fed Proc 39, 60–5.

WHO (1957). General Principles Governing the Use of Food Additives. First Report of the Joint FAO/WHO Expert Committee on Food Additives. WHO Tech Rep Ser No. 129.

Chemical index

AAF. *See* Acetylaminofluorene
Abamectin, 284
ABP. *See* Androgen-binding proteins
Acetaminophen, 31, 32, 34, 68, 173, 328
Acetone, 101, 204
Acetozolamide, 128
2-Acetylaminofluorene, 36
Acetylaminofluorene (AAF), 60, 91, 112
Acetylate sulfanilamide, 62
Acetylcholine (ACh), 55, 214, 220, 279, 282, 288
Acetylcholinesterase (AChE), 50, 218, 354, 357, 366
    inhibitors, 68, 205, 278, 354
Acetyl coenzyme A, 31
Acetylesterases, 30
Acetyl ethyl tetramethyl tetralin (AETT), 221
Acetylsalicylic acid, 12, 328
Acetylsulfapyridine. *See* Sulfapyridine
ACh. *See* Acetylcholine
AChE. *See* Acetylcholinesterase
Acid phosphatase, 188
Acids, 17, 204
Acridine, 194
Acrylamide, 207, 219, 220, 356, 357
Acrylamide-A, 228
Acrylonitrile, 269, 281, 357
ACTH, 53, 214
Actinomycin, 152, 220
Actinomycin D, 128
Actinomycin-M, 228
Adenosine triphosphate (ATP), 46, 173, 236
Adenylate cyclase activity, 186
ADH. *See* Antidiuretic hormone
Adrenergic β-receptor agonists, 236, 241
Adriamycin. *See* Doxorubicin
AETT. *See* Acetyl ethyl tetramethyl tetralin
AETT-M, 228
Aflatoxins, 68, 153, 176, 270, 271
Aflatoxin B, 93
Aflatoxin B1, 7, 34, 64, 66, 88, 90, 270, 370
Aflatoxin-8,9-epoxide, 90, 270

Agar, 276
Aglycone, 35
AHH. *See* Aryl hydrocarbon hydroxylase
Ah receptors, 48, 55, 155
Alachlor, 245
Alanine aminotransferase (ALT), 82, 176
Alanosine-N, 228
ALAS. *See* Δ-Aminolevulinic acid synthetase
Albumin, 82, 158, 185, 309
Alcohol, 128, 217
Alcohol dehydrogenase, 36
Alcohol-N, T, 228
Aldehyde dehydrogenase, 36
Aldicarb, 245, 279, 292
Aldrin, 279, 282, 292, 354, 355
Algae, 343, 344
Alginic acid, 276
Aliphatic nitriles, 35
Aliphatic oxidation, 28
Alkalies, 204
Alkali metals, 265
Alkaline earth metals, 265
Alkaline phosphatase (AP), 82, 176, 188
Alkylating agents, 52, 112, 231, 232
Alkyl epoxides, 92
Alkyl mercury compounds, 18, 272
Alkylphenol, 245
Alkylphenol polyethoxylates (APEs), 246, 253
Alloxan, 205
Allyl alcohol, 180
Allylamine, 235, 239
ALT. *See* Alanine aminotransferase
Aluminosis, 167
Aluminum, 163, 164, 217, 323
    abrasives, 167
    dust, 167
Aluminum-N, 228
Aluminum oxide, 293
Amaranth, 18, 276
Amine oxidation, 29
Amines, 244

Amino acid nitrogen, 284
Amino acids, 16, 284, 311
Amino acids, 244
Aminoazo dyes, 34, 91
Aminobenzoic acid derivatives, 194, 196
7-Aminobutyric acid (GABA), 214
Aminoglycosides, 184, 185, 186
δ-Aminolevulinic acid dehydratase, 306, 307
Δ-Aminolevulinic acid synthetase (ALAS), 306, 307
6-Aminonicotinamide, 130, 221
6-Aminonicotinamide-BV, 228
Aminotriazole. See Amitrole
Amitriptyline, 180
Amitrole, 245, 280, 283, 372
Ammonia, 162, 183
Amoxicillin, 153
Amphotericin-B, 184, 186
Anabolic agents, 263, 269, 270
Anatase, 298
Anatoxin-C, 228
Anatoxin-S, 220
Androgen-binding proteins (ABP), 230
Androgens, 95, 128
Angiotensin, 53, 160
Aniline, 60
    disposition of, 13, 14
    tumors, 6
ANIT (α-naphthylisocyanate), 174, 176
Anthracene, 194
Anthracycline antibiotics, 237, 240, 241
Anthraquinone dyes, 98, 194
Antibiotics, 237, 269
Anticaking agents, 276
Anticholinesterases, 205, 211
Anticoagulants, 197, 281, 360
Antidiuretic hormone (ADH), 183, 186
Antigen-presenting cells (APC), 150
Antimetabolites, 52
Antineoplastic drugs, 235, 237
Antipyrine, 61
ANTU (α-naphthylthiourea), 281
AP. See Alkaline phosphatase
APC. See Antigen-presenting cells
APEs. See Alkylphenol polyethoxylates
Aromatic amines, 30, 50, 93
Aromatic carboxylic acids, 31
Aromatic hydrocarbon toluene, 145
Aromatic hydroxylation, 29
Arsenate, 152

Arsenic, 51, 91, 92, 96, 128, 164, 196, 231, 238, 245, 272, 305, 310, 318, 344
    contamination, 272
Arsenic-BV, 228
Arsenic trioxide, 152, 281
Arachidonic acid, 244
Arthropods (jellyfish), 196
Artificial sweeteners, 266
Arylacetic acids, 31
Arylcarbamates, 360
Aryl epoxides, 92
Arylesterases, 30
Aryl hydrocarbon hydroxylase (AHH), 69
Aryl-substituted acrylic acids, 31
Asbestos, 162, 163, 164, 339–340
    fibrosis, 340
Ascorbic acid, 276
Aspartame, 276
Aspartate, 214
Aspirin, 328, 329, 330, 331
ATP. See Adenosine triphosphate
Atrazine, 88, 245
Atropine, 55, 68, 205
Azaserine, 50, 180
Azathioprine, 95, 98, 152
Azide, 216
Azide-N, 228
Azinphosmethyl, 62, 279, 292, 354, 355
Azo dyes, 16
Azorubine, 276

BAP. See Benzo[a]pyrene
BaP-7,8-diol-9,10-epoxide, 91
BaP-7,8-epoxide, 91
Barbiturate-N, 228
Barbiturates, 216
Baygon. See Propoxur
Benomyl, 281
Benzene, 16, 27, 34, 39, 62, 91, 98, 136, 350, 352, 353
Benzimidazoles, 360
Benzo[a]pyrene (BaP), 153, 196, 199, 232
Benzoates, 153
Benzocaine, 194
Benzoic acid, 276
    disposition of, 13, 14
Benzyl penicillin, 269
Beryllium, 152, 154, 167, 172, 194, 310, 311, 318–319, 354
Beta-BHC, 245

BHA. *See* Butylated hydroxyanisole
BHT. *See* Butylated hydroxytoluene
Bicarbonate (HCO_3^-), 183
Bilirubin, 177
Biogenic amines, 160
Bisphenol A (BPA), 245, 246–247
Bipyridyls, 280, 359
Bismuth, 308, 323
Black widow spider venom, 220
Bleomycin, 165
Blue asbestos (crocidolites), 163
Boron compounds, 162
BPA. *See* Bisphenol A
5-BrdU (5-bromo-deoxyuridine), 118
Brominated vegetable oils (BVO), 235, 238, 268
Bromobenzene, 173, 176, 184, 186, 352
Bromobenzene epoxide, 33, 34
Bromosulfophthalein, 177
Bromotrichloromethane, 34
Brookite, 298
BTEX. *See* Xylene
Busulfan, 165, 205, 232
Butyl-benzyl phthalate, 247
Butylated hydroxyanisole (BHA), 61, 267, 276
Butylated hydroxytoluene (BHT), 267, 276
BVO. *See* Brominated vegetable oils

C_{60}. *See* Fullerenes
Ca. *See* Calcium
Cadmium, 96, 98, 141, 184, 185, 232,
    239, 245, 272, 307, 308, 309, 311,
    316–317, 354
Cadmium oxide, 164, 167
Calcium (Ca), 16, 187, 236
Calcium citrate, 276
Calcium gluconate, 276
Captan, 194, 280
Captopril, 153
Ca^{2+} pump, 173
Carbamate insecticides, 279, 282
Carbamates, 248, 357
    propham, 280
Carbamazepine, 180
Carbarsone, 180
Carbaryl, 152, 156, 218, 245, 279, 282–283,
    284, 292, 354, 355
Carbides, 163, 167
Carbofuran, 152, 279
Carbon-based nanomaterials, 293
Carbon black, 296, 299

Carbon dioxide, 21, 36, 60, 160
Carbon disulfide (CS_2), 180, 207, 239, 357
Carbon fullerenes, 293
Carbon monoxide, 16, 50, 207, 216, 221, 239
Carbon monoxide-N, 228
Carbon nanomaterials, 293
Carbon tetrabromide, 173
Carbon tetrachloride (CCl_4), 16, 36, 39,
    51, 65, 67, 136, 172, 173, , 180, 184,
    186, 350, 352
Carboxy-hemoglobin, 357
Carboxylesterases, 30
Carbromide, 235
Carcinogenic chemicals, 372–373
Cardiotonic drugs, 235
Carotene, 276
Carrageenans, 15
Casein, 309
Cataractogenic chemicals, 205, 211
Cathepsin, 140
Ca^{2+} transporting ATPase, 48
CCl_4. *See* Carbon tetrachloride
CdSe compounds, 293
CdTe compounds, 293
Cellulose derivatives, 276
Cement dust, 164, 355, 356
Cerium oxide, 293
Cephaloridine, 184, 186
Chloramphenicol, 63, 237
Chlordane, 152, 245, 279, 292, 354, 355
Chlordecone, 284
Chlorfenvinphos, 279, 292
Chlorine, 162, 167, 306
Chloroaliphatics, 360
Chlorobenzenes, 360
4 [3(7-Chloro-5,11-dihydrodibenz *[b,e]*
    [1,4]-oxyazepin-5-YL)propyl]-
    1- piperazineethanol dichloride, 211
Chlorofenvinphos, 35
Chloroform, 16, 40, 61, 104, 152, 173, 176,
    180, 184, 186, 343, 350
Chlorophenoxy compounds, 280
Chlorophyll, 276
Chloropicrin, 281
Chloropropham, 280
Chloroquine, 47, 165, 204, 206, 207, 209
Chlorothiazides, 194, 196
Chlorphentermine, 165
Chlorpromazine, 174, 176, 180, 194, 195, 196,
    204, 211, 269

Chlorpropamide, 195
Chlorthiazide, 180
Chocolate, 153, 270
Cholesterol, 244
Cholinesterases, 30
Chondroitin sulfates, 192
Chromium, 91, 96, 152, 154, 165, 184, 185, 310, 311, 312, 319
Cigarette smoke, 164
Cimetidine, 330, 331, 332
Ciguatoxin, 271
Cisplatin, 184, 186, 310
CK. See Creatine kinase
Clioquinol, 207, 219
Clioquinol-A, 228
Coal dust, 163, 164, 167, 355
Coal tar derivatives, 194, 196
Cobalt, 236, 310, 322
Cocaine, 128
Coke oven emissions, 164, 167, 355
Concanavalin A, 156
COPROD. See Coproporphyrinogen oxidase
Copper, 196, 311, 322
Copper oxide, 293
Coproporphyrinogen oxidase (COPROD), 307, 315
Corrosive agents, 52
Corticosteroids, 153, 156, 205, 211, 244
Cotton dust, 164, 167
Coumestrol, 245
Creatine kinase (CK), 82
Creatinine, 82, 188
C-S lyase, 186
CS₂. See Carbon disulfide
Cyanide, 216, 221
Cyanide-N, BV, 228
Cycasin, 35, 40, 93, 180
Cycloheximide, 180
Cyclohexylamine, 35, 231, 266
Cyclophosphamide, 152, 165
Cyclosporin, 184, 186
Cyclosporin A, 95
Cylindrospermopsin, 344
CYP19. See Cytochrome P450 enzyme aromatase
Cytochalasin B, 172
Cytochrome-linked monooxygenases (oxidases), 28
Cytochrome P-450 (CYP-450) enzymes, 28, 36, 62, 67, 160, 170, 185, 351

Cytochrome P450 enzyme aromatase, 255
Cytotoxicants, 95

2,4-D, 144, 280, 354, 355
Daidzein, 245
Daunorubicin, 237
DBCP. See 1,2-Dibromo-3-chloropropane
p,p'-DDD, 245
p,p'-DDE, 245, 248
DDT, 19, 43, 63, 64, 79, 144, 219, 231, 232, 245, 252, 254, 278, 279, 282, 283, 285, 292, 354, 355
o,p'-DDT, 248
p,p'-DDT, 245
DDT-C, 228
Decalin, 61, 62, 184
Decabromodiphenyl ether, 248
DEET. See N,N-diethyl-m-toluamide
Deoxynivalenol, 51, 153, 185, 270
DEHP. See Di(2-ethylhexyl) phthalate
DEPC. See Diethyl pyrocarbonate
DES. See Diethylstilbestrol
Desferal, 211
Detergents, 164, 204
DFP. See Diisopropyl fluorophosphate
Di(2-ethylhexyl) phthalate (DEHP), 247
Di(n-butyl) phthalate, 247
Di(n-octyl) phthalate, 247
Dialkyl nitrosamines, 180
Diazepam, 152, 180
Diazinon, 279, 292, 354, 355
Dibenzofurans, 253
1,2-Dibromo-3-chloropropane (DBCP), 231, 232, 245, 283
Dicarboximides, 280
Dichlorobenzene, 180
Dichloro-diphenyl trichloroethane. See DDT
2,6-Dichloro-4-nitroaniline, 211
2,4-Dichlorophenoxyacetic acid (2,4-D), 245
Dichlorvos, 278, 279, 292
Dicofol, 245
Dieldrin, 19, 63, 64, 152, 155, 176, 245, 279, 292
Diesel exhaust particles, 31, 93, 153, 162, 164
Di(2-ethylhexyl) phthalate, 95, 247, 343
Diethyl phthalate, 247
Diethyl pyrocarbonate (DEPC), 267
Diethyl sulfate, 112
Diethylstilbestrol (DES), 20, 43, 95, 126, 129, 131, 245, 251, 270

5α-Dihydrotestosterone, 254
1,25-Dihydroxyvitamin D3, 183
Diisopropyl fluorophosphate (DFP), 282
Dimercaprol, 67, 306
Dimethoate, 279, 292
Dimethylnitrosamine, 180
Dimethylnitrosamine (DMN), 180, 186
Dimethyl sulfoxide (DMSO), 17, 101, 206, 211
Dimethylthiocarbamates, 280
Dinitro-*o*-cresol, 280
Dinitrophenol, 50, 62, 205
2,4-Dinitrophenol (DNP), 205, 211
Dinocap, 284
Dinoseb, 129
Dioxane, 350, 353
Dioxins, 140, 176, 248, 253
Diphenylhydantoin, 129. *See also* Phenytoin
Diphtheria toxin, 54, 220
Diphtheria toxin-M, 228
Dipterex. *See* Trichlorfon
Diquat, 152, 165, 180, 211, 280, 284, 354, 355
Disulfoton, 279, 292
Disulfiram, 36, 207
Di-Syston. *See* Disulfoton
Dithiocarbamates, 360
DMN. *See* Dimethylnitrosamine
DMSO. *See* Dimethyl sulfoxide
DNP. *See* 2,4-Dinitrophenol
Doxorubicin, 152, 215, 217, 237
Doxorubicin-N, 228

EDB. *See* Ethylene dibromide
Eicosanoids, 244
Elemental phosphorus, 281
Emetine, 235
β-Endorphin, 214
Endosulfan, 245
Endrin, 292
Entero-Vioform. *See* Clioquinol
EPN. *See* O-Ethyl-*o*-(4-nitrophenyl)
phenylphosphonothioate
EPN-A, 228
Ergot, 62, 271
Ergot alkaloids, 238
Erythromycin, 153, 176
Erythromycin estolate, 180
Erythromycin lactobionate, 174
Estradiol, 95, 180, 232, 270
17β-Estradiol, 254, 256
Estrogen, 98, 136, 141

Ethacrynic acid, 180
Ethambutol, 207
Ethanol, 35, 36, 145, 171, 174, 235, 352
Ethidium bromide, 220
Ethidium bromide-M, 228
Ethinyl estradiol, 174
Ethionine, 171, 180
Ethylbenzene, 69, 340
Ethylene, 16
Ethylene-bis-dithiocarbamates, 280, 283
Ethylenediamine, 194
Ethylene dibromide (EDB), 281, 283
Ethylene glycol, 60, 352
Ethylmethane sulfonate, 117
Ethylnitrosourea, 64, 112
17α-Ethynyl estradiol, 256

Febantel, 269
Fenbendazole, 269
Fenitrothion, 35
Fenofibrate, 95
Fentichlor. *See* 2,2-thiobis(4-chlorophenol)
Finasteride, 245
Flavones, 66
Floxacillin, 153
Fluoride, 343
Fluorinated agents, 360
Fluoroacetamide, 281
Fluoroacetic acid, 50
Fluorocarbons, 237
5-Fluorouracil, 16, 130, 152
Flutamide, 245, 256
Folic acid, 174, 205
Folpet, 280
Formaldehyde, 338, 339
Fullerenes, 293, 299, 301
Fumonisin B, 176, 180
Fumonisin B1, 271
Furans, 248
Furazolidone, 235
Furosemide, 34, 180
Fusarium solani, 163

G-6-PD. *See* Glucose-6-phosphate
dehydrogenase
GABA. *See* 7-aminobutyric acid
Galactosamine, 180
Galactose-1-phosphate uridylyl transferase, 205
Gamma-BHC (lindane), 245
Genistein, 245

Gentamicin, 184
Glazing agents, 276
Glucans, 163
Glucose, 187, 211, 216, 311
Glucose-6-phosphate dehydrogenase (G-6-PD),
    82, 130
    deficiency, 61
Glucuronide conjugates, 20, 63
Glutamate, 215, 217
Glutamate-N, 228
Glutathione, 173, 176
Glutathione conjugation, 31–33
Glutathione S-tranferases, 31, 45
Glycine, 31, 214, 220, 315
Glycols, 184, 187
Glycosides scillaren- A and -B, 281
Glyphosate, 284
Gold, 152, 155, 184, 185, 293, 295,
    311, 323
Gossypol, 232, 233
Guanethidine, 232
Guthion. *See* Azinphosmethyl

Halogenated hydrocarbons, 93, 144–145,
    184
Halogenated salicylanilides, 195
Haloperidol, 232
Halothane, 21, 34, 153, 175, 180
HCB. *See* Hexachlorobenzene
HCN. *See* Hydrocyanic acid
HCO_3^- . *See* Bicarbonate
Heme synthetase (HS), 307, 315
Heptacholor, 245, 292
Heptachlor epoxide, 245
Herbicides, 277, 280, 354, 359
Hexacarbons, 219
Hexachlorobenzene (HCB), 141, 281
Hexachlorobutadiene, 184
    damages, 186
Hexachlorophene, 221, 222, 231
Hexachlorophene-M, BV, 228
Hexane, 204, 207, 219, 350
Hexobarbital, 60, 62, 63
Holocrine, 197
HS. *See* Heme synthetase
Hyaluronic acid, 192
Hydralazine, 153, 236, 239
Hydrazides, 31
Hydrazines, 31
Hydrocyanic acid (HCN), 50

Hydrogen fluoride, 168
Hydroquinone, 61, 184
Hydroxychloroquine, 206
5-Hydroxytryptamine, 29
25-Hydroxy-vitamin D3, 183
Hyperglycemic drugs, 332

IDPN. *See* β, β -Iminodiproprionitrile
IDPN-A, 228
IgD immunoglobulins, 151
IgE antibody, 153
IgG-producing plaques, 157
IgM immunoglobulins, 151
IL. *See* Interleukins
Imidazolines, 331, 332
β, β -Iminodiproprionitrile (IDPN), 218
Imipramine, 180
Immunoglobin A, 185
Immunoglobins (Ig family), 151
Immunoglobulin E, 356
Immunosuppressants, 155, 184
Immunosuppressive drugs, 95
Indigotine, 276
Indoles, 66
Indomethacin, 180
Insecticides, 278–280, 292
Interleukins (IL), 151
Iodoacetic acid, 211
Ionizable toxicants, 12
Ipomeanol, 163
4-Ipomeanol, 47
Iproniazid, 68, 173, 180
Iron, 16, 308, 315, 322, 331
Iron oxides, 168, 293
Isocyanates, 164, 168
Isoniazid, 31, 68, 173, 176, 180, 221, 222
Isopropanol, 67
Isoproterenol, 236
^{132}I-triolein, 157

K. *See* Potassium
Kainic acid-N, 228
Kanamycin, 47, 185, 186
Kaolin, 163, 168, 355

Lactate dehydrogenase (LDH), 82, 188
Lactones, 92
LDH. *See* Lactate dehydrogenase
Lead, 6, 16, 152, 184, 220, 221, 238, 245, 272,
    273, 305–306, 314–316, 308, 354

Lead-MS, 228
Lecithin, 276
Leptophos, 282
Leptophos-A, 228
Lindane, 292, 354, 355
Linuron, 232
Lipids, 51–52
Lipopolysaccharide, 113
Liposomes, 296
Lithium, 235, 311
Lithocholate, 172
Loperamide, 330, 332
Losulazine, 232
Luciferin substrate, 254
Lysolecithin-M, 228
Lysozyme, 150, 317

Magnesium (Mg), 186, 265
Magnesium sulfate, 331
Malathion, 279, 282, 285, 292, 354, 355
Malondialdehyde (MDA), 298
Maltase, 188
Mancozeb, 283
Maneb, 152, 280, 283
Manganese, 311, 322
Mannitol, 12
3-MC. *See* 3-Methylcholanthrene
MDA. *See* Malondialdehyde
Melanin, 47
Melphalan, 165
Mepazine, 180
Mephenytoin, 211
6-Mercaptopurine, 152, 180
Mercapturic acids, 357
Mercuric chloride, 353
Mercury, 155, 184, 186, 238, 245, 273, 312–314, 354
Methacholine, 55
Methandrolone, 180
Methanol, 350
Methimazole, 180
Methionine, 174
   enkephalin, 214
   sulfoximine, 211
Methomyl, 245, 279
Methotrexate, 152, 165
Methoxsalen, 211
Methoxychlor, 232, 245, 292, 354, 355
2-Methoxyethanol, 152
Methoxyflurane, 180, 184, 186

Methoxypsoralens, 196
Methylazoxymethanol, 35
Methylcholanthrene, 152
3-Methylcholanthrene (3-MC), 68, 113, 232
Methylcyclopentadienyl manganese tricarbonyl (MMT), 6
Methyldopa, 152
α-Methyldopa, 180
Methylene chloride, 350
4,4-Methylenedianiline, 206
Methylene tetrafolate reductase, 45
3-Methylindole, 32
Methyl mercury, 24, 46, 152, 207, 217, 306
Methyl mercury-N, BV, 228
Methylmethane sulfonate (MMS), 232
Methyl *n*-butyl ketone, 207, 350
Methyl *n*-butyl ketone-A, 228
Methyl sulfoxime, 221
Methysergide, 235
Mevinphos, 279, 292
Mg. *See* Magnesium
Microcystins, 173, 344
β_2-Microglobulin, 317
Mimosine (leucenol), 211
Minoxidil, 239
Mipafox, 282
Mirex, 245, 284
Mitomycin, 165
Mitomycin C, 110
MMT. *See* Methylcyclopentadienyl manganese tricarbonyl
MNU. *See* N-Methyl-N-nitrosourea
Molybdenum, 322
Monoamine oxidase, 29
Monocrotaline, 163, 238
Monosaccharides, 16
Monosodium glutamate (MSG), 153, 268
Mono-(2-ethylhexyl) phthalate (MEHP), 247
MSG. *See* Monosodium glutamate
Mucopolysaccharides, 192
Mycotoxins, 270

Na. *See* Sodium
Nabam, 280, 283
N-Acetylcysteine (mercapturic acid) derivatives, 31
N-Acetyl-l-cysteine *S*-conjugates, 357
N-Acetyl transferases, 31
NAD, 173
NADP, 173

NADPH cytochrome P-450 reductase, 28
Nano zinc oxide (ZnO), 293, 298
Naphthalene, 211
2-Naphthylamine, 60, 100
α-Naphthylisocyanate, 176
α-Naphthylthiourea, 360
N-Arylsuccinimides, 185
Neomycin, 186, 194
N-Heterocyclic compounds, 281
N-Hexane, 207, 225, 350
N-Hexane-A, 228
N-Hydroxy derivatives, 91
Nickel, 152, 153, 155, 168, 194, 311, 312,
     319, 354
Nickel carbonyl, 162
Nicotine, 69, 232
Nicotine-C, 228
Nissl substances, 217
Nitrates, 267, 343
Nitric oxide (NO), 214, 239
Nitrilotriacetic acid (NTA), 95
Nitrites, 267
Nitrobenzol, 207
Nitrofen, 245
Nitrogen dioxide (NO_2), 337–338
Nitrogen mustards, 152, 232
Nitrogen oxides, 16
Nitrosamides, 92
Nitrosamines, 61, 93, 129, 267
Nitrosoureas, 92
N-Methylcarbamic acid, 279
N-Methyl-N-nitrosourea (MNU), 48
N,N-diethyl-m-toluamide (DEET), 59,
     288–289
N(Nitrosomethyl)urea, 180
NO. See Nitric oxide
NO_2. See Nitrogen dioxide (NO_2)
Nodulins, 344
Nomifensine, 153
N-Phenyl-β-hydrazinopropionitriles, 211
NTA. See Nitrilotriacetic acid
Nutraceuticals, 7

O_3. See Ozone
O_6-Alkyl-guanine, 48
O-Aminophenol, 60
Ochratoxin A, 92, 271
Ochratoxins, 153, 271
OCT. See Ornithine carbamoyl transferase
Octabromodiphenyl ether, 248

Octylphenol, 245
O-Ethyl-o-(4-nitrophenyl)
     phenylphosphonothioate (EPN), 282
Olefins, 34
Oleoresins, 276
Omethoate, 35
Orange RN, 268
Organic solvents, 207, 350–351
Organic solvents-A, 228
Organic tin compounds, 152
Organochlorine (OC) insecticides, 63, 248, 272,
     279, 281, 284, 354
Organochlorine pesticides, 156
Organochlorines, 359
Organomercurials (thimerosol), 194
Organophosphate AChE inhibitor, 55, 68
Organophosphate insecticides, 282
Organophosphate pesticides, 144, 282
Organophosphates, 359
Organophosphorus insecticides, 35, 62, 354
Organotin compounds, 252
Organotin-N, 228
Organotins, 217
Ornithine carbamoyl transferase (OCT), 176
Ouabain, 71, 221
Oxalic acid, 60. See Glycols
Oxfendazole, 269
Oxides of nitrogen, 168
Oxychlordane, 245
Oxyphenisatin, 180
Oxyphenylbutazone, 165
Oxytetracycline, 269
Oxytocin, 214
Ozone (O_3), 168, 337–338

PAH. See P-aminohippuric acid
PAHs. See Polycyclic aromatic hydrocarbons
P-Aminohippuric acid (PAH), 189
P-Aminophenol, 60
P-Aminosalicylic acid, 176, 180
Papaverine, 180
Paracetamol, 328, 330
Paradichlorobenzene, 211
Paraquat, 34, 51, 152, 165, 217, 280,
     284, 355
Parasympatholytic agents, 205
Parathion, 35, 62, 245, 292, 354, 355
Parathion-methyl, 279, 292
PB. See Pyridostigmine bromide
PBB. See Polybrominated biphenyls

P-Bromophenol, 34
PbS compounds, 294
PbSe compounds, 294
P-Chlorophenylalanine, 206
PCNB. *See* Pentachloronitrobenzene
P-Nonylphenol, 245
PBDEs. *See* Polybrominated diphenyl ethers
PBDE-47, 248
PBDE-99, 248
PCB. *See* Polychlorinated biphenyls
Penicillamine, 153, 186
Penicillin, 153, 187, 195, 239
Pentabromodiphenyl ether, 248
Pentachloronitrobenzene (PCNB), 245, 280
Pentachlorophenol, 245
Pentachlorophenol (PCP), 152, 281
PCP. *See* Pentachlorophenol
Perchloroethylene, 145, 162, 168
Perfluorooctanoic acid (PFOA), 152
Perfluorooctanesulfonate (PFOS), 152
Peptides, 244
Permethrin, 288–289
Perphenazine, 180
PFOA. *See* Perfluorooctanoic acid
PFOS. *See* Perfluorooctanesulfonate
Phalloidin, 172
Phenanthrene, 194
Phenindione, 180
Phenobarbital, 68–69, 113
Phenols, 197, 248
Phenolics, 360
Phenolsulfonphthalein (PSP) excretion test, 189
Phenothiazines, 194, 235
Phenoxyacids, 360
Phenylbutazone, 165, 180
Phenytoin, 176, 180, 235
Phosgene, 168
Phosphates, 276, 343
3-Phosphoadenosine-5'-phosphosulfate, 30
Phosphorus, 172, 173, 180
Phthalate esters, 247–248, 343
Phthalates, 245, 356
Phthalimide derivatives, 280
Phytohemagglutinin, 156
Piperonyl butoxide, 68, 279
Plant extracts, 276
Platinum, 152, 153, 196, 311, 311
Poison ivy, 194
Poison oak, 194
Polybrominated biphenyls (PBB), 34, 152, 342

Polybrominated diphenyl ethers (PBDEs),
    245, 248
Polycarbonate resins, 245
Polychlorinated biphenyls (PCB), 19, 34, 66, 68,
    113, 152, 180, 197, 245, 254, 272, 341–342
Polycyclic aromatic hydrocarbons (PAHs),
    69, 93, 232, 248
Polycyclic hydrocarbons, 91, 99
Polyribocytidylic acid, 211
Polyriboinosinic acid, 211
Polystyrene latex, 16
Polyvinyl chloride (PVC), 247
Ponceau 2R, 268
Potassium (K), 265
P-Phenylenediamine, 194
Practolol, 153
Primaquine, 61
Probenecid, 20, 153
Procainamide, 153
Procarcinogens, 93
Procymidone, 284
Prolactin, 141
Promazine, 180
Promethazine, 195
Prontosil, 29
Propellants, 276
Propionic acid, 276
Propoxur, 279, 292
Propranolol, 197
Propylene glycol, 235
Prostaglandins, 160
Proteins, 174, 244
Psoralens, 110, 196
PSP. *See* Phenolsulfonphthalein
Puromycin, 180, 185
Putrescine, 29
PVC. *See* Polyvinyl chloride
Pyrethroids, 152, 245, 248, 359
Pyrethroids-C, 228
Pyridine, 194
Pyridostigmine bromide (PB), 288
Pyrrolizidine alkaloids, 35, 93, 180

Quartz, 163
Quietidine (1, 4-bis(phenylisopropyl)-
    piperazine·2HCl), 211
Quinine, 153

R1881. *See* 5α-dihydrotestosterone
Radiogallium, 323

Radon, 96
Raloxifene, 245
Rapeseed oil, 235, 238
Retinoic acid, 56
Retinoids, 129
Retinol-binding protein, 317
Riboflavin, 276
Rodenticides, 61, 281, 360
Rotenone, 220, 279
Rutile, 298

Saccharin, 266, 276
S-Adenosylmethionine (SAM), 31
Safrole, 66, 93, 180
Saline laxatives, 332
SAM. *See* S-Adenosylmethionine
Saxitoxin, 219, 271, 344
Saxitoxin-C, 228
Schradan (octamethyl pyrophosphoramide), 64
SDH. *See* Sorbitol dehydrogenase
Selenium, 321
Serum aspartate aminotransferase (AST or SGOT), 82
Serum thyroid-stimulating hormone, 256
Serum thyroxin (T4), 248, 256
Sevin. *See* Carbaryl
SGOT. *See* Serum aspartate aminotransferase
Silica, 168, 355
Silicone, 141, 142
Silver, 296, 299
SKF 525 A, 68
Smog, 204, 338
SO_2. *See* Sulfur dioxide
Sodium arsenite, 152
Sodium fluoroacetate, 281
Sodium (Na), 16, 265
Sorbic acid, 276
Sorbitol dehydrogenase (SDH), 176
Spironolactone, 232
Steroids, 180, 244
Streptomycin, 165, 186, 237
Streptozotocin, 205, 211
Strontium-90, 47
Strychnine, 360
Styrene, 51, 91, 245
Substilisin, 153
Succinyl coenzyme A (CoA), 315
Sugars (glucose, galactose, xylose), 211
Sulfaethoxypyridazine, 211

Sulfanilamide, 29, 180, 194–195
Sulfapyridine, 184, 186
Sulfate, 173
Sulfate conjugates, 20
Sulfate esters, 92
Sulfites, 153
Sulfonamides, 19, 31, 180, 187, 196, 239
Sulfur dioxide (SO_2), 16, 165, 168, 267, 268, 276
Sulfur oxides, 337, 340
Suspended particulate matter, 337, 340

T4. *See* Serum thyroxin
2,4,5-T. *See* 2,4,5-trichlorophenoxyacetic acid
Talc, 168, 355
Tamoxifen, 245
Tannic acid, 172, 180
Tartrazine, 153, 267, 276
Taurocholate, 172, 174
TBA. *See* Thiobarbituric acid
TCDD. *See* 2,3,7,8-Tetrachlorodibenzo-p-dioxin
TDI. *See* Toluene diisocyanate
Tellurium-BV, M, 228
Temik. *See* Aldicarb
Testosterone propionate, 256
Tetanoplasmin, 220
Tetanoplasmin-C, 228
2,3,7,8-Tetrachlorodibenzo-*p*-dioxin (TCDD), 48, 56, 133, 152, 155, 197, 343
Tetrachloroethane, 173, 180
Tetracyclines, 172, 180, 184, 196, 237
12,0-Tetradecanoyl phorbol 13-acetate (TPA), 56, 153
Tetraethyl lead, 308, 316
Tetramethyl lead, 316
Tetrodotoxin, 219, 271
Tetrodotoxin-C, 228
Thalidomide, 6, 129, 130
Thallium, 16, 205, 207, 211
Thallium-A, 228
Thallium sulfate, 281
Thiabendazole, 180
Thiazides, 194–195
Thioacetamide, 180, 211
Thioamides, 93
Thiobarbituric acid (TBA), 177
Thiobendazole, 281
2,2-Thiobis(4-chlorophenol), 195
Thiopental, 12
Thiophanates, 360

Thioridazine, 180
Thioureas, 281
Thiram, 280, 354, 355
Thyroxine, 141
Tin, 168, 307
T-independent antigens, 157
TiO_2, 293, 298, 299
Titanium, 306, 323
TNT. See 2,4,6-Trinitrotoluene
TOCP. See Tri-o-cresyl phosphate
Tolbutamide, 153
Toluene, 69, 165, 204, 350, 351
Toluene diisocyanate (TDI), 153, 154, 164, 194, 356
Total serum testosterone, 256
Toxaphene, 245
TPA. See 12,0-Tetradecanoyl phorbol 13-acetate
Trans-nonachlor, 245
Trenbolone acetate, 270
Triazines, 360
Tributyltin, 252
Tributyltin chloride, 245
Trichlorfon, 279, 292
Trichloroethene, 155
Trichloroethylene, 34, 67, 152, 172, 180, 350
1,1,2-Tricholoroethylene, 95
Trichlorofon, 282
Trichloromethyl radical CCl_3, 173
2,4,5-Trichlorophenoxyacetic acid (2,4,5-T), 245
Trichothecenes, 271
Tricresyl phosphate, 216
Tricyclic antidepressants, 235, 237
Triethyltin, 220–222, 311
Triethyltin-M, BV, 228
Trifluralin, 245
Triglycerides, 82, 173
Trihalomethanes, 343
2,4,6-Trinitrotoluene (TNT), 211
Tri-o-cresyl phosphate, 207
Tri-o-cresyl phosphate (TOCP), 225, 282
Tri-o-cresyl phosphate (TOCP)-A, 228
Triparanol, 165, 197, 205, 211, 220
Triparanol-M, 228
Tris-(4-chlorophenyl)-methanol, 248

Tritiated water, 255
Tryptophan, 244
Tyrosine, 211, 244
UDP-glucuronyl transferase, 30
Ureas, 360
Urethane, 34, 180
Uridine-5'-diphospho-α-d-glucuronic acid, 30
UROD. See Uroporphyrinogen decarboxylase
Uroporphyrinogen decarboxylase (UROD), 315

Valproic acid, 129, 180
Vanadium, 168
Vasopressin, 214
Vegetable gums, 276
Vinblastine, 232
Vinclozolin, 248
Vincristine, 219
Vincristine-A, 228
Vinyl chloride, 34, 91, 176, 180, 269, 356
Vioform. See Clioquinol
Vitamin A, 331, 332
Vitamin B_{12}, 174
Vitamin D, 331–332
Vitamin K, 140, 281, 331, 332
Vitamins A, 140
Vitamins C, 309
Vitamins D, 309

Warfarin, 281

Xanthines, 66
Xylene, 69, 162

Zearalenone, 245, 248, 271
Zinc, 322
Zinc phosphide, 281, 360
Zinc protoporphyrin, 357
Zineb, 280, 283
Ziram, 280
Zirconium, 311, 311
ZnO. See Nano zinc oxide
ZnS compounds, 293
ZnSe compounds, 293
Zoxazolamine, 177, 180

Subject index

Aberrations chromosomal, 116
ABP. *See* Androgen-binding proteins
Absorption
  gastrointestinal tract, 15–16
  pH effect, 12–13
  respiratory tract, 16
  skin, 17
  toxicants ionized and nonionized, 15–17
Acceptable daily intake (ADI), 264, 265, 270,
     363–367
  definition, 363–364
  exposure acceptability, 366–367
  procedures for estimating, 364–366
Acetylation, 31
Acetylcholinesterase (AChE) inhibitors,
     278–279, 282
AChE. *See* Acetylcholinesterase
Active transport, 14, 15
Acute toxicity studies, 74–80
  evaluation of data, 77–78
  experimental design, 75
  multiple endpoint evaluation, 76–77
  observation and examination, 76
  signs of, 78–80
Additive, 67
ADH. *See* Antidiuretic hormone
ADI. *See* Acceptable daily intake
Adipose tissue, 19
AFLD. *See* Alcoholic fatty liver disease
Age factors, 63–65
Ah receptor, 55
Air pollutants, 335–341
  asbestos, 339–340
  current condition, 336
  formaldehyde, 339
  indoor, 339–341
  outdoor, 337
  past disasters, 11, 335–336
  photochemical oxidants, 337–339
Alcoholic fatty liver disease (AFLD),
     171–172
Allergic reaction, 44, 153–154, 164

Alveolar air, 16
Amine oxidation, 29
Amino acid conjugation, 31
Amphibian metamorphosis assay, 255
Anabolic agents, 269–270
Anaerobic metabolism, 46
Analgesics, 186
Analytical toxicology, 2
Anaphylaxis, 153
Androgen-binding proteins (ABP), 230
Androgen receptor binding assay, 254
Aneuploidy chromosomal, 116
Angiosarcoma, 175–176
Aniline tumors, 6, 87
Animal drug residues, 269–270
Anoxia, 216, 350
Antagonism, 67
Antigen-antibody interaction, 44
Antigen-presenting cells, 150
Antimetabolites, 52
Antineoplastic drugs, 235, 237
Antioncogenes, 91
APEs. *See* Alkylphenol polyethoxylates
Apoptosis, 92
Appendix, 150
Aqueous humor, 204–205
Arc welder's lung, 168
Area postrema, 215
Areas under the curve, 24
Aromatase assay, 255
Arrhythmias, 237
Aryl hydrocarbon hydroxylase, 69
Asbestosis, 339–340
Aspergillus, 113
Aspergillus flavus, 270
Asthma, 63, 66, 153, 162, 164, 194, 284, 298,
     315, 339, 354, 356
Astrocytes, 214, 221, 223
Ataxia telangiectasia, 110
Atherosclerosis, 239
Atypical hyperplasia, 103
Autoimmune diseases, 44, 145, 155, 314

Autoimmune reactions, 149
Autoimmune syndrome, 153
Autoimmunity, 44, 155
Axonopathy, 215, 217–218
Azoospermia, 232

Bacillus subtilis, 119, 164
Bacillus thuringiensis, 280
Bacteria, 119
Balkan endemic nephropathy (BEN), 185
Barbiturate coma, 216
Barriers, 17–18
Basophils, 150, 151
Bauxite lung, 167
BBB. *See* Blood-brain barrier
B cells (B lymphocytes), 151
    deficiency, 158
BEN. *See* Balkan endemic nephropathy
Benign tumors, 103
Bergsucht (Paracelsus), 3
Berylliosis, 318
BHA. *See* Butylated hydroxyanisole
BHT. *See* Butylated hydroxytoluene
Biliary functions, 20–21
Biliary passages, 170
Binding, 18–19
Bioaccumulation, 285
Bioactivation, 33–35, 39–41, 47, 90–91
Biochemical asphyxia, 50
Biochemical effects, 44
Biological indicators, 309–310
Biological markers. *See* Biomarkers
Biological monitoring, 356–357
Biologic membrane, 13
Biomagnification, 285
Biomarkers, 309–310
    metals, 309–310
    new, 188
    of carcinogenesis/human cancers, 108
    of exposure, 140–141
    reproductive system, 235
Biotransformation, of toxicants
    complexity
        sensitivity in children, 36–37
        sensitivity in elderly, 37
    general considerations, 27–28
    phase I reactions
        hydrolysis, 30
        oxidation, 28–29
        reduction, 29

phase II reactions
    acetylation, 31
    amino acid conjugation, 31
    epoxide formation, 33–34
    free radical and superoxide formation,
        34–35
    G.I. tract, 35
    glucuronide formation, 30
    glutathione conjugation, 31–33
    methylation, 31
    N-hydroxylation, 34
    other pathways, 35
    sulfate conjugation, 30
Black-foot disease, 238
Black lung disease, 164
Blockade, of renal and biliary tubules, 52
Blood analysis, 24, 188
Blood-brain barrier (BBB), 17–18, 64, 214–215
Blood clotting mechanism, 206
Blood-nerve barrier (BNB), 215
Blood-testis barrier (BTB), 231
Blood urea nitrogen (BUN), 188
Blood vessels
    endothelial damage, 238
    fibrosis, 239
    hypersensitivity reaction, 239
    increased capillary permeability, 238
    toxic effects, 238–239
    tumors, 239
    vasoconstriction, 238–239
    vasodilatation, 238–239
B lymphocytes, 156
BNB. *See* Blood-nerve barrier
Bowman's capsules, 183
Breast-feeding
    alcohol, 145
    benefits of, 138–140
    biomakers of exposure, 140–141
    cancer, 139
    food allergies, 139–140
    halogenated hydrocarbons, 144–145
    immune system, 138–139
    lead, 143–144
    mercury, 142–143
    psychological bonding, 140
    silicone, 142
    solvents, 145
    toxicants, 141–145
Bronchioles, 160–161
BTB. *See* Blood-testis barrier

Bulk laxatives, 332
BUN. *See* Blood urea nitrogen

Calcium homeostasis, 173
Cancer. *See also* Carcinogenesis
  liver, 175–176
  lung, 164
  prostate, 232
  reproductive system, 255–256
  skin, 196, 199
Carcinogenesis, 87–104
  categories
    genotoxic carcinogens, 92–94
    nongenotoxic carcinogens, 94–97
  definition and identification, 87–88
  evaluation, 102–104
  historical background, 87
  human carcinogens, 97, 98
  mode of action, 89–92
    bioactivation, 90–91
    conversion and progression, 92
    initiation, 91
    interaction with macromolecules, 104
    promotion, 91
  target organs, 97, 98
  test for, 97–102
  weight of evidence, 88–89
Carcinogenicity, 266–267
Cardiac arrhythmias, 237
Cardiomyopathy, 236–237
Cardiovascular (CV) system toxicology,
      229–241
  cardiotoxic drugs and chemicals, 235
  structure, 235–236
  testing for toxicity, 240–241
  toxic effects on heart
    cardiac arrhythmias, 237
    cardiomyopathy, 236–237
    interference with nucleic acid synthesis, 237
    myocardial depression, 237
    others, 238
  toxic effects on blood vessels
    degenerative changes, 239
    endothelial damage, 238
    fibrosis, 239
    hypersensitivity reactions, 239
    increased capillary permeability, 238
    tumors, 239
    vasoconstriction and vasodilatation,
        238–239

Cataract, 205–206
Cell-mediated immunity, 156–157
Cell-mediated system, 115
Cell membrane, 51
  Carrier-mediated transport and, 14–15
  filtration and, 14
  peroxidation of, 162
Cell-membrane-associated antigens, 150
Cell membrane derangement, 51
Cell transformation, 97
Cellular damages, 162
Cellular edema, 162, 221–222
Cellular necrosis, 163
Central nervous system (CNS), 213–225
Chemical antagonism, 67
Chemical carcinogenesis, 87, 89
Chemical distribution, in organs
  adipose tissue, 19
  binding and storage, 18–19
  blood-brain barrier, 17–18
  bone, 19
  brain, 17–18
  kidney, 19
  liver, 19
  placental barrier, 18
  plasma proteins, 18
Chemical interaction, 67–69
Chemosis, 212
Chinese restaurant syndrome, 268
Chloracne, 197, 273, 280, 342
Chlorinated aromatic hydrocarbons, 341–344
Cholestasis, 174
Cholinergic receptors (ChR), 53
Cholinesterases, 30
ChR. *See* Cholinergic receptors
Chromatid break, 117
Chromosomal effects, 111, 116–118
Chronic alcoholism, 221
Chronic toxicity studies, 73–84, 80–83. *See also*
      Long-term toxicity studies
Chrysanthemum cinerariaefolium, 279
Cigarette smokers, 67
Ciliary body, 204–205
Cirrhosis, 174–175
Clara cells, 47, 161, 163
Clinical laboratory test, 82
Clinical toxicology, 2
Clostridium botulinum, 220, 267, 271
Clostridium tetani, 220
CNS. *See* Central nervous system

CNS damage, 216
Co-carcinogens, 94
Codex Alimentarius Commission, 262
Coenzymes, 51
Collagen, 51, 163, 192
Competitive antagonism, 67
Complement system, 152
Conjugation reactions, 30–33
Conjunctiva redness, 212
Contact urticaria, 195–196
Contaminants, 270–273
Conventional toxicity studies, 73–84
  acute toxicity studies, 74–80
  categories, 73–74
  good laboratory practice, 83–84
  rat strains in, 74
  short term and long term, 80–83
  usefulness, 73
Conventional toxicology, 2
Cornea, 204
Corrosive agents, 52
Corundum smelter's lung, 167
Covalent binding, 52
Creatinine, 188
Cutaneous cancer, 196, 199
CV. *See* Cardiovascular system toxicology
Cyanobacterial blooms, 173
Cyanotoxins, 344
Cyclamates, 266
Cystic fibrosis, 109
Cytochrome P-450, 28, 36, 170, 173
Cytokines, 151
Cytoskeleton, 48, 51, 96
Cytotoxicants, 95

Decalin-induced hyalin droplet
    nephropathy, 62
Defense mechanisms, 161
Definitive assessment, 103
  Dose-response relationship, 103
  general consideration, 103
  reproducibility of the results, 103
  tumor incidence, 103
Degradation reactions, 28–30
Delayed effects, 43, 133
Delayed hypersensitivity, 194
Delayed neuropathy, 218
Demyelination, 220
Dendrimers, 294
DEPC. *See* Diethyl pyrocarbonate

Dermatotoxicants, 193–197
  primary irritation, 193
  sensitization reaction, 194
Derris elliptica, 280
Descemet's membrane, 202
Developmental toxicology, 6, 125–134
  embryology, 126–127
  evaluation of teratogenic effects
    categories and relative significance, 133
    extrapolation of humans, 133–134
  historical background, 125–126
  mode of action
    deficiency of energy supply and osmolarity,
      129–130
    inhibition of enzymes, 130
    interference with nucleic acids, 129
    others, 130
    oxidative stress, 130
  teratogens, 127–129
    of special interest, 130–132
  testing procedures
    administration of chemical, 132
    animals, 132
    observations, 132–133
Distal axonopathy, 218–219
Distribution, 17–19
DNA
  adducts, 112
  characteristics, 112
  damage, 91, 119
  human cancer and, 110
  metals and, 96
  mutagenicity and, 109, 119
  mycotoxins, 270
  recombination, 118–119
  repair, 118–119
  replication of, 117–118
Dominant lethal test, 118
Dose-effect relationship, 45, 46, 78, 103
Dose-response relation, 45, 46, 79, 313
Down's syndrome, 109
Draize test, 198
Drosophila melanogaster, 114, 116
Drug receptors, 53
Drugs, 128

Edema, 118–119
Edward's syndrome, 109
Effective renal plasma flow (ERPF), 189
Electromyography, 223

Electrooculography, 209
ELISA. *See* Enzyme–linked immunosorbent
assay
Embryology, 126–127
Embryonic stage, 126
Emphysema, 164
Endocrine disruptors, 244–248
adverse effects of, 252–254
bisphenol A, 246–247
evaluation of, 254–257
free radical production, 249–250
molecular mechanism of, 248–251
nuclear receptor–mediated carcinogenicity,
250–251
on humans, 253–254
on wild life species, 252–253
phthalate esters, 247–248
polybrominated diphenyl ethers, 248
Endocrine system
Alkylphenol polyethoxylates (APEs), 246
endocrine disrupting chemical, 244–245
endocrine disruptors, 244–248
Hershberger assay, 256–257
in-vitro assay, 254–255
in-vivo assay, 255–256
Test Guideline 407 (TG407), 257
uterotrophic assay, 256
Endocytosis, 15
Endoneural edema, 221
Endothelial damage, 238
Environmental factors, 66–67
Environmental pollutants, 335–344
Environmental toxicology, 2
Enzyme–linked immunosorbent assay
(ELISA), 157
Enzymes
induction, 69
inhibition of, 50
interference with, 129
Epidemiological studies, 349
Epidermal adnexa, 196–197
Epoxide formation, 33–34
ERPF. *See* Effective renal plasma flow
Escherichia coli., 113, 119
Estrogen receptor binding assay, 254
Estrogen receptor transcriptional activation
assay, 254
Eukaryotic microorganisms, 113–114
Eutrophication, 344
Excretion, 19–21

biliary, 20–21
gastrointestinal tract, 21
lungs, 21
sweat and saliva, 21
urinary, 20
Excretion rate, saccharin, 24
Experimental design
acute toxicity, 75
dosage, 76, 81
duration, 81
long-term toxicity, 80–83
number of animals, 76, 80
route of administration, 75–76, 81
species, 80
Extracellular edema, 221
Eye irritation, grading of, 212
Eye, toxicology of, 202–209
evaluation, 209
site of effects
cornea, 204
iris, aqueous humor, and ciliary body,
204–205
lens, 205–206
optic nerve, 206–207
retina, 206
structure of, 202–203
testing
electrooculography, 209
gross examination, 207–208
histological and biochemical examinations,
209
ophthalmoscopy, 208
visual perimetry, 208–209
visual-evoked responses, 209

Facilitated diffusion, 15
Fanconi's anemia, 110
FAO. *See* Food and Agricultural Organization of
the United Nations
FAS. *See* Fetal alcohol syndrome
Fatal neurological syndrome, 323
Fatty liver disease (FLD), 171
FEMA. *See* Flavor and Extract Manufacturers'
Association
Female pubertal assay, 255–256
Female reproductive system, 232–233
Fetal alcohol syndrome (FAS), 145
Fetal stage, 126
Fetal toxicity, 133
Fibrosis, 163–164

Fibrotic lung lesions, 152
Filtration, 14
Fish short-term reproduction assay, 255
Flavor and Extract Manufacturers' Association
    (FEMA), 266
FLD. *See* Fatty liver disease
Fluorescent-plus-Giemsa technique, 118
FOB. *See* Functional observational battery
Follicle-stimulating hormone (FSH), 232, 235
Food additives and contamination
    classification, 263
    contaminants
        metals, 272–273
        mycotoxins, 270
        neurotoxins, 271
    definition, 262–263
    indirect
        animal drug residues in human food,
            269–270
        packaging materials, 268–269
    toxicologic testing and evaluation, 264–266
    types, 266–268
Food allergies and lactation, 139–140
Food and Agricultural Organization of the
    United Nations (FAO), 373
Food contaminants, 263
Forensic toxicology, 2
Free radical formation, 34–35
Free radical production, 249–250
FSH. *See* Follicle-stimulating hormone
Fumigants, 281
Functional antagonism, 67
Functional effects, 43–44
Functional observational battery (FOB), 222
Fungicides, 280–281
Fusarium solani, 163

Ganglion cells, 202, 206
Gap junction, 95
Gene mutation, 112–115
Generally recognized as safe (GRAS), 262–263,
    266, 269
Genotoxic carcinogens, 92–94
German measles, 127
Germ cells, 117
GFR. *See* Glomerular filtration rate
Glial cells, 220–221
Glomerular filtration rate (GFR), 188
Glomeruli, 185
Glucuronide formation, 30

Glutathione conjugation, 31–33
Glycosuria, 187
Good laboratory practice, 83–84
Gonyaulax, 219
G-protein coupled receptors, 53–54
Gram-negative bacteria, 156
GRAS. *See* Generally recognized as safe
Gulf War Syndrome, 287–289

Helper cells, 150
Hemangiosarcoma, 239
Hematological examination, 82
Hematopoietic system, 315, 352
Hepatic necrosis, 172–173
Hepatitis viral–like, 175
Hepatocytes, 170, 173, 174, 176
Hepatotoxicants, 176
Herbicides, 280
Heritable effects, 122
Heritable translocation test, in mice, 118
Hershberger assay, 256–257
HIV. *See* Human immunodeficiency virus
Holocrine, 197
Hormesis, 45
Hormone receptors, 53
Hormones, 95
Host-mediated assay, 114
Human cancer with chromosomal aberrations,
    110
Human glomerulonephritis nephropathy, 185
Human immunodeficiency virus (HIV), during
    breast–feeding, 139
Human recombinant assay, 255
Humoral immunity, 157
Hyperosmolarity, 183
Hypersensitivity reactions, 52, 153–154
Hypothalamus-pituitary-testis axis, 232
Hypoxia, 129, 236

Idiosyncratic reactions, 44–45
Immediate effects, 43
Immune system, toxicology of
    components of system
        B cells, 151
        Langerhans cells, 151
        macrophages, 151
        natural killer (NK) cells, 151
        polymorphonuclear (PMN) cells, 150
        soluble mediators, 151–152
        T cells, 150

immunotoxicants
  impact, 153–156
  major, 152–153
Immunoglobins, 151
Immunosuppression, 155–156
Immunosuppressive drugs, 95
Immunotoxicities
  cell-mediated immunity, 156–157
  functions of bone marrow, 157
  functions of macrophages, 157
  humoral immunity, 157
  immunocompetence tests, 156
Implantation, 232–233
Indirect food additives, 263, 268–270
Infections, 127
Inhalation toxicology
  effects on upper respiratory tract, 164–165
  toxicants, 161–165
Insecticides, 278–280
  botanical, 279–280
  carbamate, 279
  organochlorine, 279
  organophosphates, 278–279
Interactions, 67–69
Interference with impulse conduction, 219
Interference with synaptic transmission, 220
Interleukins, 151
Intracellular receptors, 55
Intramuscular injection, 15
Intraperitoneal injection, 15
In-vitro assay, 254–255
In-vivo assay, 255–256
Irreversible effects, 43
Itai-itai disease, 6, 11, 318

JECFA. See Joint FAO/WHO Expert Committee
    on Food Additives and Contaminants
JMPR. See Joint FAO/WHO Meeting of Experts
    on Pesticide Residues
Joint FAO/WHO Expert Committee on Food
    Additives and Contaminants (JECFA),
    264, 265, 362–364, 373
Joint FAO/WHO Meeting of Experts on
    Pesticide Residues (JMPR), 264, 373

Kaolinosis, 168
Kidney
  nephrons, 5, 181
  non-excretory functions, 183
  renin, 183

secretion, 183
structure of, 181
tubular resorption, 183
Kidney toxicology, 181–189
  binding chemicals, 19
  nature of, 189
  nephrotoxicants, 183–187
  nonexcretory functions, 183
  renal failure, 186
  testing procedure, 187–189
Klinefelter's syndrome, 109

Lactation, 137–145
  adverse infant conditions protected by,
      137–138
  benefits
    food allergies, 139–140
    immune system, 138–139
    protection from cancer, 139
    psychological bonding, 140
    biomarkers of exposure, 140–140
    importance and necessity of, 137
Lactation index, 234
Langerhans cells, 151, 192
LD_{50}, 74–80, 286
Leber's optic neuropathy, 220
Lens, 205–206
Lethal mutation, 232
Lethal synthesis, 50
Leukemia, 162
Leukoencephalopathy, 216
Leydig cells, 230, 232, 235
LH. See Luteinizing hormone
Ligand-receptor complex, 53–55
Limit test, 74
Lipids, 51–52
Liver necrosis, 172–173
Liver toxicology, 170–177
  clinical biochemical tests for, 176–177
  complications, 170
  effect on subcellular organelles in liver cells,
      172
  hepatotoxicants, 176
  types of injury
    carcinogenesis, 175–176
    cholestasis, 174
    cirrhosis, 174–175
    fatty liver (steatosis), 171–172
    liver necrosis, 172–173
    viral-like hepatitis, 175

Local effects, 42
Local irritation, 162
Long-term carcinogenicity studies, 99–102
  animals, 100
  doses, 101
  inception and duration, 100
  observation and examination, 101
  route of administration, 100
  treatment groups, 101
  tumors, reporting of, 102
Long-term toxicity studies, 73–84, 80–83
Loop of Henle, 181, 183–184, 186
LT_{50}, 75
Lung cancer, 164
Lungs
  allergic reaction, 164
  cancer, 164
  fibrosis, 163–164
  pneumoconiosis, 163
Luteinizing hormone (LH), 232
Lymphocyte proliferation, 156
Lymphocytes, 149–152, 154–157
Lymphoid hypoplasia, 158
Lymphokines, 150–151

Macrophages, 150–152, 157
Male pubertal assay, 255–256
Male reproductive system, 231–232
Malformations, 133
Mammalian cells
  cytogenetic studies and, 116–117
  DNA repair and, 118–119
  in culture, 114–115
  in vitro transformation, 119–120
  testing procedures and, 114–115
Mass poisoning, 11
Maximally tolerated dose (MTD), 101
Maximization test, 198
Mechanism of action, 48–49
Mechanistic models, 369–371
Mechanistic toxicology, 2
Median lethal dose, 74
Melanocytes, 192
Memory cells, 151
Metabolic imbalance, 128
Metabolic syndrome, 171
Metal-based nanomaterials, 293–294
Metal fume fever, 322
Metals, 305–323
  arsenic, 318

beryllium, 318–319
biological indicators/biomarkers, 309–310
Cadmium, 96, 98, 141, 184, 185, 232,
  239, 245, 272, 307, 308, 309, 311,
  316–317, 354
  effects on the respiratory system, 317
  and hypertension, 317
  occurrence in nature, 316
  toxicity, 317
chromium, 319
common effects
  carcinogenicity, 310
  immune function, 310
  kidney, 311
  nervous system, 311
  respiratory system, 312
factors affecting, 308–309
lead, 6, 16, 152, 184, 220, 221, 238, 245, 272,
  273, 305–306, 308, 314–316, 354
  carcinogenicity of, 316
  environmental levels, 314
  exposure on infants and young
    children, 315
  human exposure, 335, 357
  and kidney functions, 316
  levels, in milk, 143–144
  major industrial uses, 315
  and nervous system, 315–316
  organic compounds, 316
  other effects, 316
  toxicity, 315–316
mercury, 155, 184, 186, 238, 245, 273,
  312–314, 354
  anthropogenic activities, 312
  chloride, 215
  compounds, 221
  daily intake and effect, 312
  elemental form of, 312
  human exposure, 357
  levels, in milk, 142–143
  poisoning, 3
  toxicity, 312–314
  vapor, 311
nickel, 319
occurrence, 304
risk and benefit considerations, 319–323
site of action, 306–308
uses and human exposure, 305–306
Methemoglobin, 50, 64
Methylation, 31

MFO. *See* Microsomal mixed–function oxidase
Microbial tests
  in vitro, 113–114
  in vivo, 114
Microcephaly, 127–129
Microcystis aeruginosa, 344
Micronucleus test, 117
Microsomal mixed–function oxidase (MFO),
  28, 65–66
Microsomal oxidation, 28–29
Microsome mediated, 115
Microsomes, 28
Minamata disease, 6, 11
MMT. *See* Methylcyclopentadienyl manganese
  tricarbonyl
Modifying factors
  chemical interaction
    as toxicologic tools, 69
    characteristics of enzyme induction, 69
    mechanism of action, 68
    type of interaction, 67–68
  environmental factors, 66–67
  general considerations, 59
  host factors
    age, 63–65
    diseases, 66
    gender, hormonal status, and pregnancy,
      62–63
    nutritional status, 65–66
    species, strain, and individual, 60–62
Molecular target, 49–52
Monitoring, 356–357
Monokines, 151
Monosomy, 116
Morphologic effects, of toxicants, 43–44
Morphologic examination, for neurotoxicity,
  223
Mouse spot test, 115
MSG. *See* Monosodium glutamate
MTD. *See* Maximally tolerated dose
Multigeneration reproduction studies,
  233–234
Mutagenesis, 109–122
  categories of, 110–111
  chromosomal effects
    dominant lethal test in rodents, 118
    heritable translocation test in mice, 118
    in vitro tests, 116–117
    in vivo tests, 117
    insects, 116

    sister chromatid exchange (SCE),
      117–118
  DNA repair and recombination
    bacteria, 119
    mammalian cells/UDS, 119
    yeasts, 119
  evaluation
    election of test systems, 120
    significance of results, 121–122
  gene mutations
    eukaryotic microorganisms, 128
    frame-shift mutation, 112
    insects, 114
    mammalian cells in culture, 114–115
    microbial tests in vitro, 113–114
    microbial tests in vivo, 114
    prokaryotic microorganisms, 113
    tests in mice, 115
  health hazards, 109–110
  tests, 102
    in vitro transformation of mammalian cells,
      119–120
    nuclear enlargement test, 120
Myelinating cells, 220
Myelinopathy, 216
Myelin sheath, 220–221
Myocardial contraction, 236
Myocardial depression, 237

NADH methemoglobinemia reductase,
  deficiency of, 44–45
NAFLD. *See* Non-alcoholic fatty liver disease
Nanocomposites, 294
Nanomaterials
  carbon-based, 293
  dendrimers, 294
  exposure sources, 294–295
  metal-based, 293–294
  nanocomposites, 294
  physicochemical properties of, 295
  toxicities of, 296–300
  types of, 293–294
  usage and effects of, 296
Nanotoxicity, 293–301
  cancer, 299
  cell cycle arrest, 301
  endocrine disruption, 300
  free radical generation, 301
  immunotoxicity, 299–300
  inflammation, 301

Nanotoxicity (*Continued*)
  mechanisms of, 300–301
  mitochondrial perturbation, 301
  mutation, 299
  neurotoxicity, 300
  pulmonary diseases, 298
  reproductive toxicity, 300
  skin toxicity, 298
Natural killer (NK) cells, 151
NBR. *See* NCI-Black Reiter
NCI-Black Reiter (NBR), 62
Nephritis, 153–155, 185–187
Nephrons, 5, 181
Nephrotoxicants, 183–187
Nervous system, toxicology of, 213–226
  behavioral studies, 223–225
  cells and appendages, 213–214
  central nervous system, 213
  evaluation, 225–226
  nerve barriers, 214–215
  neurotransmitters, 214
  peripheral nervous system, 213
  testing
    electrophysiologic examinations, 223
    functional observational battery (FOB), 222
    morphologic examinations, 223
    neurologic examinations, 222–223
  toxic effects
    axonopathy, 217–220
    blood vessels and edema, 221
    cellular edema, 221–222
    glial cells and myelin, 220–221
    neuronopathy, 216–217
Neurotoxins, 271
Neurotransmitter receptors, 53
Neurotransmitters, 214
Neurospora, 113
N-Hydroxylation, 34
NK. *See* Natural killer cells
NK-cell activity, 155
NOAEL. *See* No-observed-adverse-effect level
Non-alcoholic fatty liver disease (NAFLD), 172
Noncarcinogenic chemicals, 372
Noncompetitive antagonism, 67
Non-excretory functions, 183
Nongenotoxic carcinogenesis, 94–97
Nonmicrosomal oxidation, 29
Nonmicrosomal reductions, 29
No-observed-adverse-effect level (NOAEL), 45, 73, 81, 83, 350

Nuclear engagement test, 120
Nuclear receptor-mediated carcinogenicity, 250–251
Nucleic acids, 52
  inhibition of, 130
Null cells, 151

Occupational toxicology, 2, 347–357
  effects
    carcinogenesis, 353
    CNS depression, 351
    hematopoietic system, 352
    interactions, 351
    irritation, 351
    kidney functions, 352
    liver functions, 352
    nervous system, 352
    testicular degeneration and cardiovascular (CV) abnormalities, 353
  exposure limits, 348–350
  monitoring, 356–357
  toxicants
    gases, 355
    metals, 353–354
    organic solvents, 350–351
    particulate matter, 355
    pesticides, 354
    plastics, 356
Oncogene, 91
Onco-suppressor gene, 91
Oocytes, 229, 231, 232
Ophthalmoscopy, 208
Optic nerve, 206–207
Osmolarity, 187
Osmolarity teratogens, 129–130
Osteomalacia, 317
OTC. *See* Over-the-counter products
Over-the-counter preparations, 327–332
  adverse consequences, 329–332
  prevalence, 328–329
Over-the-counter (OTC) products, 7
Oxidases, 28
Oxidative stress, 130
  by cigarette smoke, 164, 169

Packaging Materials, 268–269
Paired feeding, 82
Paracelsus. *See* Bergsucht (Paracelsus)
Parkinson's disease, 217, 220, 284
Particulate matter, 340

Passive diffusion, 12–13
PBPK. *See* Physiologically based
  pharmacokinetic models
PBTK. *See* Physiologically based toxicokinetic
  models
Percutaneous absorption, 17
Perfused male reproductive tracts, 235
Peripheral axonopathy, 286
Peripheral nerves, 223
Permissible exposure limits
  scientific basis, 349–350
Peroxidation, of polyenoic fatty acids, 51
Peroxisome proliferators, 95
Pesticides, 277–289
  adverse effects of pesticides, 277–278
  categories of pesticides
    fumigants, 281
    fungicides, 280–281
    herbicides, 280
    insecticides, 278–280
    rodenticides, 281
  Gulf War syndrome, 287–289
  occupational exposure to, 278
  properties
    bioaccumulation, 285
    biomagnification, 285
    carcinogenicity, 282–283
    hypersensitivity reactions, 284
    nervous system, 281–282
    renal effects, 284
    teratogenicity and effects on reproductive
      functions, 283–284
  testing, evaluation and control, 285–287
  value of pesticides, 277
  Peyer's patches, 150
Phagocytosis, 15
Pharmacokinetics, 231
Phase I reactions, 28–30
Phase II reactions, 30–33
Phenol sulfonphthalein excretion test, 189
Phocomelia, 125, 129
Photochemical oxidants, 337–339
Phototoxicity, 198
Physiologically based pharmacokinetic (PBPK)
  models, 21–23
Physiologically based toxicokinetic (PBTK)
  models, 23
PII. *See* Primary irritation index
Pinocytosis, 15, 16
Placental barrier, 18, 125

Plasma cells, 151
Plasma proteins, 18
PMN. *See* Polymorphonuclear cells
Pneumoconiosis, 163, 298
Poisoning, methyl mercury,142, 310
Poisons, 3
Pollutants
  air, 335–341
  environmental, 335–344
  soil and water, 341–344
Polycythemia, 236
Polymorphonuclear cells, 150
Polyploidy, 116
Potentiation, 67
Precarcinogens, 93
Predifferentiation stage, 126
Preliminary assessment, 102
  carcinogenicity test, 102
  chemical structure, 102
  mutagenicity, 102
Primary irritation index (PII), 197
Probability models, 369
Prokaryotic microorganisms, 113
Promoters, 94–96
Proteinuria, 187
Proto-oncogene, 91
Proximal axonopathy, 218
Proximal tubules, 185–186
Psychological bonding and breast-fed infants,
  140
Pulmonary effects
  allergic reaction, 164
  edema, 162–163
  fibrosis, 163–164
  local irritation, 162
  lung cancer, 164
Pulmonary fibrosis, 163

Radiation, 127
Rats and mice
  altered foci, 99
  breast cancer test in, 99
  pulmonary tumors in, 99
  skin tumors in, 99
Reactive oxygen species (ROS), 31, 34–35
Receptors
  drug, 53
  functional categories, 53
  G-protein coupled receptors, 53–54
  historical notes, 52–53

Receptors (*Continued*)
  hormone, 53
  in toxicology, 55–56
  intracellular, 55
  neurotransmitter, 53
  signal transduction, 53–55
  toxic effects, 49, 52–56
Recessive gene disorders, 109
Recombination of DNA, 118–119
REF. *See* Renal erythropoietic factor
Reference dose (RfD), 363–364
Regulatory toxicology, 2
Renal clearance, 189
Renal erythropoietic factor (REF), 183
Renin, 183
Repair mechanism, 48
Reproductive system toxicology, 5, 229–235
  biomarkers and, 235
  female system, 232–233
  male system, 231–232
  perfused male reproductive tracts, 235
  pesticides, 232
  pharmacokinetics, 231
  process and organs, 229–230
  sperm count and, 234
  studies multigeneration, 233–234
  toxicants, 231–233
Resorption, 133
Respiratory system, 160–165. *See also*
    Pulmonary effects
  defense mechanisms, 161
  function of, 160
  pulmonary effects, 162
  structure of, 160
  systemic effects, 161
  toxicants and, 161–165
Response
  graded, 45–46
  hormesis, 45
  quantal, 45–46
Retina, 206
Reversible effects, 43
RfD. *See* Reference dose
Risk
  assessment, 104, 371
  estimation of, 367–368
  models for estimating, 368–371
  virtually safe dose, 368–371
Rodenticides, 281
ROS. *See* Reactive oxygen species

Saccharomyces cerevisiae, 113, 119
Salmonella typhimurium, 113
Saxidomas giganteus, 219
SCE. *See* Sister chromatid exchange
Schizosaccharomyces, 113
Sebaceous glands, 197
Secondary carcinogens, 97, 372
Secretion, 183
Selenium, 321
  deficiency, 321
  exposure, 321
Sertoli cells, 230–232
Sex-linked recessive lethal test, 114
Short-term and long-term toxicity studies,
    80–83
  evaluation, 83
  experimental design, 80–81
  laboratory tests, 82
  observation and examination, 82
  postmortem examination, 82–83
Sick Building Syndrome, 339–344
Sickle-cell anemia, 109
Signal transduction, 53–55
Silicosis, 163
Sister chromatid exchange (SCE), 117–118
Skin
SLE. *See* Systemic lupus erythematosus
Social factors, 67
Soil and water pollutants, 341–344
  inorganic ions, 343–344
  microcystins, 344
  neurotoxins, 344
  phthalate esters, 343
  synthetic chemicals, 341–343
Solid state carcinogens, 96
Specific locus test, 115
Spermatid, 229, 231–232
Spermatozoa, 230, 232
Spina bifida, 128–129
Steatosis, 171–172
Steroidogenesis assay, 255
Structural proteins, 51
S. typhimurium, 121
Subacute myelo-opticoneuropathy, 207
Subacute toxicity studies, 73, 80–83. *See also*
    Short-term and long-term toxicity
    studies
Subcellular effects, 48
Sulfate conjugation, 30
Superoxide formation, 34–35

Suppressor gene, 91
Sweat glands, 197
Synergistic effects, 67
Systemic effects, 42–43, 161
Systemic lupus erythematosus (SLE), 44

Target organs, 46–48, 97
  biotransformation, 47–48
  distribution, 46–47
  repair mechanism, 48
  selective uptake, 47
  sensitivity of the organ, 46
T cells, 150
Tay-Sachs disease, 109
Teratogenic effect, evaluation of, 133–134
Teratogens, 127–129
  of special interest, 130–132
  teratogenic effect, 133–134
Teratology, 6
Test Guideline 407 (TG407), 257
Testicular tumor, 232
Testing procedure. *See specific tests*
  behavioral tests in, 223–225
  cardiovascular system and, 240–241
  contact urticaria and, 198–199
  cutaneous cancer and, 199
  developmental toxicity, 132–133
  eye and, 207–209
  kidney toxicology and, 187–189
  liver toxicology, 176–177
  nervous system toxicology, 222–223
  photoallergy and, 198
  phototoxicity and, 198
  skin toxicology, 197–199
TG407. *See* Test Guideline 407
Therapeutic drugs, 269
Therapeutic index, 3
Thiamine kinase, 51
Threshold limit value (TLV), 348
Thyroid-stimulating hormone (TSH), 283
Tier systems, 4
Time-weighted average (TWA), 348
T-lymphocytes, 150, 155–156
TLV. *See* Threshold limit value
Tm. *See* Transport maximum
Tolerance models, 369
Toluene, maternal exposure to, 145
Toxicants. *See also* specific Toxicants
Toxic effects, 42–56. *See also* Modifying
    factors, of toxic effects

general considerations, 42
mechanisms of action, 48–49
molecular targets
  coenzymes, 51
  lipids, 51–52
  nucleic acids, 52
  others, 52
  proteins, 49–51
receptors
  functional categories, 53
  historical notes, 52–53
  significance, 55
  structure and signal transduction, 53–55
SPECTRUM
  allergic and idiosyncratic reactions,
    44–45
  graded and quantal responses, 45–46
  immediate and delayed effects, 43
  local and systemic effects, 42–43
  morphologic, functional, and biochemical
    effects, 43–44
  reversible and irreversible effects, 43
target organs
  biotransformation, 47–48
  distribution, 46–47
  repair mechanism, 48
  selective uptake, 47
  sensitivity of the organ, 46
Toxicity. *See also* specific Toxicity
  vs. other considerations, 7
Toxicity studies
  acute
    data evaluation, 77–78
    dosage and number of animals, 76
    experimental design, 75
    multiple endpoint evaluation, 76
    observations and examinations, 76
    route of administration, 75–76
    uses of LD_{50} values and signs of toxicity,
      78–80
  categories, 73–74
  good laboratory practice, 83–84
  importance of selection of rat strains, 74
  short-term and long-term
    evaluation, 83
    experimental design, 80–81
    laboratory tests, 82
    observations and examinations, 82
    postmortem examination, 82–83
  usefulness, 73

Toxicological evaluation, 361–374
  acceptable daily intake (ADI/RfD)/safety
    assessment, 363–367
    assessment of exposure acceptability,
      366–367
    definitions and usage, 363–364
    estimating procedure, 364–366
  carcinogenic chemicals, 372–373
  historical development, 361–362
  international perspective, 373
  mathematical models, 367–371
  noncarcinogenic chemicals, 372
  risk assessment, 371
  risk estimation, 368–371
Toxicology. *See also* specific Toxicology
  challenges and successes, 6–7
  clinical, 2
  conventional, 2
  definition of, 1
  developmental, 6
  early developments in, 3
  environmental, 2
  forensic, 2
  function of, 5
  future prospects in, 7–9
  mechanistic, 2
  occupational, 2
  purpose of, 1
  recent developments in, 3–5
  regulatory, 2
  reproductive, 5
  risk assessment, 2–3
  scopes, 1–3
  subdisciplines in, 2–3
  system, 4
  tier systems in, 4
Transformation cell, 97, 119–120
Transgenerational diseases, 251–252
Transport maximum (Tm), 187
Traveler's diarrhea, 207
Trisomy, 116
TSH. *See* Thyroid-stimulating hormone
Tumor incidence, 103
Tumors, of blood vessels, 239

Tubular resorption, 183
TWA. *See* Time-weighted average

UDS. *See* Unscheduled DNA synthesis
Ultraviolet light, 196
Uncoupling agents, 50
UNEP. *See* United Nations Environment
    Program
United Nations Environment Program (UNEP),
    373
Unscheduled DNA synthesis (UDS), 119
Urinalysis, 82, 187–188
Urine
  acidifying capacity, 188
  concentration test, 187
  dilution test, 187
  enzymes, 188
  new biomarkers, 188
  production of, 181–183
  volume, 187
U.S. Federal Food, Drug, and Cosmetic
    Act, 262
Uterotrophic assay, 256
Uticarial reaction, 195–196

Vasoconstriction, 238–239
Viral-like hepatitis, 175
Virtually safe dose (VSD), 368–371
Visual perimetry, 208–209
Vitamin A, deficiency, 66
Vitamin K, deficiency, 177
Voltage-gated channels, 53–54
VSD. *See* Virtually safe dose
Water pollutants, 341–344
Weight of evidence, 88–89
WHO. *See* World Health Organization
Wilson's disease, 322
Workplace monitoring, 356
World Health Organization (WHO), 264, 373
Xenobiotic-metabolizing enzymes, 68, 170
Xenobiotics, 27, 249
Xeroderma pigmentosa, 110

Yeasts in mutagenesis tests, 119